GENDER, RACE, CLASS, AND HEALTH

GENDER, RACE, CLASS, AND HEALTH

Intersectional Approaches

Amy J. Schulz

Leith Mullings

EDITORS

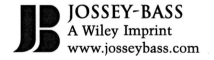

JOSSEY-BASS
A Wiley Imprint
www.josseybass.com

Published by Jossey-Bass
A Wiley Imprint
989 Market Street, San Francisco, CA 94103-1741   www.josseybass.com

Jossey-Bass books and products are available through most bookstores. To contact Jossey-Bass directly call our Customer Care Department within the U.S. at 800-956-7739, outside the U.S. at 317-572-3986, or fax 317-572-4002.

Jossey-Bass also publishes its books in a variety of electronic formats. Some content that appears in print may not be available in electronic books.

Library of Congress Cataloging-in-Publication Data

Gender, race, class, and health : intersectional approaches / Amy J. Schulz, Leith Mullings, editors.
    p. ; cm.
    Includes bibliographical references and index.
    ISBN-13: 978-0-7879-7663-7 (alk. paper)
    ISBN-10: 0-7879-7663-6 (alk. paper)
    1. Health and race—United States. 2. Racism—Health aspects—United States. 3. Health—United States—Sex differences. 4. Social status—Health aspects—United States. 5. Economic status—Health aspects—United States. 6. Discrimination in medical care—United States. 7. Health status indicators—United States. 8. Equality—Health aspects—United States. 9. Minorities—Medical care—United States. 10. Women—Medical care—United States. I. Schulz, Amy J. II. Mullings, Leith.
    [DNLM: 1. Health Status—United States. 2. Minority Groups—United States. 3. Delivery of Health Care—United States. 4. Prejudice—United States. 5. Sex Factors—United States. 6. Social Class—United States.
WA 300 G325 2006]
RA448.4.G46 2006
362.1089—dc22   2005028724

FIRST EDITION
PB Printing   10 9 8 7 6 5 4 3 2

Contents

TABLES AND FIGURES

TABLES

FIGURES

ACKNOWLEDGMENTS

This book was made possible by the generous contributions of many individuals and organizations. The initial idea for this book emerged out of the Gender, Race and Health reading group co-sponsored by the Institute for Research on Women and Gender and the Center for Research on Ethnicity, Culture and Health between 2000 and 2002. Students and faculty involved with that group initiated the idea of bringing together scholars from the social sciences working on the topic of intersectionality with scholars from public health working to address racial disparities in health. Out of these discussions emerged the idea of creating and edited book that would bring together leading scholars from a variety of disciplines and perspectives to examine the contributions of intersectional frameworks to efforts to address health inequalities.

After agreeing to take on this responsibility, Amy Schulz invited Leith Mullings to co-edit this book, and the resulting volume reflects the joint intellectual contributions of the editors as well as the contributing scholars. We worked together to convene the group of leading scholars whose work is reflected here and to engage them in a year-long process of review, critique and dialogue. With much support from multiple arenas, the contributing the authors who so graciously shared their time and insights in writing the chapters. Nearly all of the chapter authors participated scholars met forin a week-end-long review and critical discussion of early versions of all of the chapters in this book. Chapters were reviewed and discussed critically by the entire group, with regard to potential contributions to the central goal of the edited volume: bringing together theoretical and empirical work from the humanities, social sciences, and public health to inform theory and inform efforts to understand and eliminate inequalities in health.

The process focused on encouraging dialogue, and synthesis within and across disciplines and paradigms in order to crystallize key issues while at the same time engaging in broader dialogue aboutrelated to the intersections of gender, race, class, sexuality, and other axes of inequality and their implications for health. The chapters that appear in this volume have been shaped by this interdisciplinary dialogue, and reflect both commonalities and points of tension that emerged out of these differing perspectives and approaches. The opportunity to work with a group of such engaged and committed scholars was one that will remain a highlight of both our careers

Those conversations were made possible by the foresight, commitment, and grant-writing ability of Abigail Stewart, in her role as director of the University of Michigan Institute for Research on Women and Gender between 1995 and 2002, as well as ongoing support from Sherman James and, later Harold (Woody) Neighbors as directors of the Center of Research on Ethnicity, Culture and Health. Particular thanks also to Edna Viruell-Fuentes, who was instrumental in developing the initial vision for this effort and in conceptualizing and implementing the Think Tank at the University of Michigan that laid the groundwork for subsequent work on this book. We are indebted to their vision and unfailing support throughout this process. We also thank the Office of the Vice President for Research at the University of Michigan which contributed funding for this effort and graciously extended the funding period to allow the work for this book to develop to fruition.

We are indebted toalso thank the friends and colleagues who have had an impact on the analyses presented here. These include the members of the Race, Class, Gender and Health Reading Group (2000–2002) who were instrumental in the events that lead up to deciding to create the book. We have been most fortunate to have worked with, learned from, and been inspired by many colleagues from both public health and the social science communities as this volume has unfolded. We especially thank Keri Norris for assistance with background research; Debbie Barrington and Summer Wood for invaluable assistance capturing the conversations as the chapter authors engaged in critical discussions and feedback on the early draft chapters; and Elizabeth Baker, who was a generous discussant at the conference.

An edited book such as this involves considerable organizational skills and attention to details. We owe tremendous thanks to Alicia Fenty, Mindy Finnigan, Lynda Fuerstnau, Janet Malley, and Patty Smith for their ongoing support and assistance with a seemingly unending array of budgetary and administrative tasks, and to Peg Lourie, whose careful editing on draft chapters was invaluable.

We have been most fortunate to work with Andy Pasternack, a senior editor at Jossey-Bass. His knowledge of the publishing process, flexibility, and ongoing thoughtful contributions were instrumental in guiding our efforts. We thank Seth Schwartz, assistant editor at Jossey-Bass, and production editor Justin Frahm and copyeditor Beverly H. Miller for their assistance. We also appreciate the thoughtful comments of the anonymous reviewers of our book proposal.

Finally, we are grateful for family who instilled and nurtured in us a commitment to social justice and to friends and family who continue to support and encourage us in this work. We could not have completed this book without you.

Leith Mullings
Amy J. Schulz

THE EDITORS

Amy J. Schulz is research associate professor, with joint appointments in the Department of Health Behavior and Health Education and the Institute for Research on Women and Gender, and associate director of the Center for Research on Ethnicity, Culture, and Health at the University of Michigan. She completed her doctorate in sociology in 1994, and has published on the social production of health disparities in urban contexts, with a particular focus on the impact of race-based residential segregation and class inequalities on health, and on individual and collective efforts to sustain health within urban contexts with limited economic resources. In addition, she has published on processes of racialization expressed in U.S. Indian policies, Navajo women's strategies of resistance to those processes, and the reproduction of racial and class inequalities through differential access to genetic information and medical technologies. Schulz has participated in several community-based participatory research and intervention efforts designed to address racial and socioeconomic disparities in health in urban communities and has published widely on this topic. She has taught courses on qualitative research methods and participatory action research; facilitated working groups on race, gender, and health; and currently cofacilitates a graduate seminar, Eliminating Racial/Ethnic Disparities in Health.

Leith Mullings, is Presidential Professor of Anthropology at the Graduate Center of the City University of New York. She completed her doctorate in Anthropology at the University of Chicago. Before accepting a full-time position at the Graduate Center, she directed the Program in Medical Anthropology at the Sophie Davis School of Biomedical Education at City College. One of her recent projects, a multiyear ethnographic study of gender and reproductive health in central Harlem, was funded by the Centers for Disease Control and Prevention. The project used participatory research techniques, involving community residents in research design and implementation. She has presented this research in various venues involving practitioners, policymakers, politicians, academics, and community residents. Her book on this work, coauthored with Alaka Wali, *Stress and Resilience: The Social Context of Reproduction in Harlem,* has been widely distributed by the Centers for Disease Control and Prevention to researchers and practitioners around the country.

Her other books include *On Our Own Terms: Race, Class and Gender in the Lives of African American Women* (1997); and *Let Nobody Turn Us Around: Voices of Resistance, Reform and Renewal, An African America Anthology* (2000, coedited with Manning Marable). She has written articles on stratification, ethnicity, race, gender, health, globalization, participatory research, and public policy. In 1997, she received the Prize for Distinguished Achievement in the Critical Study of North America from the Society for the Anthropology of North America. She is currently serving as a member of the executive board of the American Anthropological Association.

THE CONTRIBUTORS

Mary K. Anglin is associate professor in anthropology and holds a joint appointment in the Department of Behavioral Science in the College of Medicine at the University of Kentucky. Her research interests include feminist perspectives on health and social justice, as well as ethnographies of gender, ethnicity, and class in southern Appalachia. Her book, *Women, Power, and Dissent in the Hills of Carolina* (2002), concerns women's factory labor in southern Appalachia.

Marianne P. Brown was director of the University of California at Los Angeles's Labor Occupational Safety and Health (LOSH) Program from 1984 until her retirement in 2004. Currently she has the title of associate at LOSH. She was a lecturer in the School of Public Health's Department of Community Health Sciences and the Center for Occupational and Environmental Health from 1980 to 2004. Brown received a B.A. in psychology and a master's degree in public health from the University of California, Berkeley. Previous positions include project director of Project CHIP for the American Cancer Society and program director of community cancer prevention at the UCLA Jonsson Comprehensive Cancer Center.

Cleopatra Howard Caldwell, is associate professor in the Department of Health Behavior and Health Education at the School of Public Health and co-associate director for the Program for Research on Black Americans, Institute for Social Research, University of Michigan. Her research is focused on intergenerational family influences on the psychological well-being of adolescent parents; improving adolescent health and well-being through strengthening nonresident African American father-son relationships; and racial identity, family relationships, and the mental health status of

African American and Caribbean black adolescents. She has published on culturally competent research methods within African American communities, black churches as community support systems, and community-based research. In addition, she has served as a Congressional Science Scholar and a health policy analyst for U.S. Congressman J. Roy Rowland and a policy fellow in the office of U.S. Congressman Sander Levin.

Jessie Daniels is project director at the Center for Community and Urban Health at Hunter College, City University of New York, where she also teaches in sociology and urban public health. She directs a program that addresses the needs of young men leaving Rikers Island, New York City's largest jail. Daniels's research focuses on the social and political intersections of race, class, and gender, as in her first book, *White Lies* (1997). Currently she is the Scholar in Residence at the International Center on Tolerance Education, where she is writing on the effects of Internet technology on discourse, information, and social justice around race, gender, and class. She received her Ph.D. from the University of Texas-Austin.

Bonnie Thornton Dill is professor and chair of the Department of Women's Studies and director of the Consortium on Race, Gender and Ethnicity at the University of Maryland. Her research focuses on intersections of race, class, and gender, with an emphasis on African American women and families. Her publications have been reprinted in numerous collections and edited volumes. Among Dill's recently published works are "Between a Rock and a Hard Place: Motherhood, Choice and Welfare in the Rural South," in *Sister Circle: Black Women and Work* (S. Harley and others, eds., 2002), and "Poverty in the Rural U.S.: Implications for Children, Families and Communities," in *Blackwell Companion to Sociology* (edited by J. Blau, 2001). She is the recipient of several awards, including the Jessie Bernard Award and Distinguished Contributions to Teaching Award (American Sociological Association) and the 2001–2002 Robin Williams Jr. Distinguished Lectureship (Eastern Sociological Society).

Nicholas Freudenberg is Distinguished Professor of Urban Public Health at Hunter College, City University of New York, and has worked with community organizations and health agencies in New York City for more than thirty years. He currently directs a program in New York City for male adolescents returning from incarceration. He is an investigator for the Harlem Urban Research Center and a member of its Community Action Board and its Policy Work Group, and he has served as an adviser to the New York City Departments of Health and Correction on the health needs of people returning from incarceration. He received his Dr.P.H. degree from Columbia University.

H. Jack Geiger is the Arthur C. Logan Professor Emeritus of Community Medicine at the City University of New York Medical School. Most of his professional career has been devoted to the problems of health, poverty, and human rights. He is the initiator of the community health center network in the United States and directed the first two centers, in the Mississippi Delta and inner-city Boston. A member of the Institute of Medicine, he was the 1998 recipient of the IOM's Lienhard Award for "outstanding contributions to minority health" and the Sedgwick Memorial Medal of the American Public Health Association. He completed his M.D. at Western Reserve University School of Medicine.

Barbara Guthrie is associate professor of nursing and women's studies and associate faculty researcher at the Center for Group Dynamics, Institute for Social Research at the University of Michigan. She has over twenty-five years of experience working to promote the health of girls from diverse ethnic and social backgrounds. Her research has focused on examining the impact of broad sociopolitical and contextual influences on adolescent girls' initiation of health-compromising behaviors such as substance use and abuse and early sexual activity. The results have provided the foundation for several gender- and ethnic-responsive health programs specifically designed for female adolescents. She received her Ph.D. from New York University in 1987 and was inducted as a fellow into American Academy of Nursing in 2003.

James S. Jackson is the Daniel Katz Distinguished University Professor of Psychology; professor of health behavior and health education, School of Public Health; director of the Institute for Social

Research; and research professor and past director of the Program for Research on Black Americans, Institute for Social Research, all at the University of Michigan. He is past chair of the Section on Social, Economic, and Political Sciences of the American Association for the Advancement of Science and a member of the Institute of Medicine. He is the principal investigator of over two dozen funded National Institutes of Health grants and is directing the most extensive social and health survey on the black American population ever conducted: the National Survey of American Life and Across Generations and Across Nations family study supported by the National Institute of Mental Health, National Institute of Aging, and National Institute on Drug Abuse.

Pamela Braboy Jackson is associate professor of sociology at Indiana University and was an assistant professor of sociology at Duke University from 1993 to 2000. She publishes in mainstream areas of sociology, focusing particularly on persistent racial inequality in health outcomes. Her three broad research areas are the study of social roles, minority group status (especially race and gender tokenism), and the relationship between family dynamics and other social institutions. She received her Ph.D. in social psychology from Indiana University.

Emily Martin is professor of anthropology at New York University. Her research interests include the anthropology of science and medicine, gender, money and other measures of value, and the ethnography of work in China and the United States. She has published numerous books and articles, including *The Woman in the Body: A Cultural Analysis of Reproduction* (1987), which won an award from the Society for Medical Anthropology. Martin has also been awarded a Guggenheim Fellowship and a Spencer Foundation Grant for her work. She received her Ph.D. from Cornell University.

Sandi Morgen combines her position as director of the Center for the Study of Women in Society (CSWS) with a position as a professor in the Anthropology Department at the University of Oregon, Eugene. In addition, she directs the CSWS Women in the Northwest Research Initiative, the main project of which for the past five years has been an in-depth study of welfare restructuring in Oregon. Her most recent books include *Into Our Own Hands: The Women's Health Movement in the U.S., 1969–1990* (2002) and Work, Welfare, and Politics (coedited with Margaret Hallock, 2002). She received her Ph.D. from the University of North Carolina at Chapel Hill.

Cheryl Mwaria is an associate professor of anthropology and the director of Africana studies at Hofstra University. She has conducted research in Africa, the United States, and Cuba and has published on health-related issues in those areas. Currently she is completing a manuscript on African American women with disabilities and serving as a board member of the American Ethnological Society. She received her Ph.D. in medical anthropology from Columbia University.

Lynn Weber is the director of the Women's Studies Program and professor of sociology at the University of South Carolina. Cofounder of the Center for Research on Women at the University of Memphis, her research and teaching have explored the intersections of race, class, gender, and sexuality for over twenty years. Since the publication in 2001 of *Understanding Race, Class, Gender, and Sexuality: A Conceptual Framework,* her work has focused on bringing the insights of intersectional scholarship to the problem of persistent social inequalities in health. With Deborah Parra-Medina, she recently published "Intersectionality and Women's Health: Charting a Path to Eliminating Health Disparities," in *Advances in Gender Research.* Weber is also coauthor of *The American Perception of Class* (with Reeve Vanneman, 1988).

David R. Williams is at the University of Michigan, where he serves as the Harold W. Cruse Collegiate Professor of Sociology, a senior research scientist at the Institute for Social Research, and a professor of epidemiology in the School of Public Health. His research interests are in the trends and determinants of socioeconomic and racial differences in mental and physical health. In 1995, he received an Investigator Award in Health Policy Research from the Robert Wood Johnson Foundation. In 2001, he was elected a member of the Institute of Medicine. He holds a master's degree in public health from Loma Linda University and a Ph.D. in sociology from the University of Michigan.

Ruth E. Zambrana, Ph.D., is professor and graduate director in the Women's Studies Department; director of research of the Consortium on Race, Gender and Ethnicity at the University of Maryland, College Park; and adjunct professor of family medicine at the University of Maryland, Baltimore, School of Medicine, Department of Family Medicine. Her work focuses on the intersections of gender, race/ethnicity, socioeconomic status, and institutional factors and health disparities, with an emphasis on Latino women and children. Two books include *Health Issues in the Latino Community* (coeditor with Marilyn Aguirre-Molina and Carlos W. Molina, 2001) and *Drawing from the Data: Working Effectively with Latino Families* (2003). Her recent work focuses on domains of patient-centered care and chronic conditions among women of color. She has published extensively in her field, serves on several editorial boards, and is currently working with the Health Information Workgroup of the Centers for Disease Control and Prevention and is a member of the Health Equity Champions work group. She received her Ph.D. from Boston University.

GENDER, RACE, CLASS, AND HEALTH

PART ONE

INTERSECTIONALITY AND HEALTH

CHAPTER ONE

INTERSECTIONALITY AND HEALTH
An Introduction

Leith Mullings, Amy J. Schulz

Health disparities based on race/racism, class, and gender/sexism are matters of life and death. They express, in differences of both quality and length of life, the unequal structuring of life chances. Efforts to reduce or eliminate persistent health disparities offer among the most important opportunities to improve the health of residents of the United States, and are rightfully a high priority for public health and social science scholars.

Theoretical and empirical efforts to understand and address disparities in health have emerged in multiple arenas and among scholars and practitioners working within public health, as well as scholars located in the social sciences and humanities. While these scholars all focus on understanding and eliminating health disparities, they bring diverse perspectives and insights to an understanding of the topic and to potential solutions. Yet there are relatively few opportunities for dialogue and mutual exchange across the disciplines and paradigms that inform this work. In this book, we have brought together an interdisciplinary group of scholars from the social sciences and public health to examine the ways that gender, race, and class are mutually constituted and interconnected. Our goal is to inform theory, research, and practice focused on the elimination of health disparities.

THE CHALLENGE

The domain of health disparities has become an arena for asserting and contesting explanatory paradigms about difference, inequality, health, and illness. Until recently, mainstream interpretive frameworks in medicine and health research attributed racial disparities in disease—particularly those that remain after adjusting for socioeconomic indicators—to biological, genetic, cultural, or lifestyle choice differences between racial groups (for early critiques of these approaches, see Cooper and David, 1986; Kreiger and Bassett, 1986; Mullings, 1984). Notions of race that are based on a typological approach to human variation—with the implication that genetic differences related to race are a major factor in explaining disease disparities—continue to pervade the literature. In 1996, Williams wrote that while most current research in racial disparities "has abandoned blatant racist ideology . . . much of it still assumes that racial variations in disease are due to underlying differences in biology" (p. 493); that racial taxonomies are meaningful classifications of genetic differences; and that genes determining race also determine the number and type of health problems.

The cultural or lifestyle explanatory paradigms, sometimes barely concealing notions of culture of poverty and deviance, can be equally problematic. Alleged cultural traits, behaviors, or beliefs, frequently implicitly or explicitly considered to be associated with racial groups, are often seen as constant, unchanging, and independent of social and historical processes. Analyses that construct culture or lifestyle in this manner simply substitute an essentialized notion of culture for race, with little attention to the structure of constraints within which people make lifestyle choices (Mullings, 1989). Such constructions have been critiqued by social science and public health scholars and practitioners, who have pointed to the ways in which they locate the cause of health disparities within individuals or groups rather than in sets of social relations, as well as their ineffectiveness as a basis for interventions to improve health (Gottlieb and McLeroy, 1994; Stokols, 1996; Krieger, 1999; Mullings, 1989).

In the past few years, there have been significant strides in understanding the social construction of race. In the biological and social sciences, evolutionary biologists, anthropologists, and sociologists have problematized the assumption that discrete races exist and that traits conventionally defined as racial are commensurate with data on biological variation. Among cultural anthropologists and sociologists, emphasis has shifted to understanding the social construction of race, that is, the "force of history, power, and political economy in constructing and reconstructing the boundaries, categories, institutional configurations, and experiences of race" (Harrison, 1998, p. 610). Social constructionist approaches to race are concerned with how race is made: the conditions of conquest, slavery, segregation, and inequality that gave rise to the emergence of racial classification in western Europe and the United States and the institutions that produce and reproduce inequality from difference. These directions suggest that it is analysis of the social context of inequality that tells us why race is such an important predictor of health status.

Although this direction is promising, the way in which class and race intersect with gender to produce health continues to be a challenge for theory and policy (see Krieger and Fee, 1994). Recent developments in the social science literature have attempted to address the ways in which women's and men's lives are constituted by the structural forces of class, race, and gender.

Confronting the essentialism of the early second-wave feminist frameworks, intersectionality theory was developed most prominently by black feminist social scientists emphasizing the simultaneous production of race, class, and gender inequality, such that in any given situation, the unique contribution of one factor might be difficult to measure (see Mullings, 1997, for a discussion of the intersectional tradition among black feminist scholars). This framework—an advance over earlier models that assumed that advantage and disadvantage simply accumulate, for example, to produce double jeopardy—suggests that the content and implications of gender and race as socially constructed categories vary as a function of each other. Thus, the very meaning of *manhood* may vary when applied to one's own racial group as compared to another group; similarly, the meaning of a given racial category may vary for men and for women. Feminist and other scholars have argued that we need to examine the ways in which race and gender are mutually defining (see Fine, Powell, Weis, and Wong, 1997; Ferber, 1998; Hermann and Stewart, 2000; Brodkin-Sacks, 1989): for example, whiteness and blackness are gendered, and masculinity and femininity are "raced" within particular cultural contexts. Despite these major advances in theorizing intersectionality, the social science literature tends to be fairly abstract: it is often difficult to pinpoint how the interaction, articulation, and simultaneity of race, class, and gender affect women and men in their daily lives, and the ways in which these forms of inequality interact in specific situations to condition health.

The challenge we now encounter is how to understand the ways in which gender, race, and class relations intertwine and are expressed in disparate chances for health, illness, and well-being. To this end, we have brought together an interdisciplinary group of social scientists and public health scholars to produce this book, which examines the ways in which gender, race, and class relations are mutually constitutive and interconnected and, ultimately, how those interconnections work to produce disparities in morbidity and mortality. The scholars who have contributed to this book include those who have been at the forefront of theorizing the intersections of gender, race, and class and those who have engaged in efforts to understand and address (dare we say eliminate) persistent racial, socioeconomic, and gender disparities in health in the United States. Our goal in assembling this diverse group of contributors has been to engage scholars in a critical dialogue that informs social science theorizing and empirical research, bridges gaps between theory and practice, and informs and enhances continued efforts to eliminate the social inequalities that drive persistent disparities in health.

Together, contributors to this book examine the malleability of race, gender, and class as socially constructed categories as well as the obdurate nature of inequalities structured around these concepts in the United States. In keeping with paradigms that emphasize that race is socially constructed, rather than a biological or genetic characteristic of individuals, race is conceptualized in this book as relations between groups rather than as something that people of color "have" and whites do not. Similarly, gender is considered to be a set of social relations rather than an attribute of individuals. As a result, rather than organizing the book around the health status and concerns of particular racially or ethnically defined groups, or genders, the chapters in this book have been selected because of their contribution to understanding how gender, race, and class structure social relationships in ways that produce differentials in health and disease.

In accordance with the idea that gender, race, and class are social relationships reproduced within local contexts, this book includes a number of in-depth case studies intended to examine how intersections of gender, race, and class influence health within particular contexts. While traditional epidemiological methods are useful in forming and testing predictive models, the emphasis on independent, discrete variables within epidemiological models limits their explanatory capacity for disentangling complex phenomena. In contrast, ethnographic or case study accounts are notably useful in terms of providing detailed accounts that illustrate complex social relationships and dynamics in some depth and contribute to an understanding not only of relationships between concepts, but of the processes and the meanings that those processes and relationships hold. Such understandings are essential if we are to move beyond documenting relationships toward apprehending the ways that these relationships are created and maintained, and thus understanding the ways that they may be modified to reduce disparities in health.

To consider how analyses might be transformed by considering the health effects of racial/ethnic, gendered, and class-based inequality, the book takes up four overarching questions. First, we consider the ways that historical and contemporary social, cultural, and institutional contexts shape knowledge and thus how we understand illness, health, and inequality. Second, we consider how race, class, gender, and health inequalities are produced within particular social contexts, in order to gain a better understanding of commonalities as well as differences in these patterns as they emerge in various locations. Third, we consider the ways that institutions differentially structure health care and access to health care on the basis of race, class, and gender. Finally, we consider the question of the potential for the reduction or elimination of inequalities in health outcomes through day-to-day resistance, planned intervention, and organized social movements.

RACE, CLASS, GENDER, AND KNOWLEDGE PRODUCTION

Analysis of how the paradigms that guide research influence our understanding of racial disparities and health is a theme that emerges in several of the chapters. What are the implications of emphasis on measurement and quantification, the widespread acceptance of individuals as units of analysis, and the search for independent and proximate causes for our understanding of health and illness? In Chapter Two, Lynn Weber examines this topic explicitly in her analysis of the differences between biomedical research paradigms and intersectional frameworks. She points to the manner in which biomedical frameworks for analysis may serve to homogenize difference or complexity by, for example, separating race from socioeconomic status and gender as discrete, rather than mutually constitutive, concepts. Furthermore, she probes the ways in which biomedical research paradigms emphasize gender, race, and class as characteristics of individuals rather than as social relations, contributing to explanations for health disparities that are disconnected from the historical, social, and political processes from which they emerge. She describes the potential contributions of feminist intersectional frameworks to efforts to attain equity in health. This theme is also taken up in some detail by Sandi Morgen in Chapter Fourteen, who notes the emergence of new and critical analyses of knowledge production out of the women's movement's critiques of the limits of analyses grounded solely in gender, race, or class without an understanding of the ways that they are mutually constitutive.

Conceptualizations of illness and health change significantly through historical periods, shaped by such nonbiomedical structural issues as the organization of work. Emily Martin, in Chapter Three, traces the manner in which views of moods and mood disorders are transformed in different historical periods and interrogates the ways interpretations of mental illness and mental health are gendered, raced, and classed in specific historical contexts. She particularly probes the implications of these changing constructions over time for understanding racial differences in diagnosis of mental health conditions, as well as the differential meanings of these conditions when applied to different racial groups at different points in time. Asking whether "the categories into which psychiatry divides disorders themselves already have cultural assumptions embedded in them," she invites us to consider the implications for efforts to reduce or eliminate racial disparities in the treatment of mental health, suggesting that such efforts must move beyond simply improvements in the way health care is delivered to address the underlying cultural assumptions themselves.

Martin's analysis of the racialized, gendered, and classed interpretations of health and mental health leads us to be wary of the reification of culture. While it is important to recognize the culture history of populations (for example, Mullings describes the Sojourner Syndrome as history in culture in Chapter Twelve), stereotypical conceptualizations of culture may substitute for race in describing a fixed, unchanging, bounded, homogeneous set of values, meanings, and behaviors. In this sense, culture becomes biologized or essentialized, reducing heterogeneous, complex, and contingent behaviors and values to a heritage passed down unchanged from generation to generation. This book underscores the need for a more dynamic, complex, and nuanced notion of culture. Analysis of cultural beliefs and practices must be located in the broader context within which individuals and groups live their lives if we are to understand their relationships to, and interactions with, broader social, political, and economic contexts. Chapter Seven by Ruth Zambrana and Bonnie Dill and Chapter Eight by Marianne Brown examine the ways that behaviors considered out of a social context may be attributed to "cultural" or "lifestyle" factors, failing to understand the ways that they are structured by social, economic, or political contexts. Thus, processes of creating knowledge that emphasize individual attributes or characteristics without analysis of the contexts within which they emerge offer only a partial understanding of the social factors that contribute to health disparities.

In keeping with this emphasis on understanding how the ways in which knowledge is created influence what it is we think we know, several chapters explicitly examine conceptualizations of the content, context, and boundaries of social groups. Zambrana and Dill call our attention to the nuances of language, with a discussion of the labels *Hispanic* and *Latina* and *Latino* and the ways that these labels position groups differentially in relation to histories of

colonization. Continuing their discussion of the problems associated with the content and boundaries of social groups, these
authors consider in detail the relatively recent gendered, racial,
and ethnic construct of *Latina* and how this category can function
to homogenize Latinas and Latinos, overlooking differences associated with modes of incorporation, race, socioeconomic status, and
place of residence. Their discussion of the complexities and prob-
lematics of determining the boundaries of racial or ethnic groups,
as well as understanding the ways that labels reflect historical and
contemporary group relations, is critical to an understanding of
how assumptions of race or ethnicity can shape knowledge about
health disparities.

Whiteness too requires interrogation, and in Chapter Four,
Jessie Daniels and Amy Schulz examine the ways that whiteness is
constructed within the literature on racial disparities in health,
with particular attention to the recent surge of interest in genetic
explanations for racial inequalities in health. They probe the ways
in which varying constructions of whiteness, and more broadly
race, serve to highlight or conceal the social, political, and economic processes through which groups are racialized. They argue
that an emphasis on race as an explanatory variable, without examination of the relationships between race, social class, and gender
within local social and political context, serves to obscure the heterogeneity within and overstate differences between racial groups,
reifying racial categories and obscuring the social, political, and
economic processes that shape health disparities.

Race, Class, Gender, and Health

Analyses incorporating social constructionist approaches to race
have emerged recently in medicine, public health, and epidemiology. While by no means dominant (see, for example, Burchard
and others, 2003; Phimister, 2003), this approach builds on an epidemiological tradition demonstrating that economic disparities
frequently, but not always, explain racial disparities in health and
illness (Krieger, 1999). In addition to addressing the nonequiva-
lence of measuring socioeconomic status across race and ethnicity (Williams, 1996) by finding more accurate ways of assessing
economic differences such as the measurement of wealth, studies

emphasizing social constructionist approaches also seek to identify health consequences that may arise from disparities other than solely economic ones, for example, those generated by racism. Extending this work an additional step toward an intersectional analysis, Pamela Jackson and David Williams examine in Chapter Five the complex distribution of health and disease that emerges when categories of race/ethnicity, gender, and socioeconomic status are considered simultaneously. For example, that race complicates and can disrupt relationships between socioeconomic status and health has particular implications when considering health among middle-class African Americans (Jackson and Williams; see also Mullings in Chapter Twelve).

Zambrana and Dill write that "race, ethnicity, and geography matter; they are all determinants of access to social capital or social resources." Their chapter, and Chapter Twelve by Mullings, demonstrate the ways in which the social production and maintenance of inequality are reflected in such variables as housing, neighborhood, employment, access to and quality of health care, and funding for research and how these affect health. Furthermore, the chapters by Zambrana and Dill and by Brown consider the ways that immigration status may complicate health. Low-skilled immigrant workers in the United States enter a workforce already stratified by race, sex, age, ethnicity, and education. They may also face special work-related hazards and injuries, particularly in situations where their undocumented status makes them reluctant to report injuries or seek health care. In Chapter Eight, Marianne Brown describes how the health of immigrant workers in California is conditioned by both gender and immigrant status, influencing both the extent to which they are exposed to occupational hazards and their knowledge of and willingness to draw on supports for worker safety. Relationships between immigration status and length of residence in the United States and health are multifaceted, and implications for health vary. In contrast to the occupational hazards experienced by immigrants that Brown describes, Jackson and Williams note that foreign-born black women have a lower incidence of low-birth-weight babies when compared to black women born and raised in the United States, and Zambrana and Dill describe data indicating that among Latinas, being born in the United States is associated with elevated risk for mental health problems. Each of these diverse results may speak to the health effects of residence within contexts permeated by racism.

Furthermore, the ways in which social groups and individuals are represented—how they are viewed and stereotyped by the society—and the dominant group's behavior, practices, and expectations as influenced by these depictions, also have implications for health. Stereotypes of Latinas as immigrants, as unable to speak English, as unable to articulate their symptoms, and as having too many children (Zambrana and Dill); media portrayals criminalizing young men of color or portraying communities as deficient and with few assets or strengths (Amy Schulz, Nicholas Freudenberg, and Jessie Daniels in Chapter Thirteen); or negative racial stereotypes widely held by the majority population simultaneously with the denial of the existence of current racism (H. Jack Geiger in Chapter Nine), all enter into research as well as policy formation in health. These stereotypes serve to turn the lens toward racialized groups or communities, while obscuring the role of racism as a contributing factor to racial disparities in health.

RACE, CLASS, GENDER, AND HEALTH CARE

Studies in medicine, epidemiology, and public health, interrogating the role of racism in producing health risks, seek to identify the pathways through which racism has an impact on health status. These include structural racism that operates at the societal level, privileging some groups and denying others access to the resources of society; institutional racism, which operates through organizational structures; and interpersonal racism, expressed in individual interactions (see Jones, 2000; Kreiger, 1999; LaViest, 1996). This work speaks to the need to continue tracking health data by race in order to measure the biological effects of the social construction of race. The work of Muntaner and others (2001) on racist beliefs among a cohort of students from which epidemiologists are drawn and Geiger's analysis (2003) of health provider and institutional racism are excellent examples of this approach. After reviewing 150 representative studies, Geiger notes, "The preponderance of the evidence strongly suggests that among the multiple causes of racial and ethnic disparities in American health care, provider and institutional bias are significant contributors" (p. 440).

Institutions structure health care by race, class, and gender at various levels. Martin's case study of mood disorders in Chapter Three demonstrates how race, class, and gender structure diagnosis as well as treatment. Geiger reviews the "robust and credible" evidence—in studies controlled for such variables as insurance status, income and education, age, gender, stage, and severity of disease—of differences in the "quality, intensity, and comprehensiveness" of medical care provided to people of color. Focusing on a particular medical context, access to clinical trials, Cheryl Mwaria suggests in Chapter Ten that prescreening by physicians, which frequently involves implicit and unwarranted assumptions about patients based on race, gender, and class, may lead to prejudgment about whether patients will understand or follow protocols. Despite health care providers' widespread assumptions that people of color do not participate in clinical trials due to mistrust of the medical care system, she reports evidence that many patients of color in the hospital where she conducted her ethnographic work valued the opportunity to participate in such trials. Mwaria suggests instead that gatekeeping by physicians plays a substantial role in maintaining differential access by race, class, gender, and ethnicity to clinical trials. This may deny people of color access to cutting-edge medical care and assistance with coverage.

National social movements around health have been effective in intervening in knowledge production and delivery of health care. However, these too are shaped by race and class hierarchies. Drawing on material from in-depth interviews with women describing their experience of diagnosis and initial treatment of breast cancer, in Chapter Eleven, Mary Anglin considers gender as "part of a web of relationships that constitute social location and cultural identities" and probes how the contexts of diagnosis, treatment, and illness are shaped by gender, race, and class. She examines these experiences for their implications for the incorporation of the racial and class diversity of women affected by breast cancer, noting that the national breast cancer movement primarily reflects the concerns of a constituency whose position affords them access to the medical system and advanced technological medicine. Anglin concludes that the inability to incorporate the diversity of those affected renders the national breast cancer movement less effective.

RESISTANCE, DISRUPTION, AND TRANSFORMATIONS

The development of strategies for survival and transformation within the context of pervasive inequalities structured around race, class, and gender, and their implications for health, is another theme that emerges from this literature. Scholars have examined the ways that responses to experiences of oppression can serve to exacerbate (James and others, 1992; Mullings and Wali, 2001) or to reduce (Sellers, Caldwell, Schmelke-Cone, and Zimmerman, 2003; Caldwell and others, 2004) the negative health effects of those inequalities. Some have suggested that relationships among these survival strategies and health may be influenced by the particular context within which they are enacted (James and Thomas, 2000; Dressler, Bindon, and Neggers, 1998; Mullings and Wali, 2001).

Strategies that resist or seek to disrupt oppressive social relations may emerge at many levels, ranging from households to communities to social movements. Cleopatra Caldwell, Barbara Guthrie, and James Jackson probe in Chapter Six the implications of confrontations with processes of racialization in the United States for identity formation and indicators of health and well-being among African American and Caribbean American youth. African American families, for example, play a key role in socializing females toward an "extended definition of self," which emphasizes the "importance of maintaining immediate and extended family connectedness," and socializing males to present a "cool" demeanor when confronted with personal assaults. Similarly, Leith Mullings coins the term *Sojourner Syndrome* to describe strategies among African American women, ranging from women-centered networks to community organizing. She suggests the need to explore the health consequences of this "transformative work," which spans the domains of household, work, and community. Schulz, Freudenberg, and Daniels explore how constructions of race, class, and gender create unequal life opportunities in two distinctly different contexts: New York City and East Los Angeles. In each case study, they examine the emergence of unequal social relations within the particular context, examining histories of residential patterns, labor force, and educational and criminal justice systems as well as the contributions of media portrayals and racialized imagery to inequalities. They then describe both individual and collective actions taken by community residents alone and in conjunction with public health professions, as part of efforts to maintain and promote health "within the context of inequalities."

Social movements can emerge from the activities of everyday life, as is clear in the women's health care movement. Morgen describes the development of the women's health care struggle into a movement in the context of the civil rights movement and second-wave feminism. This emergent movement organized alternative models of health care delivery, challenged pharmaceutical and hospital equipment companies, and intervened in national, state, and local policy. Bringing us full circle to where we began in this book (see Weber, Chapter Two), activists and other nonacademics confronted and challenged the knowledge production process. Women of color, in particular, incorporated an intersectional analysis of health, asserting the mutually constitutive nature of race, class, and gender, thereby providing an alternative analysis of health, illness, and health care. Morgen argues that it was grassroots activists equipped with "movement-grounded theory" who played a major role in elaborating an intersectional analysis of health inequalities.

Chapters by Martin and Anglin, as well as the chapter by Morgen discussed above, suggest that social movements have the potential to inform the conceptual lens, practice, policy, and politics of public health. Several authors in this book suggest that the language of health disparities has significant connotations and implications: a need to measure rather than act for change (Weber); carrying a "faint connotation of moral concern," stronger than "differences, but weaker than inequity" (Geiger); and "mut[ing] the urgency and costs of social injustice" (Morgen). The chapters in this book lead us to the language and analysis of health *inequalities,* which shifts our gaze from those most negatively affected toward the broad structures of inequality. A critical, intersectional analysis can provide a framework for analyzing the health effects of racial/ethnic, gendered, and class-based inequalities in the United States and help provide a theoretical foundation for claiming health as a human right.

References

Brodkin-Sacks, K. "Toward a Unified Theory of Class, Race and Gender." *American Ethnologist*, 1989, *16*, 534–550.

Burchard, E. G., and others. "The Importance of Race and Ethnic Background in Biomedical Research and Clinical Practice." *New England Journal of Medicine*, 2003, *348*(12), 1170–1175.

Caldwell, C., and others. "Racial Discrimination and Racial Identity as Risk or Protective Factors for Violent Behaviors in African American Young Adults." *American Journal of Community Psychology*, 2004, *33*(1–2), 91–105.

Cooper, R. S., and David, R. "The Biological Concept of Race and Its Application to Public Health and Epidemiology." *Journal of Health Politics, Policy and Law*, 1986, *11*, 97–116.

Dressler, W. W., Bindon, J., and Neggers, Y. H. "John Henryism, Gender, and Arterial Blood Pressure in an African American Community." *Psychosomatic Medicine*, 1998, *60*, 620–624.

Ferber, A. L. *White Man Falling: Race, Gender and White Supremacy.* Lanham, Md.: Rowman & Littlefield, 1998.

Fine, M., Powell, L., Weis, L., and Wong, L. M. (eds.). *Off-White: Readings on Race, Power and Society.* New York: Routledge, 1997.

Geiger, J. H. "Racial and Ethnic Disparities in Diagnosis and Treatment: A Review of the Evidence and a Consideration of Causes." In B. D. Smedley, A. Y. Stith, and A. R. Nelson (eds.), *Unequal Treatment: Confronting Racial and Ethnic Disparities in Health Care.* Washington, D.C.: National Academy Press, 2003.

Gottlieb, N. H., and McLeroy, K. R. "Social Health." In J. S. Harris (ed.), *Health Promotion in the Workplace.* Albany, N.Y.: Delmar, 1994.

Harrison, F. "Introduction: Expanding the Discourse on 'Race.'" *American Anthropologist*, 1998, *100*(3), 1–19.

Hermann, A., and Stewart, A. J. *Theorizing Feminism.* (2nd ed.) Boulder, Colo.: Westview, 2000.

James, S. A., and Thomas, P. E. "John Henryism and Blood Pressure in Black Populations: A Review of the Evidence." *African American Research Perspectives*, 2000, *6*(3), 1–10.

James, S. A., and others. "Socioeconomic Status, John Henryism, and Blood Pressure in Black Adults: The Pitt County Study." *American Journal of Epidemiology*, 1992, *135*(1), 59–67.

Jones, C. P. "Levels of Racism: A Theoretic Framework and a Gardener's Tale." *American Journal of Public Health*, 2000, *90*(8), 1212–1215.

Krieger, N. "Embodying Inequality: A Review of Concepts, Measures, and Methods for Studying Health Consequences of Discrimination." *International Journal of Health Services*, 1999, *29*(2), 295–352.

Krieger, N., and Bassett, M. "The Health of Black Folks: Disease, Class and Ideology in Science." *Monthly Review—An Independent Socialist Magazine*, 1986, *38*, 74–85.

Krieger, N., and Fee, E. "Man-Made Medicine and Women's Health: The Biopolitics of Sex/Gender and Race/Ethnicity." In E. Fee and N. Krieger (eds.), *Women's Health, Politics, and Power: Essays on Sex/Gender, Medicine, and Public Health*. Amityville, N.Y.: Baywood Publishing, 1994.

LaViest, T. A. "Why We Should Continue to Study Race . . . But Do a Better Job: An Essay on Race, Racism and Health." *Ethnicity and Disease*, 1996, *6*, 21–29.

Mullings, L. "Minority Women, Work and Health." In W. Chavkin (ed.), *Double Exposure: Women's Health Hazards on the Job and at Home*. New York: Monthly Review Press, 1984.

Mullings, L. "Inequality and Afro-American Health Status: Policies and Prospects." In W. Van Horne (ed.), *Race: Twentieth Century Dilemmas—Twenty-First Century Prognoses*. Milwaukee: University of Wisconsin Institute on Race and Ethnicity, 1989.

Mullings, L. *On Our Own Terms: Race, Class and Gender in the Lives of African American Women*. New York: Routledge, 1997.

Mullings, L., and Wali, A. *Stress and Resilience: The Social Context of Reproduction in Central Harlem*. New York: Kluwer/Plenum, 2001.

Muntaner, C., and others. "Racial Ideology and Explanations for Health Inequalities Among Middle-Class Whites." *International Journal of Health Services*, 2001, *31*(3), 659–668.

Phimister, E. G. "Medicine and the Racial Divide." *New England Journal of Medicine*, 2003, *348*(12), 1081–1082.

Sellers, R. M., Caldwell, C. H., Schmelke-Cone, K. H., and Zimmerman, M. A. "Racial Identity, Racial Discrimination, Perceived Stress, and Psychological Distress Among African American Young Adults." *Journal of Health and Social Behavior*, 2003, *44*, 302–317.

Stokols, D. "Translating Social Ecological Theory into Guidelines for Community Health Promotion." *American Journal of Health Promotion*, 1996, *10*(4), 282–298.

Williams, D. "Race/Ethnicity and Socioeconomic Status: Measurement and Methodological Issues." *International Journal of Health Services*, 1996, *26*(3), 483–505.

PART TWO

RACE, CLASS, GENDER, AND KNOWLEDGE PRODUCTION

CHAPTER TWO

RECONSTRUCTING THE LANDSCAPE OF HEALTH DISPARITIES RESEARCH

Promoting Dialogue and Collaboration Between Feminist Intersectional and Biomedical Paradigms

Lynn Weber

Hierarchies of health and illness across race, ethnicity, social class, socioeconomic status, and gender have been continually reproduced for a century in an ever-changing array of diseases, illnesses, and adverse health conditions (Aday, 2001; Adler and Newman, 2002; Hofrichter, 2003; House, 2002; House and Williams, 2000; Robert and House, 2000a; Shim, 2000; Smedley, Stith, and Nelson, 2003). In recent years, finding new approaches to reducing or eliminating these health disparities has become a priority for national health agencies, politicians, health advocates, and researchers, and increased funding has been allocated for this purpose.[1] Yet the bulk of the research to date has not varied significantly from its historical patterns, dominated by the biomedical paradigm and the psychosocial and biobehavioral approaches that emulate it. This apparent contradiction between political and scientific concern about the longstanding problem of health disparities, on the one hand, and continued funding and support for traditional nominally effective approaches, on the other, raises key questions about the structure of the scientific enterprise and the potential for alternative paradigms to engage intellectually with dominant paradigms, to generate new knowledge, and to shape policy about health disparities.

In the past thirty years, feminist scholarship on the intersections of race, class, gender, sexuality, and other dimensions of difference has advanced knowledge and reshaped views of the nature and consequences of these systems of social inequality (Acker, 2000; Baca Zinn and Dill, 1996; Collins, 2000a; Davis, 1981; Glenn, 2000; Mann and Grimes, 2001; Weber, 2001; Zambrana, 1987). During this time, intersectional scholarship has become one of the leading approaches to the study of gender in women's studies and ethnic studies and in gender studies within traditional disciplines (Howard and Allen, 2000). Yet feminist intersectional research remains largely marginalized in the academy and public policy—as are other critical public health approaches to health disparities that differ in significant ways from the biomedical paradigm: ecological (Bent, 2003; McLeroy, Bibeau, Steckler, and Glanz, 1988; Glanz and others, 1995; Parra-Medina and Fore, 2004), technoscience (Clarke and Olesen, 1999; Shim, 2002), social capital (Wallack, 2000), community-based participatory research (McLeroy and others, 2003; Merzel and D'Afflitti, 2003; Minkler and Wallerstein, 2003; Wallerstein and Bernstein, 1988; Wallerstein and Sanchez-Merki, 1994), and social justice (Hofrichter, 2003).

The aim of this chapter is to reconfigure the terrain of health disparities scholarship by highlighting the unique contributions of feminist intersectional approaches to knowledge that derive from their critical assumptions, methods, and orientations to research. However, if we hope to significantly change the landscape that constitutes health science and policy on health disparities, merely identifying the contributions to be made by intersectional and related critical scholarships is not enough. To produce a deeper understanding of the ways that differentials of power perpetuate health disparities and to effect change in the practice of science and policy, these approaches must also be in a position to engage in critical exchange with dominant paradigms on a more equal footing. To that end, the chapter concludes by identifying some promising areas of convergence in understandings and approaches across dominant and critical paradigms and by suggesting ways to facilitate a more balanced and effective dialogue and collaboration among dominant, feminist intersectional, and other critical paradigms addressing health disparities.

DOMINANCE OF THE BIOMEDICAL PARADIGM

Most scholarship on health disparities that is considered mainstream in the social sciences and biomedical science and that receives the lion's share of research funding emerges from the biomedical paradigm and the psychosocial and biobehavioral approaches that emulate it—each of which employs a positivist epistemology. With the massive national investment in biomedical research and related medical interventions and treatments, it is almost unnecessary to note that applications of the biomedical model have improved the health of the population and of many individuals. Research that extends the biomedical model to incorporate biobehavioral traits such as health-related behaviors (for example, smoking, exercise, diet; Ainsworth and others, 1991; Cockerham, 2000; Crespo and others, 2000; Harrell and Gore, 1998; Lynch, Kaplan, and Salonen, 1997; Smedley and Syme, 2000) and individual-level psychosocial characteristics and processes such as social supports, self-esteem, stress of discrimination, and perceptions of mastery and control (House, Landis, and Umberson, 1988; Mirowsky, Ross, and Reynolds, 2000; Schulz and others, 2000) has also increased our knowledge of the disease process and has supported interventions that work for individuals (Lantz and others, 1998)

Although there are important variations among these types of studies, they typically employ standards reflecting the ideals of a positivist biomedical paradigm and share common assumptions, conceptualizations, and methodologies. Driven primarily by a goal of knowledge accumulation, researchers assume a stance of affective neutrality and objectivity. They value and reinforce a hierarchical relationship between themselves and the subjects of their research, playing the role of the "expert" who controls all aspects of the research process. Methods emphasize measurement and quantification and employ individuals as units of analysis in large-scale surveys or randomized controlled trials (LeCompte and

Schensul, 1999). Within this paradigm, health disparities research commonly conceives and measures social inequalities as resource differences among individuals (for example, who has more education or income), not as group dynamics (for example, which groups have power over others). One goal of analyses is to separate the independent effects of social inequalities (for example, race or gender or socioeconomic status) from one another and from other determinants of health. Furthermore, even when researchers acknowledge the importance of macrosocial forces, analyses typically seek to identify the more proximate causes, such as health behaviors, social supports, cultural values, and stress, that mediate between these social inequalities and individual health outcomes (Adler and Newman, 2002; Mirowsky, Ross, and Reynolds, 2000; House, 2002). Consequently, proximate causes become the primary targets for intervention, typically leaving broader systems of social inequality unanalyzed and unaddressed.

In contrast, feminist intersectional scholarship, driven foremost by the pursuit of social justice, takes a researcher stance of engaged subjectivity and reflexivity—critically reflecting throughout the research process on the impact of the social locations of the researchers and the researched. A collaborative relationship more closely resembling a partnership between researchers and researched is seen as ideal. Methods focus less on measurement and quantification and more on identifying and holistically representing meanings in the lives of the researched and in institutional arrangements. Multimethod approaches are valued, often mixing ethnographic, historical, community-based qualitative approaches with surveys and other tools. Inequalities are conceived as social constructions situated in social contexts and structures beyond the individual—in societies, institutions, communities, and families—and are characterized as power, not simply resource, differences between dominant and subordinate groups. The primary analytical goal is not to separate the effects of inequalities from other determinants of health or to identify more proximate causes of health inequalities. Instead, it is to explicate the processes through which multiple social inequalities of race, gender, social class, and other dimensions of difference are simultaneously generated, maintained, and challenged at the institutional and individual levels, shaping the health of societies, communities, and individuals. And finally, broad systems of inequality become the targets for intervention, including systems outside the health arena that nonetheless determine health, such as the economy, jobs, education, and the law (Fonow and Cook, 2005; for a more complete comparison of these paradigms, see Weber and Parra-Medina, 2003).

The biomedical and feminist intersectional paradigms are not only different; they are differently situated in the health disparities research and policy landscape. The biomedical paradigm clearly dominates the health science terrain, as evidenced by the paucity of alternative critical approaches receiving significant funding, appearing in prestigious publication outlets, and informing public policy. A recent Institute of Medicine report, *The Future of the Public's Health in the Twenty-First Century* (2002), points to the dominance of the biomedical paradigm as a cause of the gap between U.S. health-related expenditures—roughly 13 percent of our gross domestic product, more than any other industrialized nation—and our health status, which lags behind many nations: "The vast majority of health care spending, as much as 95 percent by some estimates, is directed toward medical care and biomedical research. However, there is strong evidence that behavior and environment are responsible for over 70 percent of avoidable mortality, and health care is just one of several determinants of health" (Institute of Medicine, 2002, p. 2).

In a recent review of feminist methodology in the academy and public policy, Mary Margaret Fonow and Judith Cook (2005) note, "At this time in the United States, traditional methodologies remain highly valued, while many other countries rely more on qualitative and consensus studies in setting their public policy agendas and enacting corresponding legislation. The current U.S. Congress is calling for, and in some cases requiring, very narrow 'scientific' research designs and protocols that focus on 'proving' cause and effect—a troubling and obviously political move."

A search of the CRISP database of information on all biomedical research (the term used for all health science, including social science) projects funded by the National Institutes of Health,

Centers for Disease (CDC), and other federal agencies revealed that in the past ten years, thirty-nine unique projects included the term *health disparities* in the title or abstract.[2] Thirty-five of those (90 percent) are squarely situated in the positivist biomedical paradigm: all the projects employ survey or experimental designs and quantitative methodologies, with individuals as units of analysis and with race, socioeconomic status, and gender measured as individual traits. They all seek either to track (not necessarily explain) differences in health outcomes across some measure of social inequality (most commonly race/ethnicity), for example, in oral health, drug use, smoking, or cardiovascular disease, and/or to uncover proximate, mediating causes between social inequalities and health outcomes.

While none of the remaining four studies emerged from an intersectional paradigm, they diverge from the positivist biomedical ideal in critical ways that are shared with intersectional research. These studies approach the researcher-researched relationship as reciprocal and collaborative and engage with community-based organizations in Detroit (Schulz and others, forthcoming), poultry workers in North Carolina (Arcury, 1996), a parent-teacher collaboration in schools (McClowry, 1998), and rural women workers (Lipscomb, 2000). They also employ qualitative as well as quantitative methods and conceptualize social inequalities as power relationships, not solely as resource differences.

Publication data on health disparities reveal a similar pattern of dominance by the biomedical paradigm. For example, Weber and Parra-Medina (2003) reviewed articles on health disparities in physical activity and cardiovascular disease published since 1990 and found that all studies were more reflective of than divergent from the basic tenets of the biomedical paradigm. Here too, however, two recent studies diverge in key ways from the biomedical by taking an ecological approach and taking into account social context factors beyond the individual (Crespo and others, 2000; King and others, 2000). Not surprisingly, however, since these more critical studies are also funded by agencies wedded to the biomedical paradigm, they remain largely shaped by the assumptions and practices of that paradigm. For example, they emphasize measurement and quantification, search for independent and proximate causes of social inequalities, and, perhaps most important, fail to explicitly incorporate a critical analysis of unequal power relations.

LIMITATIONS AND BIAS IN THE BIOMEDICAL PARADIGM

Although a vibrant science almost by definition requires a free space for the balanced exchange of ideas and critical dialogue, the dominance of the biomedical paradigm has inhibited such an ideal. As Collins, an intersectional scholar, notes (2000a, p. 275), "Mainstream science operates as such a powerful discourse and set of social practices that, to many, it appears to be invincible." It is so powerful and ubiquitous, in fact, that even many feminist scholars whose work is deeply critical of mainstream science unwittingly contribute to its dominance by simply rejecting science out of hand and refusing to engage in dialogue at all. Postmodernist theories, for example, have become popular in feminist circles in part because, by minimizing the importance of science's power over the intellectual landscape, these theories simultaneously avoid addressing the role of power relationships in shaping feminists' own critical knowledge (Collins, 2000a). In the end, while comfortably isolating postmodernist scholars from critical self-reflection on the role of class, race, sexuality, gender, and national power in shaping their own theories and research, these approaches do little to challenge science for its biases.

The dominance of the biomedical paradigm has resulted in health science and policy that are infused with the biases of the paradigm—biases that a vibrant critical exchange among diverse perspectives in a balanced scientific landscape would more effectively critique and, ideally, reduce or eliminate. To this end, feminist intersectional and critical public health scholars continue to highlight the biases of positivist biomedical science in a variety of arenas (for example, Baum, 1995; Krieger and Fee, 1994; McLeroy and others, 2003; Minkler and Wallerstein, 2003; Mutaner and Gomez, 2002; Wallerstein and Bernstein, 1988; Wallerstein and Sanchez-Merki, 1994; Shim, 2000, 2002). For some time, scholars have questioned biomedical science's claims of value neutrality by documenting its Euro- and androcentric bias. From delineating every possible bodily difference between black slaves and whites in the nineteenth century to excluding women from clinical trials because of "hormonal interference" for most of the twentieth, physician scientists have played key roles in producing race, class, and gender hierarchies by "seeing" differences in the bodies of presumably inferior groups (Krieger and Fee, 1994; Longino, 1990; Morgen, 2002; Rose, 1994; Rosser, 1994; Ruzek, Olesen, and Clarke, 1997a). Rosser (p. 5) also notes that

> the very choice of problems for study in medical research is substantially determined by a national agenda that defines what is worthy of study—i.e., funding. As Marxist (Zimmerman and others, 1980), African-American (McLeod, 1987) and feminist (Hubbard, 1990) critics of scientific research have pointed out, the research that is undertaken reflects the societal bias toward the powerful, who are overwhelmingly white, middle- to upper-class, and male in the United States. Obviously, the majority of members of Congress, who appropriate the funds for NIH and other federal agencies, fit this description; they are more likely to vote funds for health research that they view as beneficial as defined from their perspective.

One of the more egregious and far-reaching cases of scientific bias that costs thousands of lives and has fueled race, class, gender, sexuality, and nationality hierarchies has been the HIV/AIDS epidemic. Because the first cases of AIDS identified in 1981 were among gay men, intravenous drug users, and later Haitians, the illness was attributed to "lifestyle choices," victims were stigmatized, and diagnosis, prevention, and care were impeded for these and other groups. Women were invisible in the epidemic. In many studies they were seen as "vehicles" or "vectors" of the disease. The construction of AIDS based on symptoms and manifestations in men led to defining criteria of the disease that excluded numerous conditions noted in women, including cervical cancer, pelvic inflammatory disease, and human papillomavirus, until twelve years after the disease was first diagnosed.

Furthermore, lack of knowledge among scientists of different cultural definitions of sex among Hispanic men—where men who engage in male-to-male sex do not see themselves as gay or bisexual—rendered public campaigns targeted to gay men ineffective for these groups. And dominant-culture—white, heterosexual, Christian, and middle class—political forces have controlled knowledge and information that could limit the disease by restricting sexuality education in schools. In short, biased science and its deployment in a hierarchically structured social order led to underdiagnosis, lack of care and treatment, and increased death and burden of disease among less powerful groups—women, racial and ethnic minorities, the poor, and sexual minorities (for discussions of this history, see Oppenheimer, 1992; Singer and others, 1990; Stine, 2000).

Dominant-culture science institutions such as the National Academy of Sciences (NAS) have at times acknowledged the negative impact that scientific biases and "bad science" have had in promoting racism and sexism. In 1989, it issued a statement entitled "Methods and Values in Science":

> As with hypotheses, human values cannot be eliminated from science, and they can subtly influence scientific investigations. . . . Social and personal values unrelated to epistemological criteria— including philosophical, religious, cultural, political and economic values—can shape scientific judgment in fundamental ways. . . . The obvious question is whether holding such values can harm a person's science. In many cases the answer has to be yes. The history of science offers many episodes in which social and personal values led to the promulgation of wrong-headed ideas. For instance, past investigators produced "scientific" evidence for overtly racist views, evidence we now know to be wholly erroneous. Yet at the time the evidence was widely accepted and contributed to repressive social policies. [cited in Harding, 1993, p. 342].

The statement also notes that gender biases in scientific judgments have wrongly supported the notion of a relationship between gender and scientific abilities and that this poor science has contributed to institutional policies that have caused women and minorities to be underrepresented in science, with a consequent "loss of scientific talent and diversity" (p. 343).

Despite this history, the NAS (1989) concluded that social and personal values do not necessarily harm science. For example, the desire to do accurate work and the belief that knowledge will ultimately benefit rather than harm humankind are values that contribute to the motivations and conceptual outlook of scientists. NAS cautions that scientists can conduct good science and avoid the distorting influence of their own values by trying to identify them and the effects they have on their science. It recommends that scientists study the history, philosophy, and sociology of science. Identifying and assessing the impact of our own values on our science, however, cannot be done in a vacuum. By engaging in dialogue and collaboration with others whose values and assumptions are different, our own guiding principles can be made visible, can be clarified, and can even become subject to change.

To address health disparities more effectively, with sound science, we need to open up the landscape of health disparities research so that fruitful dialogue and collaborations can take place among intersectional scholarship centered primarily in the humanities and social sciences, other critical public health approaches, and traditional positivist biomedical research. Intersectional feminism, which interrogates the institutionally structured power relations shaping the process of knowledge production itself, the social inequalities of health, and the relations between the two, is uniquely positioned to uncover the taken-for-granted assumptions of both traditions and to speak to the process through which a productive dialogue can take place.

FEMINIST INTERSECTIONAL SCHOLARSHIP: AN ALTERNATIVE PARADIGM

Because it emerged from a very different scholarly and social justice impulse than traditional biomedically driven scholarship on health and health disparities, feminist intersectional scholarship is a good place to look for a fresh critical approach to science. First, it arose primarily among women of color inside and outside the academy—not from the centers of power in the legitimized halls of academe and government, where the voices of women of color are still not well represented. Because intersectional scholarship never benefited from the vast resources that characterize those settings—grant funding, publication outlets, institutional validation, access to policymakers—it was not constrained by the traditional approaches to knowledge sanctioned in those venues. Instead, it emerged in a relatively free space to construct theory and knowledge that grew directly from the lived experiences of women of color.

Second, intersectional scholarship arose as a critique of mainstream scholarship and scholarly institutions and of the exclusionary practices of emerging interdisciplinary and critical movements, including women's studies and ethnic studies (for example, see Baca Zinn, Cannon, Higginbotham, and Dill, 1986). Consequently, it benefits from the ways that these critical scholarships opened up new intellectual spaces that allow different approaches to knowledge and research. For example, because feminist scholarship was interdisciplinary from its inception, it has had to develop strategies and skills for revealing the ways that disciplinary assumptions and research methodologies shape knowledge and for translating meanings across disciplines (DeVault, 1999; Fonow and Cook, 1991; Hesse-Biber and Yaiser, 2004; Pryse, 2000). And in challenging the racism and classism in women's studies and the sexism in ethnic studies, intersectional scholarship has also moved beyond some of the exclusive and limiting contours of those fields.

Third, it arose primarily to understand and to address the multiple dimensions of social inequality (class, race, ethnicity, nation, sexuality, and gender) manifest at both the macrolevel of institutions and the microlevel of the individual experiences of women who live at the intersections of multiple inequalities. The focus is on identifying the meanings of multiple inequalities in these women's lives and in institutions. Intersectional scholarship is thus not limited by the social science, public health, and biomedical traditions that typically examine these inequalities in separate studies and generate different theories about each dimension. Nor is it restricted by the methodological conventions dominant in health research—quantitative analyses of large-scale surveys or controlled randomized trials—that require prohibitive sample sizes in order to examine multiple dimensions of inequality in the same study. And by seeking social justice for those situated in multiply subordinated locations, intersectional scholars have looked for ways of facilitating liberatory dialogue across race, class, gender, and sexuality divides (Collins, 1998, 2000b; Pryse, 2000; Yuval-Davis, 1997).

Finally, the focus of feminist intersectional scholarship is not narrowly on health but more globally on the constructions of hierarchies of privilege and power across all social institutions, including the economy, family, education, law, religion, and media. Consequently, inquiry is not bound by the traditional biomedical emphasis on individuals or individual bodies as units of analysis and as targets of concern. Emerging from the study of broad social systems and social groups, intersectional approaches focus on the processes through which group hierarchies are created, sustained, challenged, and transformed over time and in specific locales. Individuals' experiences, particularly those of individuals situated at the intersections of multiple inequalities, are explored and valued primarily for their unique ability to shed light on broader social systems—the very arena where "health disparities" are defined.

The following sections discuss core themes in feminist intersectional approaches to understanding race, class, gender, and other dimensions of difference and provide some examples to illustrate what they might bring to the goal of eliminating health disparities.

ORIENTATION AND PURPOSE

Key differences between intersectional and biomedical paradigms are the orientations, motivations, goals, and purposes of the research. Feminist intersectional scholarship emanates from the unique social positioning of women of color and is motivated by a desire for social justice—to unmask and to challenge social inequalities. Like much of feminist scholarship more broadly, it values subjectivity, researcher engagement in the process of change, and empowerment of oppressed groups (Fonow and Cook 1991, 2005; Reinharz and Davidman, 1992; Sprague and Zimmerman, 1993). Furthermore, many intersectional scholars contend that knowledge about social inequality is itself gained in the collaborative process of acting to promote social justice (Collins, 1998, 2000b; DeVault, 1999; Mies, 1983, 1991). In advocating participatory action research, for example, Maria Mies (1983, p. 125) wrote, "Social change is the starting point of science, and in order to understand the content, form, and consequences of patriarchy, the researcher must be actively involved in the fight against it; one has to change something before it can be understood." This orientation to research differs considerably from positivist biomedical approaches but is consistent with a range of social justice–driven approaches emergent in public health research since the 1960s (cf. Freire, 1970, 1982; Hofrichter, 2003; Minkler and Wallerstein, 2003).

Intersectional scholars argue that the social location of groups situated at the intersections of multiple systems of inequality provides not only a unique but also a privileged position from which to understand those systems (Collins, 1986, 1998, 2000b; DeVault, 1999; Fonow and Cook, 1991; Guinier and Torres, 2002). Women of color and other groups that experience multiple forms of inequality often occupy social locations or "border spaces" that provide them with some access to power. Collins (1986, 1998, 2000b) uses the term *outsiders-within* to describe those who occupy a contradictory location wherein they have knowledge of dominant groups but at the same time lack the full privileges afforded true insiders. Collins (1986) contends that outsider-within intellectual communities, such as those of black women scholars, have unique advantages when they choose to use their location to investigate power arrangements in social life:

- A kind of "objectivity" that is a peculiar combination of nearness and remoteness, concern and disinterest
- A tendency for people to confide in a stranger in ways they would not with each other
- The ability of a stranger to see patterns that those immersed cannot see
- Creativity that is spurred by marginality

One contribution that intersectional scholarship can make to shifting the focus of health disparities research lies in asking new questions that emanate from the position of outsiders-within and are generated from an explicitly recognized social change agenda. Since the goal of health disparities scholarship is not only to understand the processes producing disparities but also to eliminate them, a key problem for scholars is how to bridge the gap between theory in the academy and social action. This problem is particularly acute for positivist biomedical social science, but feminist intersectional scholarship, which is empirically based (that is, resting on direct observation of behavior), not positivist (assuming distance and disengagement between researcher and researched), suggests some new pathways to such bridging.

One example of social justice–driven intersectional scholarship on health disparities is Morgen's research (2002) on the women's health movement since 1969 (see the discussion in Chapter Fourteen). Building on earlier work by Ruzek (1978), Morgen, like Ruzek, examines the movement from the perspective of an insider—one who worked to build a women's health clinic during the late 1970s that would challenge the race, class, and gender inequities in the health system. As an outsider-within—a woman academic who nonetheless participated in this movement for social change—she occupied a unique social position that enabled her to see and to interpret the everyday ways that race, class, gender, and sexual hierarchies were created, challenged, and reinforced in this setting and how they shaped the health of the women who both worked at and sought services at the clinic. Combining her personal observations with many other methods (including document analysis, key informant interviews, and questionnaires), she conveys a rich description of both the macroinstitutional forces (such as co-optation by the state and economic pressures) shaping the impact of the movement and the microlevel realities of everyday life wherein those macroforces were played out (for example, class conflicts between professional and working-class staff). From this engaged stance of the outsider-within, Morgen is able to provide a much deeper understanding of how health inequalities are reproduced and how they can be challenged.

CONTEXTUALLY SPECIFIC SOCIAL CONSTRUCTIONS

Intersectional approaches to scholarship share with other critical perspectives an analysis of race, ethnicity, class, gender, sexuality, and other dimensions of difference as systems of inequality that are socially constructed in specific historical and geographical contexts, in time and place. They are fluid, shifting group relations that nonetheless persist through time and space. Because they are shaped differently in different contexts and times, feminist intersectional research, as exemplified in work like Morgen's, investigates the historical development and change in these systems of inequality in specific communities. Health itself is viewed as a condition of communities and societies (Ruzek, Olesen, and Clarke, 1997a).[3] And intersectional research is less concerned with the search for universal laws than with building broader understandings of social inequality and health disparities from close observations of social relationships in particular sites.

The social construction of health disparities was the focus of intersectional research on the social contexts of reproduction in central Harlem conducted by Mullings and Wali in collaboration with other researchers, students, community organizations, individuals, and activists (Mullings, 2000, 2002; Mullings and Wali, 2001; see Chapter Twelve, this volume). To understand and address the disparity in infant mortality rates between African American and white women of all social classes, this collaborative undertook a multiyear, ethnographic, participatory action research study of central Harlem, a community with high infant mortality rates among African American women of all social classes.

Investigators began the research with a firm grounding in the history and current social arrangements of central Harlem. Mullings and other researchers had lived there for as many as twenty years, the Urban League was a partner from the beginning, and a community advisory board of long-time residents participated in the project throughout. This specific awareness of community history enabled researchers to identify community strengths and assets as well as deficits, to know where to observe the social stresses and strains of daily living (for example, in the struggle for safe and affordable housing), and to position themselves to learn of unanticipated critical sites (such as housing court, where women brought complaints against landlords). Because they knew and were involved in the communities being studied, researchers could observe the subtle social processes through which race, class, and gender hierarchies are reproduced and the psychological and material stresses that accompany those processes. For example, they documented the ways that media representations of life in low-income housing—even self-consciously sympathetic ones—play a role in producing public opinion and public policy that blames residents for social conditions over which they have little or no control and against which they actively work.

By engaging in a critical process of self-reflection and community involvement throughout the research process, Mullings, Wali, and their collaborators also recognize and address the ways in which the research process itself is a social construction. Like other feminist and critical public health scholars, they have challenged the notion that data exist in a one-to-one relationship with the social reality that is being studied and instead have made us more aware that the "product of any research process is a construction of, not a reflection of, what the reality is about" (Fonow and Cook, 2005; Denzin and Lincoln, 2000). For example, as a consequence of suggestions by community members, researchers constructed the descriptive data about the community to incorporate community strengths and assets (for example, the percentage of residents *not* receiving welfare, *with* college or high school educations, *employed*), not simply the reverse, as is commonly the case in studies of subordinate communities. And in their reflective preface to the book summarizing the project, Mullings and Wali (2001, p. ix) note ways that the reporting of findings in terms of "potential sources of stress and chronic strain from social, economic, and political conditions" was shaped in part by the funder's (CDC) goal of being "helpful to people in public health and related fields."

MULTILEVEL POWER RELATIONS

Perhaps the central principle undergirding intersectional conceptions of these hierarchies of difference and the primary reason they persist over time are that they are intersecting systems of power relationships—relationships of dominance and subordination—where the privilege of one group rests on the subordination of others. Power relationships exist between opposing groups where dominant groups hold power over others and use that power to secure material and social resources such as wealth, income, or access to health care and education. Power relationships also exist at both the macrolevel of institutions (as evident in structural arrangements that benefit certain groups and harm others, such as economic, political, and family policies) and the microindividual levels of interpersonal relationships (with friends, family, neighbors, and coworkers).

Groups remain dominant in a system over time because their position enables them to continue despite the will or aims of others— they have "power over" others (Townsend and others, 1999). Guinier and Torres (2002) describe three dimensions of "power over" as it is conventionally conceived. First-dimension power is exhibited in direct force or competition, typically in winner-take-all contexts—the power to win the game. Second-dimension power involves indirect manipulation of rules to shape the outcome of competition—the power to design the rules. And with third-dimension power, actors can mobilize, often through psychological means, biases, or tacit understandings, to "sell" the underlying rules and structures to the powerless. It is the power to define the discourse about the game, its significance, and why the winners won the game.

This relational conception of race, class, gender, and other social hierarchies contrasts sharply with the distributional conceptions dominant in biomedical research (Lucal, 1994, 1996; Vanneman and Weber Cannon, 1987). Distributional approaches conceive of these hierarchies as differences that are primarily centered not in their relationships to oppositional groups but rather in women's and men's bodies, in their social roles, in their material resources, and in their various cultural traditions, such as food, clothing, rituals, speech patterns, leisure activities, child-rearing practices, and sexual practices—in the things that people are, have, believe, and do. In each case, the focus of attention is typically on how the values, practices, roles, or even material resources, such as the income or property of subordinate groups, deviate from those of dominant groups. And dominant groups become the unquestioned norm—so much so that the concepts of race, class, gender, and sexuality are themselves typically seen as markers for people of color, the working classes and poor, women, and homosexuals, while whites, the middle and upper classes, men, and heterosexuals are seen as having no race, class, gender, or sexuality (Herek, 1987; Lucal, 1994, 1996). These processes of ranking, comparing, and treating dominant groups as the unmarked norm obscure the nature of race, class, gender, and sexuality as social relationships between dominant and subordinate groups and hide the role of power in producing and sustaining social inequalities. Thinking of race, class, gender, and sexuality as power relationships enables us to understand that they are not independent but rather interdependent, mutually reinforcing systems rooted in power (Collins, 1998, 2000b; Baca Zinn and Dill, 1996; Weber, 1998, 2001).

Oaks's study (2001) of the social construction of smoking during pregnancy, for example, reveals the ways that power relationships of race, class, and gender shape who smokes, why they smoke, how their smoking is interpreted by others, and the treatment accorded smokers. Oaks documents the ideological and political power that is wielded against poor and working-class women and women of color who smoke. Poor and working-class women are most likely to smoke during pregnancy and to be labeled as unfit and irresponsible mothers when they do because this image reinforces dominant-culture conceptions of their communities. Despite the fact that white mothers are significantly more likely to smoke than black mothers, the most negative attributions are made about black, particularly young black, mothers. And poor women, who are more likely to come into contact with state systems of surveillance when they are pregnant (via Medicaid and family social services, for example) are also more likely to bear the brunt of any state-sponsored interventions when women are deemed unfit. For example, although smoking has not yet sufficed to convict pregnant women for child abuse, more than two hundred women in thirty states have been prosecuted since the mid-1980s for practices during pregnancy that were deemed harmful to their fetuses, including drinking, taking drugs, and having sex (Oaks, 2001; Roth, 2000; Woliver, 2002). And in the late 1980s, child custody cases began to admit smoking as evidence of unfit parenting and to revoke custody rights to protect children from unsafe smoke-filled homes (Oaks, 2001).

By examining smoking in the contexts of these women's lives, however, Oaks (2001) reveals that the phenomenon is not as simple as either an uncontrollable addiction or a voluntary choice. Reminiscent of the contexts of reproduction in the Harlem study (Mullings and Wali, 2001), critical institutional and interpersonal power relationships shape the contexts of pregnancy for these women, producing stresses and constraints for which smoking provides some relief. First, the conditions of work and gender dynamics in the family leave poor women under great stress, with little time to rest and restore. For some, smoking is "the only time I get five minutes to myself" (Oaks, 2001, p. 197). Second, many of the women are involved in romantic relationships with partners who smoke and are surrounded by family and friends who smoke. Macrolevel policies that have isolated smokers from nonsmokers have normalized smoking in some social circles. Finally, while the women recognize the health risks, many do not trust that the "experts" are at all clear about the true risks for individuals. The increased surveillance and control by the health care and legal systems over pregnant women—especially poor women of color—in the name of protecting the rights of fetuses have posed pregnancy as a conflict between mother and fetus that is to be mediated by the state. This adversarial position contributes to a lack of trust, especially among poor women, for whom the designation of "bad mother" can have dire consequences (Oaks, 2001).

Although the reasons for smoking are varied, they can be understood in the contexts of women's lives and the power relationships within which women live. Poor women who smoke are a seriously stigmatized group. They lack first-dimension power options, choices, and control in the economic, familial, political, and health arenas. They lack second-dimension power: the power to set macropolicies and precedents that will shape the contexts of their lives. They lack third-dimension power: to shape the public interpretation of their smoking. So they are stigmatized as bad mothers, blamed for jeopardizing the health of their unborn children, and denied full access to society's valued resources.

Understanding the role of power relationships enables us to shape interventions that differ from approaches emerging from a biomedical paradigm where the focus would more likely be on changing the values, behaviors, cognitions, or even biochemical processes of individual women who smoke. When social inequalities are viewed as power relationships, the ways in which dominant groups benefit from denying others adequate child care and medical access, for example, become a focus of attention. So changes that might alter the balance of power—a living wage; shifts in workplace control; universal, affordable, quality child care; accessible public transportation; safe and affordable housing; equal access to quality education; and universal prevention-focused health care—become the preferred interventions. While the former may change the lives of those involved in targeted programs, the latter is more likely to effect change that would significantly reduce health disparities (for discussion of implications in public health, see Shim, 2000, 2002; Carter-Pokras and Baquet, 2002; Hofrichter, 2003).

Simultaneity and Connections

In some ways, the conception of structured social inequalities as interdependent, mutually constituted, integrally connected systems of inequality is the thread from which the tapestry of intersectional scholarship has been woven. Intersectional scholarship emerged from the voices of African American and other women of color whose social location at the intersections of multiple systems of oppression made any politic, practice, or scholarship that treats them as separate seem absurd (Collins, 1998, 2000b; Williams, 1991). And black women have spoken of this contradiction for a very long time—from Sojourner Truth's 1851 "Ain't I a Woman" speech (see Mullings, 2002) to the provocative title of one of the first anthologies of intersectional scholarship in the early 1980s— *All the Women Are White, All the Blacks Are Men, But Some of Us Are Brave: Black Women's Studies* (Hull, Scott, and Smith, 1982). Modern intersectional research conceives of social inequalities as interdependent and mutually constituted, *not* independent or additive; seeks complex representations of social inequalities, *not* parsimony in research models (Kneipp and Drevdahl, 2003); and seeks connections among inequalities, *not* rankings of inequalities by severity of impact.

Positivist biomedically driven scholarship on health inequalities differs in part because it has emerged from scholarly traditions that treat race, class, socioeconomic status, gender, ethnicity, and sexuality separately and that develop separate interpretations for their relationships to health. Reskin (2003) contends that this balkanized scholarship, especially in combination with the individual focus of most research, is responsible for the failure to identify the mechanisms of discrimination. The different theories generated about different sources of subordination (such as race or social class or gender) employ different sets of intervening mechanisms and "stories" to explain the relationship between a particular macroinequality and its consequences for individuals and groups. She points out that this balkanization has fostered contradictory workplace discrimination policies where people of color now have different options for redress in the face of sex or race discrimination, where women of color have to choose which one of their statuses they will argue was the source of discrimination against them if they contest employers' unfair actions, and where the outcome will likely differ depending on their choice (for a similar argument regarding domestic violence policy, see Crenshaw, 1995).

In most traditional health disparities scholarship, discrimination is a concept primarily reserved for mistreatment on the basis of race and ethnicity. Robert and House (2000a, p. 84) recently noted that socioeconomic inequalities do not fully explain the race-health relationship and suggest that "other experiences associated with race in our society, *such as discrimination* [emphasis added] . . . may also account for some race effects on health." Yet when they identified research challenges for the study of gender, socioeconomic status, and health, "discrimination" was not mentioned. Instead, Robert and House (2000a) suggested that gender research seek to understand the reasons that the relationship between socioeconomic status and health is weaker among women than among men. And they suggest that researchers should examine the connection of community socioeconomic characteristics and health, "especially for women who *do not work* [emphasis added] and may spend a substantial amount of time in their community environment" (p. 84). The clear implication in this statement is that women not in the paid labor force (and therefore not captured in traditional measurements of work) are not working and are at home in their communities—reifying the largely white and middle-class view of women as either in the paid labor force (and therefore working outside their communities) or in the home as housewives (and therefore not working but living inside their communities).

But intersectional scholarship has revealed the limits of traditional constructions of work, unmasking their hidden assumptions: that it is productive, for pay, and conducted outside the home. It has also demonstrated the inadequacy of this notion of work for explaining much of what most women in the world do and its relationship to their health (Daniels, 1987; Messias and others, 1997). In fact, intersectional scholarship reveals that women's work occurs in many sites (both inside and outside the home) and takes on many forms as yet unrecognized by traditional health research: domestic work, cottage industries, underground economy work, unpaid work in the home, and "health work"—the work of caring for and managing their family's and community's heath (Messias and others, 1997).

Research on women of color and immigrant domestic workers, for example, has problematized the notion of work "outside the home" since these women in fact work for pay "inside the homes" of largely white employers (Dill, 1994; Glenn, 1986; Hondagnu-Sotelo, 1997; Kaplan, 1987; Palmer, 1989; Rollins, 1985; Romero, 1992; Salzinger, 1991). In this case, the middle-class employer's community environment is the workplace for the employer's domestic and other workers, such as yard workers. Furthermore, domestics who work in multiple homes have no clearly defined workplace. And when low-income women work for pay in their own homes by providing, for example, day care for neighborhood children, the division between market/productive work and home/reproductive work is shattered—a division that is also shattered in the work worlds of middle-class women and men through such practices as telecommuting and job sharing. So although it emerges from analysis of the lives of marginalized people, the knowledge gained in intersectional scholarship sheds new light on and raises new questions about the ways we conceive of and investigate the lives of others, even in more privileged social locations.

One further consequence of the balkanization of research on subordination and inequality in conjunction with the positivist goal of representativeness (and large samples) is that traditional quantitative research considering more than one dimension—for example, race and socioeconomic status—typically assumes that these dimensions of inequality have additive effects on all outcomes. It implies, for example, that the consequences of racial minority status on health can simply be added to the effect of being a woman and further added to the effects of education and income to predict one's health status. Yet traditional health disparities scholarship is increasingly recognizing what intersectional and some public health traditions have consistently argued: that additivity does not hold. As Krieger and others (1993, p. 99) describe the problem, "Many studies, however, inappropriately assume that the effects of racism, sexism, and social class are simply additive. Instead, their specific combinations reflect unique historical experience forged by the social realities of life in the United States and should be studied accordingly."

RECOMMENDATIONS TO FURTHER DIALOGUE AND COLLABORATION

This analysis suggests several avenues for promoting dialogue and collaboration among intersectional, critical public health, and bio-medically derived paradigms to promote understanding and elimination of health disparities.

BEGIN DIALOGUE ON RECOGNIZED POINTS OF CONVERGENCE

Despite the biomedical paradigm's overwhelming dominance in the health research and policy landscape, the paradigm is neither monolithic nor static. Just as feminist intersectional and critical public health paradigms alter their assumptions, methods, and practice in response to critical self-reflection and to political, social, and economic contingencies (Fonow and Cook, 2005), so too do biomedical and related paradigms. Recently powerful health institutions such as the Institute of Medicine and the NIH have issued reports that call for changes to the traditional biomedical paradigm in health research, policy, and education—changes that converge with key elements of both intersectional and critical public health paradigms:

- An ecological approach to health research, policy, and education that incorporates upstream factors such as social contexts and public policies even in sectors beyond health that nonetheless shape it, such as the law, economy, education, and media
- Community-based collaborative research
- Multilevel, multimethod (including qualitative and quantitative methods), interdisciplinary research (Institute of Medicine, 1998, 2002, 2003a, 2003b; NIH, 2000, 2001, 2004; Smedley, Stith, and Nelson, 2003; Smedley and Syme, 2000)

These reports reflect growing recognition among scholars both critical of and immersed in the biomedical paradigm that understanding and reducing or eliminating health disparities requires such new directions (Breen, 2001; House, 2002; House and Williams, 2000; Kneipp and Drevdahl, 2003; Krieger, 1999; Krieger and others, 1993; Krieger, Williams, and Moss, 1997; Link and Phelan, 2000; Minkler and Wallerstein, 2003; Mullings and Wali, 2001; Robert and House, 2000a, 2000b; Ruzek, 1999; Ruzek, Olesen, and Clarke, 1997a, 1997b; Smedley and Syme, 2000; Smedley, Stith, and Nelson, 2003; Williams, 2002). And these directions represent terrain on which dialogue and collaboration can potentially take place.

INCORPORATE A POWER-RELATIONAL ANALYSIS INTO RESEARCH

Much less prevalent, although particularly important from an intersectional perspective, are calls for research that critically examines race, class, and gender health disparities as power relationships. Incorporating an explicit analysis of race, class, and gender as power relationships into health disparities scholarship is at once perhaps the most challenging and the most important contribution that intersectional and other critical scholarships can make to research and policy (Hofrichter, 2003; Israel, Schulz, Parker, and Becker, 1998; Krieger, Williams, and Moss, 1997; Minkler and Wallerstein, 2003; Navarro and Shi, 2001; Navarro, 2004). As Navarro (2004, p. 98) describes it, "We need to look for the roots of the problem (of health inequalities [sic]) in the ways that power (class, race, and gender power) is reproduced in the state, in the media, and in the value-generating systems."

Incorporating a power analysis is challenging in part because knowledge about power dynamics and the processes of change has come largely when researchers have consciously chosen to confront power hierarchies in specific social contexts, as Navarro suggests—including those hierarchies of power between researchers themselves and the communities they study. As Hall (1992, p. 22) states, "Participatory research fundamentally is about who has the right to speak, to analyze, to act." And intersectional and other critical power-based research approaches seek a collaboration that privileges and supports the voices, insights, and actions of multiply subordinated groups (Collins, 1986, 1998, 2000a; Freire, 1970, 1982; Mies, 1983, 1991; Minkler and Wallerstein, 2003).

While the IOM and NIH reports call for incorporating different methods or research designs (ecological, community-based, qualitative, multilevel) into a largely unchallenged biomedical health terrain, feminist intersectional and other power-focused traditions view these approaches less as methods and more as elements in an alternative orientation to research—a set of broad commitments guiding research practice (DeVault, 1999; Fonow and Cook, 1991, 2005; Israel, Schulz, Parker, and Becker, 1998; Reinharz and Davidman, 1992). Minkler and Wallerstein (2003, p. 5), for example, describe community-based participatory research as an orientation to research with "a heavy accent on issues of trust, power, dialogue, community capacity building, and collaborative inquiry toward the goal of social change to improve community health and well-being and eliminate health disparities."

Fruitful engagement between critical and biomedically derived traditions will therefore require understanding not only current practices but also the historical, political, social, and economic conditions that nurtured them. Intersectional and other critical traditions emerged largely to promote an explicit social justice agenda aimed at countering the dominant-culture institutions that reinforce and reproduce health and other social inequalities. Explicitly focusing research on promoting social justice is more often than not viewed within traditional biomedical science as an unscientific and illegitimate contamination of the research process. Not surprisingly, justice-driven research questions the utility of traditional research designs and analytical techniques for assessing the efficacy of their approaches and concepts. In health promotion research, for example, new orientations focus on developing social capital and community capacity and emphasize broad social and contextual influences on health. Yet the randomized controlled trial is a problematic evaluation strategy for these and other theories that target communities and are ecological and where outcomes of interest are not at the individual level (DiClemente, Crosby, and Kegler, 2002). Growing recognition of this problem is reflected in increased appreciation of and funding for assessment of macrolevel indicators of inequality as well as for the qualitative research methodologies so important to these approaches and to feminist intersectional research.

SEEK A BETTER BALANCE BETWEEN MEASUREMENT AND MEANING IN RESEARCH

While the development of new measures of macrosystemic and group-level processes is certainly a promising trend, research in the biomedical tradition can become so fixed on measurement and quantification that it impedes taking actions to eliminate hierarchies of health—actions that themselves can lead to a better understanding of these hierarchies (Collins, 1998, 2000a; Mies, 1983; DeVault, 1999). In contrast, intersectional scholarship, which has relied largely on qualitative methodologies, has often focused primarily on revealing the meaning and experience of social inequalities without documenting or assessing the efficacy of different approaches to social change. In her review of feminist methodology, DeVault (1999, p. 32) states: "Accomplishing change through feminist research and assessing whether it has occurred are, of course, quite difficult and relatively little writing addresses these problems. . . . Too often, I believe, the call for change functions as a slogan in writing on feminist methodology, and authors make assumptions about change without sufficient examination of their own implicit theories of social change."

LEVEL THE PLAYING FIELD FOR INTERSECTIONAL AND OTHER CRITICAL PARADIGMS

If we are to develop a deeper understanding of the ways that differentials of power perpetuate health disparities and to change the practice of science and policy, intersectional and other critical approaches must also be in a position to engage in meaningful exchange with dominant paradigms on a more equal footing. Promoting such an exchange will require addressing the power imbalance that exists between the traditions themselves.

Intersectional and critical public health scholars, who have identified practices that facilitate dialogue and collaboration among researchers and community members who have unequal power in the research process, suggest several principles to create a more balanced landscape. Strand and others (2003b) and other public health researchers suggest that successful partnerships require partners to share a worldview, agree about goals and strategies, have mutual trust and respect, share power, communicate clearly, understand and empathize with each other, and remain flexible. The benefits of such collaborations are many: ensuring the research focuses on an agreed-upon social-change agenda, enhancing the quality of the research, and empowering all involved by giving all participants access to the expertise of others (Strand and others, 2003a).

Many feminist communities, both here and across the globe, have sought to identify ways to bridge race, class, gender, sexuality, and disciplinary boundaries to achieve truly interdisciplinary thought and effective social action. Israeli feminist Nira Yuval-Davis, for example, credits a group of Italian feminists who went to Israel to mediate a peace discussion among Israeli and Palestinian women with developing "transversal politics," a method for bridging these barriers. Yuval-Davis (1997, p. 130) describes the method:

> The idea is that each participant in the dialogue brings with her the ROOTING in her own membership and identity, but at the same time tries to SHIFT in order to put herself in a situation of exchange with women who have different membership and identity. They called this form of dialogue "transversalism"—to differentiate from "universalism" which, by assuming a homogeneous point of departure, ends up being exclusive instead of inclusive, and [from] "relativism" which assumes that, because of the differential points of departure, no common understanding and genuine dialogue are possible at all.

By focusing the process of shifting to understand and incorporate the views of others in a rootedness born of a critical self-awareness of our race, gender, class, discipline, and other sources of identity and by employing the "shifting" skills that intersectional scholars develop as they seek to work across disciplinary boundaries, we have the potential to develop what Collins (2000a) calls principled coalitions. Such coalitions are based not on the exploitation of power differentials but on self-awareness, self-respect, and a genuine appreciation of others.

PROMOTE THE USE OF ACCESSIBLE, PLAIN LANGUAGE IN RESEARCH AND PRACTICE

A key problem in achieving this kind of balanced critical dialogue and collaboration is developing a common language. While the problems of language and translation should have been obvious to Italian and Israeli feminists, it may be equally difficult to bridge the disciplinary and paradigmatic boundaries of methods, theory, and orientation to research. Pryse (2000), in fact, argues that disciplinary methodological boundaries can be as difficult to traverse as race, class, gender, and national and cultural boundaries. Arising from an activist past, intersectional scholarship commonly calls for the elimination of disciplinary jargon and the use of widely "accessible language" (Collins, 2000a; Weber, 2001). And public health's increased emphasis on community-based collaborative research and on increasing the role of the public in setting priorities for the NIH are trends that are compatible with calls for the use of plain language in scientific reporting (IOM, 1998; NIH, 2004).

But calling for plain and accessible language is much easier than making it happen, even in feminist scholarship that explicitly aims for it. The work for this chapter, for example, required much translation and "deconstructing" of intersectional, other critical public health, and biomedical paradigms to identify the underlying orientations and assumptions as well as methods and practices that characterize these paradigms. This process requires that the translators become multilingual in order to understand the different approaches and communicate them across the paradigms to multiple audiences.

PRIVILEGE THE PERSPECTIVES OF SUBORDINATE GROUPS

Learning others' languages takes time and energy, and if it is to support a fruitful dialogue and collaboration for change, this learning requires that the participants respect each other's intellectual and social positions and histories. To do so will require that we privilege the perspectives of subordinate and marginalized groups—learn from the "outsiders within"—within both our research communities and the communities whose lives we aim to understand and to improve. Efforts to increase the numbers of women and people of color in the sciences and the health science professions, which are widespread and well funded, must not only address the economic and mentorship issues that have been common in the past but also engage the different perspectives, questions, and concerns that women of color bring to science. They must also take seriously the implications of those perspectives for how science and scientific research itself are conceptualized and practiced.

In the conclusions of her book on the women's health movement, Morgen (2002, p. 236) looks to the future and asks, "How do the various constituencies that seek a more just and equitable health care system work together?" She calls for "a movement that is politically sophisticated, racially and class inclusive, vibrant, adaptable, and willing to nourish alliances with other movements and organizations that envision a more just and equitable society." If we hope to develop a more equitable and engaged scholarship and practice to eliminate health disparities, we must promote a more inclusive intellectual landscape to support dialogue and collaboration across intersectional, critical public health, and biomedically derived paradigms.

Notes

I thank Deborah Parra-Medina and Sheryl Ruzek for reading and commenting on several versions of this chapter, and especially for input into discussions of emerging scholarship in public health research. I am indebted to my colleagues in the University of South Carolina's Women's Studies Working Papers Seminar for valuable input into the framing of this chapter: Wanda Hendricks, DeAnne Messias, Deborah Parra-Medina, Suzanne Swan, and Laura Woliver. I also appreciate the research conducted by the graduate assistants who contributed to this project: Emily Aleshire, Elizabeth Fore, Keri Norris, and Heather Smith. Finally, this work benefited tremendously from the thoughtful critique and input of the volume's editors, Leith Mullings and Amy Schulz, and from the other chapter authors.

1. For example, in July 2002, more than two thousand people attended the first National Leadership Summit on Eliminating Racial and Ethnic Disparities in Health, sponsored by the Office of Minority Health, U.S. Department of Health and Human Services. Healthy People 2010 has as one of its top two priorities eliminating racial and ethnic health disparities. And the National Institutes of Health developed a strategic

plan to reduce and eliminate health disparities by 2006 and established the National Center on Minority Health and Health Disparities (Adler and Newman, 2002; Clarke and Olesen, 1999; House and Williams, 2000; House, 2002; Krieger, 1999; Link and Phelan, 2000; National Institutes of Health, 2000, 2001; Robert and House, 2000b; Ruzek, Olesen, and Clarke, 1997b; Smedley, Stith, and Nelson, 2003; Smedley and Syme, 2000). For a discussion of multiple uses of the term *health disparities* and for their political and policy implications, see Carter-Pokras and Baquet (2002).

2. These are all the R01 projects, which tend to be the largest, best-funded, and most prestigious projects involving original research.
3. In this position, intersectional scholarship more closely reflects "what the WHO describes as the prerequisites for health: freedom from the fear of war; equal opportunity for all; satisfaction of basic needs for food, water, and sanitation; education; decent housing; secure work and a useful role in society; and political will and public support" (Ruzek, Olesen, and Clarke, 1997b, p. 14).

References

Acker, J. "Rewriting Class, Race, and Gender: Problems in Feminist Rethinking." In M. M. Ferree, J. Lorber, and B. Hess (eds.), *Revisioning Gender.* New York: Altamira Press, 2000.

Aday, L. A. *At Risk in America: The Health and Health Care Needs of Vulnerable Populations in the United States.* San Francisco: Jossey-Bass, 2001.

Adler, N. E., and Newman, K. "Socioeconomic Disparities in Health: Pathways and Policies." *Health Affairs,* 2002, *21*(2), 60–76.

Ainsworth, B. E., and others. "Physical Activity and Hypertension in Black Adults: The Pitt County Study." *American Journal of Public Health,* 1991, *81*(11), 1477–1479.

Arcury, T. "Sources of Health Disparities: Minority Poultry Workers." NIH 2R01ES008739–06, 1996–2005. [The CRISP database from which these references were obtained is the ERACommons Computer Retrieval of Information on Scientific Projects electronic databases: http://crisp.cit.nih.gov/crisp/crisp_lib.query]

Baca Zinn, M., Cannon, L. W., Higginbotham, E., and Dill, B. T. "The Costs of Exclusionary Practices in Women's Studies." *Signs: A Journal of Women in Culture and Society,* 1986, *11*(2), 290–303.

Baca Zinn, M., and Dill, B. T. "Theorizing Difference from Multiracial Feminism." *Feminist Studies,* 1996, *22*(2), 321–333.

Baum, F. "Researching Public Health: Behind the Qualitative-Quantitative Methodological Debate." *Social Science and Medicine,* 1995, *40*(4), 459–468.

Bent, K. N. "The People Know What They Want: An Empowerment Process of Sustainable Ecological Community Health." *Advances in Nursing Science,* 2003, *26*(3), 215–226.

Breen, N. "Social Discrimination and Health: Understanding Gender and Its Interaction with Other Social Determinants." Oct. 2001. http://www.hsph.harvard.edu/Organizations/healthnet/Hupapers/gender/breen.html.

Carter-Pokras, O., and Baquet, C. "What Is a Health Disparity?" *Public Health Reports,* 2002, *117,* 426–434.

Clarke, A., and Olesen, V. (eds.). *Revisioning Women, Health, and Healing: Feminist, Cultural, and Technoscience Perspectives.* New York: Routledge, 1999.

Cockerham, W. C. "The Sociology of Health Behavior and Health Lifestyles." In C. E. Bird, P. Conrad, and A. M. Fremont (eds.), *Handbook of Medical Sociology.* Upper Saddle River, N.J.: Prentice Hall, 2000.

Collins, P. H. "Learning from the Outsider Within: The Sociological Significance of Black Feminist Thought." *Social Problems,* 1986, *33*(6), 14–32.

Collins, P. H. *Fighting Words: Black Women and the Search for Justice.* Minneapolis: University of Minnesota Press, 1998.

Collins, P. H. *Black Feminist Thought.* (2nd ed.) New York: Routledge, 2000a.

Collins, P. H. "Moving Beyond Gender: Intersectionality and Scientific Knowledge." In M. M. Ferree, J. Lorber, and B. Hess (eds.), *Revisioning Gender.* New York: Altamira Press, 2000b.

Crenshaw, K. W. "Mapping the Margins: Intersectionality, Identity, Politics, and Violence Against Women of Color." In K. W. Crenshaw, N. Gotanda, G. Peller, and K. Thomas (eds.), *Critical Race Theory: The Key Writings That Formed the Movement.* New York: New Press, 1995.

Crespo, C. J., and others. "Race/Ethnicity, Social Class, and Their Relation to Physical Inactivity During Leisure Time: Results from the Third National Health and Nutrition Examination Survey, 1988–1994." *American Journal of Preventive Medicine,* 2000, *18*(1), 46–53.

Daniels, A. "Invisible Work." *Social Problems,* 1987, *34,* 403–415.

Davis, A. *Women, Race, and Class.* New York: Random House, 1981.

Denzin, N. K., and Lincoln, Y. S. "Introduction: The Discipline and Practice of Qualitative Research." In N. K. Denzin and Y. S. Lincoln (eds.), *Handbook of Qualitative Research.* Thousand Oaks, Calif.: Sage, 2000.

DeVault, M. L. *Liberating Method: Feminism and Social Research.* Philadelphia: Temple University Press, 1999.

DiClemente, R. J., Crosby, R. A., and Kegler, M. C. *Emerging Theories in Health Promotion Practice and Research: Strategies for Improving Public Health.* San Francisco: Jossey-Bass, 2002.

Dill, B. *Across the Boundaries of Race and Class.* New York: Garland, 1994.

Fonow, M. M., and Cook, J. A. (eds.). *Beyond Methodology: Feminist Scholarship as Lived Research.* Bloomington: Indiana University Press, 1991.

Fonow, M. M., and Cook, J. A. "Feminist Methodology: New Applications in the Academy and Public Policy." *Signs: A Journal of Women in Culture and Society,* 2005, *30*(4), 2211–2236.

Freire, P. *Pedagogy of the Oppressed.* New York: Seabury Press, 1970.

Freire, P. "Creating Alternative Research Methods: Learn to Do It by Doing It." In B. L. Hall, A. Gillette, and R. Tandon (eds.), *Creating Knowledge: A Monopoly?* Toronto: Participatory Research Network, 1982.

Glanz, K., and others. "Environmental and Policy Approaches to Cardiovascular Disease Prevention Through Nutrition: Opportunities for State and Local Action." *Health Education Quarterly,* 1995, *22*(4), 512–527.

Glenn, E. N. *Issei, Nisei, War Bride: Three Generations of Japanese American Women in Domestic Service.* Philadelphia: Temple University Press, 1986.

Glenn, E. N. "The Social Construction and Institutionalization of Gender and Race: An Integrative Framework." In M. M. Ferree, J. Lorber, and B. Hess (eds.), *Revisioning Gender.* New York: Altamira Press, 2000.

Guinier, L., and Torres, G. *The Miner's Canary: Enlisting Race, Resisting Power, Transforming Democracy.* Cambridge, Mass.: Harvard University Press, 2002.

Harding, S. (ed.). *The "Racial" Economy of Science: Toward a Democratic Future.* Bloomington: Indiana University Press, 1993.

Harrell, J. S., and Gore, S. V. "Cardiovascular Risk Factors and Socioeconomic Status in African American and Caucasian Women." *Research in Nursing and Health,* 1998, *21,* 285–295.

Herek, G. "On Heterosexual Masculinity." In M. Kimmel (ed.), *Changing Men: New Directions in Research on Men and Masculinity.* Thousand Oaks, Calif.: Sage, 1987.

Hesse-Biber, S. N., and Yaiser, M. *Feminist Perspectives on Social Research.* New York: Oxford University Press, 2004.

Hofrichter, R. "The Politics of Health Inequities: Contested Terrain." In R. Hofrichter (ed.), *Health and Social Justice: Politics, Ideology, and Inequity in the Distribution of Disease.* San Francisco: Jossey-Bass, 2003.

Hondagnu-Sotelo, P. "Working Without Papers in the United States: Toward the Integration of Legal Status in Frameworks of Race, Class, and Gender." In E. Higginbotham and M. Romero (eds.),

Women and Work: Exploring Race, Ethnicity, and Class. Thousand Oaks, Calif.: Sage, 1997.

House, J. S. "Understanding Social Factors and Inequalities in Health: Twentieth Century Progress and Twenty-First Century Prospects." *Journal of Health and Social Behavior,* 2002, *43*(2), 125–142.

House, J. S., Landis, K. R., and Umberson, D. "Social Relationships and Health." *Science,* 1988, *241,* 540–545.

House, J. S., and Williams, D. R. "Understanding and Reducing Socioeconomic and Racial/Ethnic Disparities in Health." In B. D. Smedley and S. L. Syme (eds.), *Promoting Health: Interventions Strategies from Social and Behavioral Research.* Washington, D.C.: National Academy Press, 2000.

Howard, J. A., and Allen, C. (eds.). "Feminisms at the Millennium." *Signs: Journal of Women in Culture and Society,* 2000, *25* (entire issue 4).

Hubbard, R. *The Politics of Women's Biology.* New Brunswick, N.J.: Rutgers University Press, 1990.

Hull, G., Scott, P. B., and Smith, B. (eds.). *All the Women Are White, All the Blacks Are Men, But Some of Us Are Brave.* New York: Feminist Press, 1982.

Institute of Medicine. *Scientific Opportunities and Public Needs: Improving Priority Setting and Public Input at the National Institutes of Health.* Washington, D.C.: National Academy of Sciences, 1998.

Institute of Medicine. *The Future of the Public's Health in the Twenty-First Century.* Washington, D.C.: National Academy of Sciences, 2002.

Institute of Medicine. *From Neurons to Neighborhoods: The Science of Early Childhood Development.* Washington, D.C.: National Academy of Sciences, 2003a.

Institute of Medicine. *Informing the Future: Critical Issues in Health.* (2nd ed.) Washington, D.C.: National Academy of Sciences, 2003b.

Israel, B. A., Schulz, A. J., Parker, E. A., and Becker, A. B. "Review of Community-Based Research: Assessing Partnership Approaches to Improve Public Health." *Annual Review of Public Health,* 1998, *19,* 173–202.

Kaplan, E. B. "I Don't Do No Windows: Competition Between Domestic Worker and Housewife." In V. Miner and H. Longino (eds.), *Competition: A Feminist Taboo?* New York: Feminist Press, 1987.

King, A. C., and others. "Personal and Environmental Factors Associated with Physical Inactivity Among Different Racial/Ethnic Groups of U.S. Middle-Aged and Older-Aged Women." *Health Psychology,* 2000, *19*(4), 354–364.

Kneipp, S. M., and Drevdahl, D. J. "Problems with Parsimony in Research on Socioeconomic Determinants of Health." *Advances in Nursing Science,* 2003, *26*(3), 162–172.

Krieger, N. "Embodying Inequality: A Review of Concepts, Measures, and Methods for Studying Health Consequences of Discrimination." *International Journal of Health Services,* 1999, *29*(2), 295–353.

Krieger, N., and Fee, E. "Man-Made Medicine and Women's Health: The Biopolitics of Sex/Gender and Race/Ethnicity." *International Journal of Health Services,* 1994, *24*(1), 265–283.

Krieger, N., Williams, D. R., and Moss, N. E. "Measuring Social Class in U.S. Public Health Research: Concepts, Methodologies, and Guidelines." *Annual Review of Public Health,* 1997, *18*, 341–378.

Krieger, N., and others. "Racism, Sexism, and Social Class: Implications for Studies of Health, Disease, and Well-Being." *American Journal of Preventive Medicine,* 1993, *9*(6, suppl.), 82–122.

Lantz, P. M., and others. "Socioeconomic Factors, Health Behaviors, and Mortality." *Journal of the American Medical Association,* 1998, *279,* 1703–1708.

LeCompte, M. D., and Schensul, J. J. *Designing and Conducting Ethnographic Research.* New York: Altamira Press, 1999.

Link, B. G., and Phelan, J. C. "Evaluating the Fundamental Cause Explanation for Social Disparities in Health." In C. Bird, P. Conrad, and A. M. Fremont (eds.), *Handbook of Medical Sociology.* (5th ed.) Upper Saddle River, N.J.: Prentice Hall, 2000.

Lipscomb, H. "Work and Health Disparities Among Rural Women." NIH 1R01ES010939–01, 2000–2005. [The database from which these references were obtained is the ERACommons Computer Retrieval of Information on Scientific Projects (CRISP) electronic databases: http://crisp.cit.nih.gov/crisp/crisp_lib.query]

Longino, H. *Science as Knowledge: Values and Objectivity in Scientific Inquiry.* Princeton, N.J.: Princeton University Press, 1990.

Lucal, B. "Class Stratification in Introductory Textbooks: Relational or Distributional Models?" *Teaching Sociology,* 1994, *22,* 139–150.

Lucal, B. "Oppression and Privilege: Toward a Relational Conceptualization of Race." *Teaching Sociology,* 1996, *24,* 245–255.

Lynch, J. W., Kaplan, G. A., and Salonen, J. T. "Why Do Poor People Behave Poorly? Variation in Adult Health Behaviours and Psychological Characteristics by Stages of Socioeconomic Life Course." *Social Science and Medicine,* 1997, *44*(6), 809–819.

Mann, S. A., and Grimes, M. D. "Common and Contested Ground: Marxism and Race, Gender and Class Analysis." *Race, Gender and Class,* 2001, *8*(2), 3–16.

McClowry, S. "Testing a Parent/Teacher Collaborative Prevention Model." NIH 2R0NR004781–06, 1998–2005. [The database from which these references were obtained is the ERACommons Computer Retrieval of Information on Scientific Projects electronic databases,: http://crisp.cit.nih.gov/crisp/crisp_lib.query]

McLeod, S. *Scientific Colonialism: A Cross-Cultural Comparison.* Washington, D.C.: Smithsonian Institution Press, 1987.

McLeroy, K. R., Bibeau, D., Steckler, A., and Glanz, K. "An Ecological Perspective on Health Promotion Programs." *Health Education Quarterly,* 1988, *15*(4), 351–377.

McLeroy, K. R., and others. "Community-Based Interventions." *American Journal of Public Health,* 2003, *93*(4), 529–533.

Merzel, C., and D'Afflitti, J. "Reconsidering Community-Based Health Promotion: Promise, Performance, and Potential." *American Journal of Public Health,* 2003, *93*(4), 557–574.

Messias, D. K., and others. "Defining and Redefining Work: Implications for Women's Health." *Gender and Society,* 1997, *11*(3), 296–323.

Mies, M. "Towards a Methodology for Feminist Research." In G. Bowles and R. D. Klein (eds.), *Theories of Women's Studies.* London: Routledge and Kegan Paul, 1983.

Mies, M. "Women's Research or Feminist Research? The Debate Surrounding Feminist Science and Methodology." In J. Cook and M. M. Fonow (eds.), *Beyond Methodology: Feminist Scholarship as Lived Research.* Bloomington: Indiana University Press, 1991.

Minkler, M., and Wallerstein, N. "Introduction to Community-Based Participatory Research." In M. Minkler and N. Wallerstein (eds.), *Community-Based Participatory Research for Health.* San Francisco: Jossey-Bass, 2003.

Mirowsky, J., Ross, C. E., and Reynolds, J. "Links Between Social Status and Health Status." In C. E. Bird, P. Conrad, and A. M. Fremont (eds.), *Handbook of Medical Sociology.* Upper Saddle River, N.J.: Prentice Hall, 2000.

Morgen, S. *Into Our Own Hands: The Women's Health Movement in the United States 1969–1990.* New Brunswick, N.J.: Rutgers University Press, 2002.

Mullings, L. "African-American Women Making Themselves: Notes on the Role of Black Feminist Research." *Souls: A Critical Journal of Black Politics, Culture, and Society,* 2000, *2*(4), 18–29.

Mullings, L. "The Sojourner Syndrome: Race, Class, and Gender in Health and Illness." *Voices,* Dec. 2002, pp. 32–36.

Mullings, L., and Wali, A. *Stress and Resilience: The Social Context of Reproduction in Central Harlem.* Norwood, Mass.: Kluwer, 2001.

Mutaner, C., and Gomez, M. B. "Anti-Egalitarianism: Legitimizing Myths, Racism, and 'Neo-McCarthyism' in Social Epidemiology and Public Health: A Review of Sally Satel's PC, M.D." *International Journal of Health Services,* 2002, *32*, 1–17.

National Academy of Science. *Being a Scientist.* Washington, D.C.: National Academy Press, 1989.

National Institutes of Health. *A Strategic Research Plan to Reduce and Ultimately Eliminate Health Disparities: Strategic Plan 2002–2006.* Washington, D.C.: National Institutes of Health, 2000.

National Institutes of Health, Council of Public Representatives. *Enhancing Public Input and Transparency in the National Institutes of Health Research Priority-Setting Process.* Washington, D.C.: National Institutes of Health, Apr. 2004.

National Institutes of Health, Office of Behavioral and Social Science Report. *Towards Higher Levels of Analysis: Progress and Promise in Research on Social and Cultural Dimensions of Health: Executive Summary.* Washington, D.C.: National Institutes of Health, Sept. 2001.

Navarro, V. "The Politics of Health Inequalities Research in the United States." *International Journal of Health Services,* 2004, *34*(1), 87–99.

Navarro, V., and Shi, L. "The Political Context of Social Inequalities and Health." *International Journal of Health Services,* 2001, *31*(1), 1–21.

Oaks, L. *Smoking and Pregnancy: The Politics of Fetal Protection.* New Brunswick, N.J.: Rutgers University Press, 2001.

Oppenheimer, G. M. "Causes, Cases, and Cohorts: The Role of Epidemiology in the Historical Construction of AIDS." In E. Fee and D. M. Fox (eds.), *AIDS: The Making of a Chronic Disease.* Berkeley: University of California Press, 1992.

Palmer, P. *Domesticity and Dirt: Housewives and Domestic Servants in the United States.* Philadelphia: Temple University Press, 1989.

Parra-Medina, D., and Fore, E. "Behavioral Studies." In B. M. Beech and M. Goodmand (eds.), *Race and Research.* Washington, D.C.: American Public Health Association, 2004.

Pryse, M. "Trans/Feminist Methodology: Bridges to Interdisciplinary Thinking." *NWSA Journal,* 2000, *12*(2), 105–118.

Reinharz, S., and Davidman, L. *Feminist Methods in Social Research.* New York: Oxford University Press, 1992.

Reskin, B. "Presidential Address: Including Mechanisms in Our Models of Ascriptive Inequality." *American Sociological Review,* 2003, *68*(1), 1–21.

Robert, S. A., and House, J. S. "Socioeconomic Inequalities in Health: An Enduring Sociological Problem." In C. E. Bird, P. Conrad, and A. M. Fremont (eds.), *Handbook of Medical Sociology.* Upper Saddle River, N.J.: Prentice Hall, 2000a.

Robert, S. A., and House, J. S. "Socioeconomic Inequalities in Health: Integrating Individual-, Community-, and Societal-Level Theory and Research." In G. L. Albrecht, R. Fitzpatrick, and S. C. Scrimshaw (eds.), *Handbook of Social Studies in Health and Medicine.* Thousand Oaks, Calif.: Sage, 2000b.

Rollins, J. *Between Women: Domestics and Their Employers.* Philadelphia: Temple University Press, 1985.

Romero, M. *Maid in the USA.* New York: Routledge, 1992.

Rose, H. *Love, Power, and Knowledge: Toward a Feminist Transformation of the Sciences.* Bloomington: Indiana University Press, 1994.

Rosser, S. *Women's Health: Missing from U.S. Medicine.* Bloomington: Indiana University Press, 1994.

Roth, R. *Making Women Pay: The Hidden Cost of Fetal Rights.* Ithaca, N.Y.: Cornell University Press, 2000.

Ruzek, S. *The Women's Health Movement.* New York: Praeger, 1978.

Ruzek, S. "Rethinking Feminist Ideologies and Actions: Thoughts on Past and Future of Health Reform." In A. Clarke and V. Olesen (eds.), *Revisioning Women, Health, and Healing: Feminist, Cultural, and Technoscience Perspectives.* New York: Routledge, 1999.

Ruzek, S., Olesen, V., and Clarke, A. "What Are the Dynamics of Difference?" In S. Ruzek, V. Olesen, and A. Clarke (eds.), *Women's Health: Complexities and Differences.* Columbus: Ohio State University Press, 1997a.

Ruzek, S., Olesen, V., and Clarke, A. (eds.). *Women's Health: Complexities and Differences.* Columbus: Ohio State University Press, 1997b.

Salzinger, L. "A Maid by Any Other Name: The Transformation of 'Dirty Work' by Central American Immigrants." In M. Burawoy and others (eds.), *Ethnography Unbound: Power and Resistance in the Modern Metropolis.* Berkeley: University of California Press, 1991.

Schulz, A., and others. "Social Inequalities, Stressors, and Self-Reported Health Status Among African American and White Women in the Detroit Metropolitan Area." *Social Science and Medicine,* 2000, *51,* 1639–1653.

Schulz, A., and others. "Social and Physical Environments and Disparities in Risk for Cardiovascular Disease: The Healthy Environments Partnership Conceptual Model." *Environmental Health Perspectives,* forthcoming.

Shim, J. "Bio-Power and Racial, Class, and Gender Formation in Biomedical Knowledge Production." *Research in the Sociology of Health Care,* 2000, *17,* 173–195.

Shim, J. "Understanding the Routinised Inclusion of Race, Socioeconomic Status and Sex in Epidemiology: The Utility of Concepts from Technoscience Studies." *Sociology of Health and Illness,* 2002, *24*(2), 129–150.

Singer, M., and others. "SIDA: The Economic, Social, and Cultural Context of AIDS Among Latinos." *Medical Anthropology Quarterly*, 1990, *4*, 72–114.

Smedley, B. D., and Syme, S. L. (eds.). *Promoting Health: Intervention Strategies from Social and Behavioral Research.* Washington, D.C.: National Academy Press, 2000.

Smedley, B. D., Stith, A. Y., and Nelson, A. R. (eds.). *Unequal Treatment: Confronting Racial and Ethnic Disparities in Health Care.* Washington, D.C.: National Academy Press, 2003.

Sprague, J., and Zimmerman, M. "Overcoming Dualisms: A Feminist Agenda for Sociological Methodology." In P. England (ed.), *Theory on Gender/Feminism on Theory.* New York: Aldine, 1993.

Stine, G. J. "Discovering AIDS, Naming the Disease." In G. J. Stined (ed.), *AIDS Update 2000.* Upper Saddle River, N.J.: Prentice Hall, 2000.

Strand, K., and others. "Methodological Principles of Community-Based Research." In K. Strand and others (eds.), *Community-Based Participatory Research and Higher Education.* San Francisco: Jossey-Bass, 2003a.

Strand, K., and others. "Why Do Community-Based Research? Benefits and Principles of Successful Partnerships." In K. Strand and others (eds.), *Community-Based Participatory Research and Higher Education.* San Francisco: Jossey-Bass, 2003b.

Townsend, J. G., and others. *Women and Power: Fighting Patriarchies.* New York: Zed Books, 1999.

Vanneman, R., and Weber Cannon, L. *The American Perception of Class.* Philadelphia: Temple University Press, 1987.

Wallack, L. "The Role of Mass Media in Creating Social Capital: A New Direction for Public Health." In B. D. Smedley and S. L. Syme (eds.), *Promoting Health: Intervention Strategies from Social and Behavioral Research.* Washington, D.C.: National Academy Press, 2000.

Wallerstein, N., and Bernstein, E. "Empowerment Education—Freire Ideas Adapted to Health- Education." *Health Education Quarterly*, 1988, *15*(4), 379–394.

Wallerstein, N., and Sanchez-Merki, V. "Freirian-Praxis in Health-Education—Research Results from an Adolescent Prevention Program." *Health Education Research*, 1994, *9*(1), 105–118.

Weber, L. "A Conceptual Framework for Understanding Race, Class, Gender, and Sexuality." *Psychology of Women Quarterly*, 1998, *22*, 13–32.

Weber, L. *Understanding Race, Class, Gender, and Sexuality: A Conceptual Framework.* New York: McGraw-Hill, 2001.

Weber, L., and Parra-Medina, D. "Intersectionality and Women's Health: Charting a Path to Eliminating Health Disparities." In V. Demos and

M. T. Segal (eds.), *Advances in Gender Research: Gender Perspectives on Health and Medicine.* Amsterdam: Elsevier, 2003.

Williams, D. R. "Racial/Ethnic Variations in Women's Health: The Social Embeddedness of Health." *American Journal of Public Health,* 2002, *92*(4), 588–597.

Williams, P. J. *The Alchemy of Race and Rights: Diary of a Law Professor.* Cambridge, Mass.: Harvard University Press, 1991.

Woliver, L. *The Political Geographies of Pregnancy.* Urbana: University of Illinois Press, 2002.

Yuval-Davis, N. "Women, Ethnicity and Empowerment: Towards Transversal Politics." In N. Yuval-Davis, *Gender and Nation.* Thousand Oaks, Calif.: Sage, 1997.

Zambrana, R. E. "A Research Agenda on Issues Affecting Poor and Minority Women: A Model for Understanding Their Health Needs." *Women and Health,* Winter 1987, pp. 137–160.

Zimmerman, B., and others. "People's Science." In R. Arditti, P. Brennan, and S. Cavrak (eds.), *Science and Liberation.* Boston: South End Press, 1980.

CHAPTER THREE

MOODS AND REPRESENTATIONS OF SOCIAL INEQUALITY

Emily Martin

How can the different modes of knowledge about race and mental health in cultural anthropology and in public health shed light on each other? In this chapter I bring what I have learned doing an ethnography in which race and mental illness played a central part up against a key public document that relies on statistical information of the kind commonly used in public health to see what each approach can learn from the other. The document, the supplement to *Mental Health: A Report of the Surgeon General* (U.S. Department of Health and Human Services, 2001), published under David Satcher's leadership, includes an extensive survey of what is understood about socioeconomic variables in relation to race and mental health. The supplement discusses the additional stress placed on members of groups who are the object of racial discrimination, of both the major institutional sort and the chronic everyday sort. It acknowledges the role of poverty in producing major stress and making mental health care affordable. The supplement spells out that whether the base rates of various kinds of mental illness are comparable for whites and African Americans (something it finds hard to sort out given available information) or higher for African Americans, it is clear that African Americans receive less medical attention for mental health and less desirable medications—for example, for depression, they are less likely to be taking newer selective serotonin reuptake inhibitors (SSRIs), which are more easily tolerated than older tricyclics.[1]

A considered anthropological response to the content of this supplement is not simple. Especially given the overall lack of attention paid to problems of mental illness, one can only welcome Satcher's efforts. Both the research it refers to and its interpretation of the research are careful, judiciously weighed, and sensitive to multiple points of view. In large part, I would want to stand with its call to make more and better treatment available for conditions that cause so much suffering, such as paranoia, panic attacks, depression, and bipolar disorder. I would certainly agree that the best treatment for such maladies should be made available to everyone it would benefit. And yet I am left with a feeling of disquiet. The supplement also raises an issue that is not dealt with so easily. Under "diagnostic issues," it states that "appropriate care depends on accurate diagnosis." Importantly, it finds that African Americans are diagnosed accurately less often than whites when they seek primary care for depression and when they are seen for psychiatric evaluation in emergency rooms. In addition, there are disparities in diagnosing such that African Americans are more often diagnosed with schizophrenia than whites and less often diagnosed with affective disorders than whites. Yet when clinicians review a sample of such cases after the initial diagnoses, the disparities by race disappear. The supplement leaves the explanation open for lack of sufficient evidence: it suggests perhaps there actually is a disparity in rates, or perhaps something in clinicians' perceptions is affecting their judgment. In this gap lies my disquiet, but also an opening. Perhaps insights from ethnographic research can suggest why categories of mental illness such as schizophrenia or mood disorders might mean something different when applied to different racial categories.

To suggest ways this open area might be more fully understood, I draw on my ethnographic research to outline some of the cultural meanings that people attach to problematic mental states, specifically moods and mood disorders, and how these meanings are inflected by race, class, and gender in the United States today.[2] My focus is on the different kinds of significance moods can have in different historical periods, particularly when race and gender are taken into account. I begin with a general description of the current popular fascination with mood states such as mania. Then I trace several trajectories of historical change in the way moods have been interpreted in the light of gender, race, and class. Finally, I return to the Satcher report to reconsider dilemmas that arise from the effort to develop diagnostic descriptions of mental illness for people in social positions differentiated by gender or race.

MOOD DISORDERS IN THE NEWS

Since the 1990s, accounts of manic-depression (also called bipolar disorder) have been flooding the press, the best-seller list, and the airwaves in the United States. Manic-depression has fueled the plot of a series of detective novels (Padgett's *A Child of Silence*, 1993, and others by Padgett), a prison escape novel (Willocks, *Green River Rising*, 1994), a southern novel (Gibbons's *Sights Unseen*, 1995), movies (*About a Boy, Pollock*), plots of television programs (*The X Files* and *ER*), and specials on MTV and PBS. Manic-depression seems to be in the process of redefinition from a disability to a strength. These new definitions, highly specific to the present social context, ignore as much as they illuminate. But this makes them no less interesting. Many books and Internet sites list famous and influential people whose diaries, letters, and other writings indicate their manic-depression played a role in the creative contributions they made to society. In support groups, I found that references to celebrities who have identified themselves as manic-depressives were common. In Orange County, where the entertainment industries are a major employer, support group members not uncommonly had direct experience with these larger-than-life manic-depressives. Some people told me they felt persisting negative images of mental illness in the media could be offset by other media accounts of manic-depressive heroes.

In the meantime, famous artists from the past said to have had manic-depression are being enlisted to help overcome stigma. At a meeting of the National Depression and Manic-Depression Association, a speaker exhorted the audience to tell others that we work in a civil rights movement for the mentally ill. "We should say this at cocktail parties and put stickers saying 'mental health advocate' on any nametag we wear. Whenever we meet a possibly helpful contact, we should send a thank-you note on cards with art by Vincent van Gogh or Georgia O'Keeffe."

The association between artistic creativity and the diagnosis of manic-depression also saturates professional psychiatry meetings I attended. At the 2000 American Psychiatric Association (APA) meeting, the extensive exhibit area for one major psychopharmaceutical used in the treatment of manic-depression featured Randy Cohen, an artist who worked on a painting throughout the conference.

By the time of the 2002 APA, the level of display in the pharmaceutical exhibit area was greatly diminished as a response to growing criticism of extravagance in the face of rising drug prices. By this time, an exhibit as elaborate as the one that included Randy Cohen was only a fond memory, and a Lilly representative told me he missed seeing Randy because it had been gratifying to witness the improvement in him as he took Zyprexa over several years. But less overt references to the link between manic-depression and creativity were still apparent. Posters showing successful treatment by SSRI antidepressants such as Celexa showed mellow women painting pictures in domestic settings. And even in the face of an agreement to reduce expenses in marketing, one pharmaceutical company, Organon, had an enormous pile of sand trucked into the convention hall, out of which craftsmen sculpted a life-sized replica of Benjamin Franklin. Whereas the link between Randy Cohen's artistic creativity and Zyprexa was unmistakable and explicit, the link between the sand sculpture and the convention, not to mention Remeron, the particular antidepressant sculpted into Ben Franklin's pedestal, was mystifying to everyone I asked, except for the obvious reference to the history of Philadelphia, the location of the APA meeting. I do not know whether anyone was aware that Ben Franklin is often used as an example of success by virtue of his manic/hyper temperament. This point is often made in literature on attention deficit hyperactivity disorder, and the success of people like Benjamin Franklin is known as the "Edison effect."

At other times, marketers' intention to link artistic creativity and manic-depression carries through to the target. At the APA dinner sponsored by Solvay, I sat across from a young doctor who practiced in the Los Angeles area. When he heard about my research, he became intently interested. He said he could offer me two anecdotes:

The first anecdote is that where I work, we get a lot of Hollywood comedians coming in. They are manic-depressives. There are two important things about this: first, they do not want their condition publicized, and second, their managers always get involved in the details of their treatment. The managers want the mania treated just so. They do not want it floridly out of control, but they also absolutely do not want it damped down too much. The second story is we had a patient who was very sick with manic-depression. He was thirty years old. Both his parents, though undiagnosed, were probably bipolar and were able to amass a huge amount of wealth. They did this through an Internet company. (You would definitely have heard of it if I could tell you its name.)

Why would a mental condition, manic-depression, involving constant shifting in emotional time and space, be undergoing such a dramatic revision in American middle-class culture? How could a condition that as recently as the first half of the twentieth century was depicted as a dreaded liability now be considered an especially valuable asset that can potentially enhance one's life? To begin to find out, I have been carrying out several years of ethnographic fieldwork in the United States, in sites on the West Coast and the East Coast. The major sites in which I did participant-observation include more than twelve support groups for psychiatric conditions such as manic-depression, which I attended regularly over several years; classes and rounds for medical students and residents in psychiatric teaching hospitals; and classes and labs for university students in neurology. Although most of my research took place as I observed ongoing social interactions in these sites, I also conducted more than eighty interviews with patient advocates, doctors, researchers, patients, and pharmaceutical employees.

MANIC CAPITAL

The historical context for the new value placed on manic-depression involves major shifts in the organization of the work economy. In the first half of the twentieth century, for example, a premium was placed on discipline and control because of the requirements of work in industrial settings. The moving assembly line, with its dedicated machinery, was oriented to efficient mass production and, eventually, to profitable mass marketing. Corporate organizations were hierarchically structured bureaucracies whose ideal employee was passive, stable, consistent, and acquiescent. Stability and solidity were stressed. Turkle (1995) observes that "earlier in this century we spoke of identity as 'forged.' The metaphor of iron-like solidity captured the central value of a core identity" (p. 179).

Since the 1970s, the internationalization of labor and markets, growth of the service economy, and abrupt decline of redistributive state services have meant that the fabric of the world has become substantially rewoven. In the United States, concentration of wealth and income at the top of the social order is more extreme than at any other time since the Great Depression, and poverty has grown correspondingly deeper. Successive waves of downsizing have picked off, in addition to the disadvantaged, significant numbers of people from occupations and classes unaccustomed to a dramatic decline in their prospects and standard of living. The imperative to become the kind of worker who can succeed in extremely competitive circumstances has intensified, and the stakes at risk for failing have greatly increased. As one sign of the unforgiving nature of the way increased competition is experienced, references to the "survival of the fittest" have increased exponentially in the news media every year since 1970.

The factory, which has often served as both a laboratory and a conceptual guide for understandings of human behavior, is also changing. The hierarchical factory of the mass production era, with its worker drones, is being replaced (mostly in the elite sectors of the global economy) with new forms: machines that process information and communicate with self-managed workers, who are invested with greater decision-making powers. Corporations are flattening hierarchies, downsizing bureaucracies, enhancing their corporate culture, becoming nimble and agile to survive in rapidly changing markets. They seek organization in the form of fluid networks of alliances, a highly decoupled and dynamic form with great organizational flexibility. Workers and managers are "evolving" with the aid of self-study, corporate training sessions, and an insistence on self-management when they are lucky enough to be employed inside a corporation, and then aggressive entrepreneurialism during the frequent periods they are now expected to spend outside. The individual is still owner of himself, but the stakes have risen and are ever changing.

Perhaps one reason for the high value now placed on mania is that the qualities of the "manic style" fit well with the kind of person frequently described as highly desirable in corporate America: always adapting by scanning the environment for signs of change, flying from one thing to another while pushing the limits of everything, and doing it all with an intense level of energy focused totally on the future.[3] I return to this line of thought below.

MANIC STYLE: IN THE NEWS AND NOT

So compellingly desirable are the depictions of manic behavior that crop up in support groups and conventions that they almost part company with the pathology of mental illness. I think they could as well be called "manic (or hyper) style" (a style that draws on the "mania" in manic-depression and on the "hyper" in attention deficit/hyperactivity disorder). Exemplars of this style are appearing on all sides, from actors and comedians like Robin Williams, Jim Carrey, or Michael Richards (*Seinfeld*'s Cosmo Kramer) to CEOs like Richard Branson (Virgin Inc.) and Jeff Taylor (Monster.com). Ted Turner is described in the magazine *GQ* as the "corporealized spirit of the age," and he appears in the *Saturday Evening Post* in a pair of photographs. In one he is a businessman, lecturing soberly behind a podium with a corporate logo, and in the other he is a wild-eyed ship's captain, fiercely gripping the helm of his yacht. The caption to the photographs notes that Turner's competition should be warned: he has stopped taking his Lithium (and so might well be about to launch a manic—and profitable—new venture) (SerVaas, 1996). Paired with the label "manic-depressive," depictions of Robin Williams as a stand-up comic or Ted Turner as a CEO are part of the movement of the category mania from an impediment to something that gives pleasure, brings rewards, and, in its inventiveness, produces forms of value. In these cases, the category mania is becoming a kind of intellectual property.

For mania to become an asset for people of substance in Hollywood or on Wall Street, it must seem stable and real. Pharmaceutical companies play a large role in conferring stability and reality on mania as a quality by investing in research to develop drugs that will dampen mania in some people or heighten it in others. The pharmaceutical part of the story is far more important than I can indicate in this context, but I will return to the thing-like quality of mania in the final section of this chapter.

At this point, I turn to a more immediate question: How do people who have the diagnosis of manic-depression but are not famous actors or CEOs respond to the presence of manics in the media? People in support groups frequently told me how important celebrated manics were for morale building. Early in my research, I visited an officer of the California patient advocacy organization whose support groups I was attending regularly. Mary and her husband, Ron, responded eagerly to my question about the number of famous people in entertainment and business who were making their diagnosis of manic-depression public:

> *Mary:* There're a lot of people with illness that know that mania has some positive aspects. If you could just control it. If you could just keep it just a little bit high but not too high. Manics are, when they are just hypomanic, really fun to be around. They are charismatic, they've got this great personality, and they are outgoing, effervescent.
>
> *Ron:* They have creativity, productivity.
>
> *Mary:* Oh, I know what I wanted to say too about the stars and the people who have come out saying that they are manic-depressive. I'm not at all surprised because this illness does seem to be linked to intelligence; people with this illness have a higher IQ on average. People are more creative, they do have more energy, so it makes perfect sense to me that they would be writers and poets and actors and actresses and CEOs. It just makes sense.

MOOD DISORDERS IN POPULATIONS

Whether on the upside or the downside of manic-depression, people are increasingly encouraged (and willing) to use "mood charts" to record daily details of their emotional experiences. Mood charts are readily available in doctors' brochures, on the

Web, in magazines and books, from patient advocacy groups and research groups. I have described these charts in detail elsewhere, with particular attention to their increasingly detailed coverage of how medication influences mood patterns.[4] Here I consider only one question: What kind of populations emerge from these record-keeping practices? Keeping a mood chart is said to be part of "mood hygiene."

In a popular book about manic-depression, Mondimore (1999) includes a picture of Hygeia, the goddess of hygiene, who, in this context, stands for "practices and habits that promote good control of mood symptoms in persons with Bipolar disorder." In the context of the image of Hygeia, Mondimore points out that research shows "just how important preventive measures can be for improving symptom control in Bipolar disorder" (p. 222). This is a powerful image because it is well known, and Mondimore emphatically reminds us how efficacious hygienic practices (cleaning water, sweeping houses, and washing bodies) were in reducing mortality and morbidity in the early twentieth century. But this is also an odd image. Hygiene reduces physical disease better the more pathogens are reduced or eliminated. What is the hygiene of moods meant to reduce or eliminate? Are the surges and dips above and below the line of "normal" meant to be reduced? If this were to happen, would emotions, feelings, and sentiments in general be reduced? Would it be more "hygienic" if they were reduced to almost nothing? Mondimore leaves unspecified the answers to these questions.

To push these questions further, I turn to the beginnings of the psychotropic drugs that are now used to manage moods. In 1978, a book edited by Frank Ayd, *Mood Disorders: The World's Major Public Health Problem,* was designed to make the mood disorder called "depression" more visible and recognizable as a public health problem. The upsurge in interest in mood disorders as a public health problem was doubtless fueled by the development of a new form of antidepression medication. Frank Ayd, coeditor of the 1978 book, ran Merck's clinical trials for its antidepressant Elavil. According to David Healy's *The Antidepressant Era* (1997), Merck bought fifty thousand copies of his book, *Recognizing the Depressed Patient,* and distributed them worldwide. This played a significant role in Elavil's success: "Merck not only sold amitriptyline, it sold an idea. Amitriptyline became the first of the antidepressants to sell in substantial amounts" (p. 76).

Why might "mood disorders" be considered a public health problem? The main reason cited is that "depression is a public health problem because it is frequent, causes distress and suffering for many patients and their families, and results in severe socioeconomic losses"(Sartorius, 1978, p. 1). The link between mood and productivity in the workplace was well entrenched in North America by the end of World War II. An early 1950s Canadian Broadcasting Corporation health education film makes clear the link between depression and lowered ability to work. Called *Feelings of Depression,* the film tells the story of John, a young man who believes he is failing at his job and, more seriously, believes his company itself is on the brink of failure. This link has been reiterated many times since, for example, in a public health poster from 1991: "Not everyone who is depressed is this visible." In this scene of a contemporary open office space, several workers are represented as immobile white plaster statues.

In more recent mass media, and some of the research that lies behind its stories, "moods," especially depression, are often associated with lack of productivity or inability to work. A spate of articles in print media, the Web, and on television look at links between moods like depression and the inability to leave the welfare rolls by finding a job. In a *60 Minutes* story on welfare and depression ("Depressed and on Welfare," 2002), Lesley Stahl begins by saying that one reason there are still 5 million people on welfare is that "a huge number of them are depressed, not just suffering from a case of the blues, but seriously medically depressed. It's an epidemic of depression among America's poor." Ronald Kessler of Harvard's School of Public Health, featured on the show, estimated that between a third and a half of people still on welfare were clinically depressed. The conversation then continued:

> *Dr. Carl Bell* The state of Illinois, bless their heart, finally
> *[of a mental* figured out that maybe the people who were
> *clinic in* going to be left on welfare were people with
> *Chicago]:* psychiatric disorders, and so maybe somebody
> ought to be here screening for that and refer-
> ring people for treatment.

> *Stahl:* So people come in for welfare, for their checks,
> to make their applications, and if somebody is
> there that perhaps spots these symptoms . . .
>
> *Dr. Bell:* You can screen them out—everybody can get a
> very simple screening form—find out who's got
> what, and then treat them.

Concern for the control of mood disorders has even spread beyond the national borders of the United States to become a global issue. In 2001, the World Health Organization (WHO) declared mental illness the main global health crisis of the year. Chief among WHO's concerns were two: the loss of productivity to the world's economies because of depressed mood and making effective pharmacological treatments more widely available. For its part, the pharmaceutical industry, by the 1990s in possession of a greater range of drug treatments, clearly envisioned a global market for these drugs (MacLennan, 2002).

In sum, a number of factors are coming together: dissemination of mood charts for individuals to track their moods on a daily or hourly basis, a strong link between mood and productivity, and interest in increasing the recognition and treatment of mood disorders on a global scale.

REVALUING MANIA

Manic-depression is said to entail a "distorted" sense of time and space: "delusions" abound in the manic phase. Objects seem to merge, to flow into each other. Shapes shift. Any ordinary thing can change into something else and then something else again. The process happens unbidden and is not necessarily sinister at all. It can be as interesting as watching things morph in a movie. The inside and outside of the self are blurred (Jamison, 1995). Thought is rapid and flighty, jumping from one thing to another (Goodwin and Jamison, 1990). As rapidly as they are described, however, these distortions become assets. In today's environment, in which linear time and space are in many ways stretching, condensing, speeding, warping, and looping, these perceptual abilities can easily seem to be talents in accord with new realities instead of irrational delusions. In general, the qualities praised fit perfectly with the kind of person frequently described as highly desirable in corporate America: always adapting, scanning the environment, continuously changing. If there is an increasing demand for restless change and continuous development of the person at all times and in many realms, then manic-depression might readily come to be regarded as normal—even ideal—for the human condition under these historically specific circumstances.

How does inhabiting such a space of flux come to seem desirable? Many people I spoke with struggled with this question. In an interview, Peter Whybrow, author of an accessible and influential book on bipolar disorder, *A Mood Apart* (1997), explained to me his view of how manic traits are being valorized:

> *PW:* I'm convinced that we have tended to deny the social values of [manic and depressive] behaviors. It's only when they go over the top and create this element of idle self- or social destruction that everybody throws up their arms and says, "Ah, this is terrible," and then stigmatizes it, which, in a peculiar way, categorizes it and distinguishes it from exactly the same behavior that doesn't reach quite these heights for some reason. My own sense is that there's a part of American culture that feeds that.
>
> *EM:* Feeds the stigmatization?
>
> *PW:* No, feeds the escalation. In fact, in the book, although I don't make it explicit, the implication is that there's something in "immigrant hubris" that's close to manic hubris. If you're sleeping four hours a night, having rapid, somewhat bizarre thoughts, on-the-edge ideas, and a few other things, you are considered to be helpful in moving an Internet company into the stratosphere . . .
>
> *EM:* Um hum . . .
>
> *PW:* . . . and conning a lot of people into giving you a lot of money. That is becoming especially very advantageous. On the other hand, if I end up saying not, "I can build this Internet company

and you should give me money because I'm
going to make you a millionaire," but just, "What
I say is significant enough that it's going to
change the world" (there is a subtle difference
of meaning here!), you immediately are seen
as a madman as opposed to an entrepreneur.

PW: I'm going to change the world with my little
company I'm making. Look at Steve Case, CEO
of America On-Line, or Jeffrey Bezos, CEO of
Amazon.com. When they're asked what they're
doing, they say, "We want to change the world"
. . . that's their standard stopping phrase. . . .

Well, you get somebody who's in the early
stages of mania who says they want to change
the world, there's no difference except the context within which they say that. One of them
says, "I'm going to change the world through
building this new marketing thing, which we
call e-commerce," and the other says, "I'm
going to change the world because I'm chosen,
and I have a better vision than everybody else."
The second person goes into the asylum, and
the first person goes to the Fortune 500, yet
there is no real difference in the early stages
of what they're saying.

The perception that mania has social value was expressed even
by people I met who have not reaped fame and fortune in their
manic-depressive lives. John, a Vietnam veteran who has been a
California support group leader for some years, is also a deeply
philosophical thinker and a kind shepherd of his support group
flock. Pondering the number of jobs he has cycled through, John
sees his frequent job changes as a reflection of his characteristics
as a person—mobile and nonlinear:

John: If you say I'm gonna move toward acting in this
new way, then I'll have to learn these new skills.
And then those skills act for you. What if these
new skills aren't worth it? Maybe I'm not making

enough effort; maybe I have to learn this other new skill. Yeah, there is a lot of drifting; it's like being a drifter in some way. Does society look down and stigmatize it because it seems aimless and you are zigzagging all over the board? But there is still value in being this way. Over and over again you have to say you have got stamina, and you have got to keep trying. It's not linear at all. Pretty much everybody has to zigzag.

EM: Is this kind of becoming mandatory today?

John: It is mandatory. It is change; it's chaos. Living with chaos is living with contradiction. Living with contradiction is to say I have these skills; I have these abilities to use them. What's gonna get me beyond the basic skills I have? What's gonna get me through the day? Skills. What's going to get me through tomorrow? Skills I don't have yet! [Laughs] . . .

EM: I like your philosophy of life.

In the next section of the interview, John begins to describe his mobile, nonlinear mode of being as connected to his manic-depression:

John: Yeah, it is definitely a philosophy of life, of the dynamics of life. Adapt, adapt, change, change, change. You can't catch a firefly: you might catch its corpse, but not the firefly itself. . . . Human beings always have to make decisions based on incomplete information. The idea, though, is to remain practical, remain open, the ability to accept something new and conditions that are new, because the world is always changing. Many times having a spike [a spike in the brain: a common way of understanding the onset of a manic or depressive episode] gives you a new perspective, an impetus to creativity. You can see ahead even if you have to go sideways. It is an environment for creativity.

If you totally eliminated the spikes, you would diminish creativity over time. The experience of having spikes is a plus and a minus; again it's a contradiction. The perspective is that having gone through a battle, you are a veteran. Just like the shamans of old, you should be praised for having survived it. There is value in it . . . like going through battle; we exalt our veterans, and at the same time we have to go on to peacetime. Manic-depression is the same as war in a way because it's the war of all sides seeing something different. Even going psychotic is like being a casualty. You can recover and have a good life, but it is still a battle. The value of it is you have seen some vistas, you've been there, and you've survived. You've seen something, and that experience should be neither exalted nor put down.

Having spikes is busting through boxes. I don't have a word for it. We would need to find an image or a metaphor. It's not linear at all.

In this section of our conversation, John is elaborating on ideals of energy and creativity that are held out for our enticement in the culture in a general way, not on his own ghastly and life-threatening experiences while he has been manic or depressed. In John's case, as for many others living under the description manic-depression, the condition can often be a source of profound suffering.

Marcy, an intense college student who approached me with a request to be interviewed after I lectured at her college, wanted to describe phenomenologically her suffering during her "racing" states and how a drug helped her:

I was having negative thoughts, and they were cycling really rapidly, and the connections between the negative thoughts would be almost just rapid-fire. And the same thing was true when I had positive thoughts; the only difference [laughs] between what they were calling mania and depression was the character of the thoughts, because either way, they were racing at breakneck speed through my head and they weren't slow enough to control in any useful way. . . .

The Depakote slowed everything down. I felt exactly the same, but slower. And when things were slower, I could control them and take them apart more easily and figure out what was going on with myself. When the thoughts were slower, I could stop them earlier in this sort of spiral and say, "Why am I thinking this? It does not make any sense. I am not going to think this; I am going to think about something else; this is absurd." And when they were fast, it was just too fast; there was nothing I could do. So in a sense, the drug worked.

However, the drug was not a simple fix for her racing thoughts because it created problems of its own:

The Depakote was sort of helping quiet that anxious manic kind of feeling, because I did not always feel so happy. A lot of time the mania just felt fast. It did not feel good, it felt too fast, so mostly I just felt out of control, which I was not really excited about. The Depakote was starting to make me feel dopey. I felt that I was sleeping in, and that the Depakote was making it difficult for me to wake up in the morning. And then I would find myself drinking, like, espresso to wake up. I thought this was like one drug on top of another, you know. I was trying to overcorrect for Depakote with caffeine.

Marcy expresses dislike of being out of control of the pace of her thoughts and also of the pace of her social interactions. Here we can see how a manic scenario that sounds like a *Sex and the City* fantasy come true can be experienced as onerous and frightening:

I was getting a lot of response from men, too much. I mean I was not answering my phone after a while. Whatever kind of energy I was giving off, I had men making passes at me. It really shocked me because I felt that they were making passes at me which were completely uninvited, and how dare they extend into my personal space. They were irritating me. I was single for the first time in four years, but this was beyond anything that any of my friends who were single appeared to be experiencing and beyond anything I've ever experienced in my entire life. These men would approach me who seemed like perfectly normal people. They were convinced that I had sent them a signal, and I am looking at them going, "Well, you're very mistaken because there was no signal." That was one of the things that made me think that there was something wrong with me.

John tells us we "have seen some vistas," and they should neither be "exalted nor put down." Peter Whybrow insists that "there is no difference except the context" between genius and derangement. Both statements are different ways of saying that the way manic states are experienced and the effect they have in the world are not fixed and invariant. There is no "thing" called mania that is, apart from its context, invariably on the side of heaven or hell, exaltation or despair. Manic experiences depend for their import on when they happen, to whom, in juxtaposition to what events and the presence of what persons. In these respects, mania is no different from any other state of mind that exists only through being experienced. Whatever the physical substrate underneath mania, whether it is in the genes or the brain or both, mania is also an experience, constituted, as are all other human experiences, by its context.

Gender Reversals

My description of the increase in contemporary positive descriptions of hyper conditions like mania is not meant to imply that appreciation for mania is altogether new. Elizabeth Lunbeck (1994) has shown that in the early twentieth century, psychiatrists generally reacted favorably to patients they diagnosed manic-depressive. As psychiatrists of the time told it,

> the story of the manic-depressive was lively, often raucously so, and entertaining. Such individuals engaged the world around them head-on, often wreaking havoc at home and driving their relations mad . . . but they did so with a verve that drew admiration. Their signal characteristics—loquacity, excitability, intense sociability, and mordant wit—differed from those of normal individuals only by virtue of their excess [p. 146].

Lunbeck also quotes E. E. Southard, a psychiatrist at the Boston Psychopathic Hospital, who supposed that "every one of us is of manic-depressive stripe" (p. 146).

But the way manic-depression was associated with gender categories in Southard's time has changed. In the early twentieth century, far more women were diagnosed with manic-depression than men, by some estimates twice as many. Lunbeck suggests that gender was encoded in the very category itself: the most salient characteristics doctors saw in manic patients were those associated in other contexts with an unbounded, out-of-control femininity that was at once frightening and alluring. Men diagnosed with manic-depression appeared to their doctors, relatives, and friends much like women: excitable, distractible, and talkative, their conduct governed less by rational considerations than by flights of fancy. In American mores more generally since the post–Civil War period, as illustrated by Louisa May Alcott's novel *Moods* (1864), a volatile temperament in adult women was a handicap for success in standard social roles and the normative definitions of femininity. Alcott's father, Amos Bronson Alcott, wrote in his letters that the volatile temperaments of his wife and daughter were "dangerous unnatural"(Schnog, 1997, p. 99). In contrast, dementia praecox (later renamed schizophrenia) was coded male: "Its stolidity, stupidness and catatonia were merely the extreme, pathological manifestations of men's naturally more stable nature, just as the periodicity that characterized the manic mimicked in a more marked form the natural periodicity of women" (Lunbeck, 1994, p. 150).

Today the gender differences for manic-depression and depression have changed. "Manic-depressive illness . . . is equally prevalent across gender," while major depression, with its immobility and numbness, is more common among women than men (Goodwin and Jamison, 1990, p. 168). It would be a mistake to make too much of such statistics, but I suspect we are observing the inception of the male manic, seen as powerful and effective despite, or, more exactly, because of, his instability and irrationality. Far from being feminized and denigrated as he was early in the century, the male manic now seems filled with potency. "Manic states . . . seem to be more the provenance of men: restless, fiery aggressive, volatile, energetic, risk taking, grandiose and visionary, and impatient with the status quo" (Jamison, 1995, p. 123). (I would add, to anticipate the next section, that manic states are more the provenance of white men.)

This change would leave the female manic no better off. In the course of her career in psychiatry, Kay Jamison notes that the extremes of mania did not sit easily with being a woman. Especially when the passion of mania tipped over into anger, it "did not seem consistent with being the kind of gentle, well-bred woman I had been brought up to admire and, indeed, continue to admire" (Jamison, 1995, p. 122). When women do manifest mania, the uneasy fit can imply weakness of a stereotypically female kind. Searching for a humorous note, a speaker at an APA session I attended said that men and women manifest mania differently: men tend to gamble and have sex, while women tend to have "mall mania"—that is, they spend money on clothes and restaurants.

Women themselves frequently describe their experience of the incompatibility between being manic and being a woman. Marcy told me:

> *Marcy:* For me the diagnosis [of manic-depression] felt like a disorder because I'm used to moving through the world in this very unhindered kind of way. Suddenly it was like I could not satisfy anyone. People were constantly disappointed in me. Everything I did was somehow less than what they had gotten from me in the past. I could not meet other people's needs at all. If I had been born with an X and a Y [chromosome], maybe none of this would have happened, because my own sensitivity to not meeting other people's needs is what finally got me upset enough to find my way into the doctor's office. Not meeting other people's needs is so unpleasant for me that I had to put a stop to that any way I could. I would have taken any drugs that they gave me if I thought that it would make it go away. The Depakote actually did; the Depakote made me more tolerable for other people, and that was fine with me.
>
> *EM:* This is fascinating . . .
>
> *Marcy:* I really believe that it would have had that effect if I took it again because I got into that energized kind of state. I did kind of think that the energy was particularly offensive to many people in a woman, and they didn't really know

why . . . but it was particularly offensive to them coming from me because I have an extremely friendly personality, and I would forget to do things when I was feeling what you would call—I don't even like the word—"hypomanic," but I guess that's it. I would forget about having other people be there in my excitement [laughs], and it was not that I was doing mean, horrible things, but when people become accustomed to you one way, this kind of change is difficult.

Race Reversals

In addition to gender reversals around mania, some shifts in racial categories may be occurring. Mania has often been associated with the irrational, out-of-control, overly emotional, racially marked person; today it can also be associated with the electrified, jubilant, hyperenergized, racially unmarked (that is, white) person. As background to this shift, historian John Corrigan found in his study of nineteenth-century American business culture that African American emotionality was constructed as outside the range of "acceptable or even human emotionality" (Corrigan, 2002, p. 243). African Americans were seen as impulsive, volatile, and prone to extreme emotional outbursts, while at the same time (and paradoxically) lacking human emotion and feeling. In the history of American expressive culture of the early twentieth century, "the primitive" marked an out-of-control and uninhibited energy culturally associated with the female, on the one hand, and the African American, on the other. Aesthetic primitivism in the 1920s could rest on "a stereotype of blackness contrived to erect white subjective potency" (Pfister, 1997, p. 190). Whites wrote about jazz at that time in the United States as a product of effects "at a level of human experience lower and more fundamental—'deeper,' in one sense—than culture" (Walser, 1997, p. 274). A Swiss commentator who wrote in 1919 described the power of jazz as emanating from a kind of ritual possession, placing possession "within a European dichotomy that strictly separates it from reason, allowing the 'depth' of these musicians to become associated with the power of nature and the thrill of barbarism" (Walser, 1997, pp. 274–275). In her autobiography, *The Words to Say It* (1983), Marie Cardinal, a white French girl who grew up in Algeria, described how her descent into madness was caused by hearing an intensely emotional trumpet song played by Louis Armstrong. Here is Cardinal's account:

> My first anxiety attack occurred during a Louis Armstrong concert. I was nineteen or twenty. Armstrong was going to improvise with his trumpet, to build a whole composition in which each note would be important and would contain within itself the essence of the whole. I was not disappointed: the atmosphere warmed up very fast. . . . The sounds of the trumpet sometimes piled up together, fusing a new musical base, a sort of matrix which gave birth to one precise, unique note, tracing a sound whose path was almost painful, so absolutely necessary had its equilibrium and duration become; it tore at the nerves of those who followed it. My heart began to accelerate, becoming more important than the music, shaking the bars of my rib cage, compressing my lungs so the air could no longer enter them. Gripped by panic at the idea of dying there in the middle of spasms, stomping feet, and the crowd howling, I ran into the street like someone possessed [pp. 39–40].

The connection here between constructions of race and mad, irrational emotion is made clear by Toni Morrison. Morrison (1993) writes that she remembers smiling when reading this passage, in part because Cardinal's recollection of the music had such immediacy and "partly because of what leaped into my mind: what on earth was Louie playing that night? What was there in his music that drove this sensitive young girl hyperventilating into the street," feeling "like someone possessed"? Morrison muses on the "way black people ignite critical moments of discovery or change or emphasis in literature not written by them" and the "consequences of jazz—its visceral, emotional, and intellectual impact on the listener," which in this case tipped Cardinal from sanity to madness, from rationality to irrationality (pp. vi–viii).

Something like Morrison's point may be behind the degree of outrage often expressed in support groups by nonwhite members when faced with life under the description of manic-depression while inhabiting a denigrated social category. Enrico explained:

I'm coming to this group for anger management. I get extremely angry at any comments about "the help," anything like that; maybe I am oversensitive. In a job interview once, they referred to me as a "green bean." At first I just thought that meant inexperienced, but later I found out that it is a term for an ignorant Mexican. I don't know what to do with the anger. I play sports, and after that incident, I played racquetball so long and hard the ball broke into pieces. Is this the best way? I think maybe I should take up boxing. I also mistrust those little boxes they want you to fill in on the employment application. Ethnic categories! Whose interest is that in? If I put "Mexican," they will think I don't speak English!

The group took this very seriously and discussed possible state agencies where a discrimination complaint could be reported. The editor of the regional association newsletter, the *Roller Coaster Times*, happened to be present, and she said she would publish the address and telephone number of the state agency in the next issue of the newsletter. But the more telling point is that extreme emotions, when exhibited by any woman or any man of color, might now be less easily tolerated than when exhibited by a white man in a position of power. As an African American colleague remarked, "A white man can be crazy like Ted Turner, but if a black man acted like that, he would be arrested."

I am asking what kinds of distinctions are created as the discursive space around the category mania opens up. Will two kinds of mania emerge: a "good" kind, harnessed by Robin Williams and Ted Turner, and a "bad" kind to which most sufferers of manic-depression are relegated? In this case, even if the value given to the irrational experience of mania increases, validity would yet again be denied to the mentally ill, and in fact their stigmatization might increase. After all, if they have, by definition, the ability to be manic or hyperactive, and if that ability comes to be seen as an important key to success, then why are they so often social and economic failures? Or will the presence of a manic style in popular culture reduce the stigmatization of manic-depression? Now that he is widely thought of as manic-depressive, could Robin Williams's performances as a stand-up comic contribute to moving the category mania away from being wholly stigmatized because his performances give pleasure, bring rewards, and in their inventiveness produce forms of value? Do his funny, madcap antics present mania to us as valuable intellectual property?

ANOTHER LENS FROM THE PAST: SPENCER AND THE CULTURE OF POVERTY

Lest we get carried away with hope that old linkages among race, gender, and irrationality might be weakening, it would be well to remember the depth and extent of their historical foundation. Amid the many ethnocentric and self-serving evolutionary schemes of the Victorian period, Herbert Spencer's stand out for explicitly and systematically spelling out positions that were only implicit in the work of others, such as John Lubbock, J. F. McLennan, and E. B. Tylor (Stocking, 1987). In 1876 Spencer articulated a picture of the stages through which all men passed in the course of evolution (Stocking, 1987, p. 225). Based on what he understood to exist among contemporary "inferior races," Spencer characterized the emotional life of primitive man as "impulsive . . . the passing of a single passion into the conduct it prompts." Closely related to this was "improvidence," which was the result of "desire go[ing] at once to gratification." Because primitive man was not able to visualize the future, he was mired in the present; because his was a "simpler nervous system," one that lacked plasticity, he was extremely conservative and unable to modify his behavior (Stocking, 1987, p. 225).

The intellectual functions of primitive man were versions of his emotional life. He had a "direct, unmediated apprehension of external nature" (Stocking, 1987, p. 225). Although he excelled at quick and detailed observation, lacking "deliberate thought," he could not form general ideas or concepts of causal relations. In sum, the savage had "the reason of a child and the instincts of a man (although not those of a civilized man, which would have been modified and constrained by reason)" (Stocking, 1987, p. 226).

One might think that the insistent critique of anthropologists like Boas in the early twentieth century would have laid these invidious distinctions to rest once and for all. But almost exactly the same set of oppositions reappeared in the middle of the twentieth century, under the guise of the culture of poverty.[5] In one striking example from 1961, anthropologist Thomas Gladwin wrote about what he called a completely disorganized and "dysfunctional sub-culture" of poverty, breeding "emotional cripples" who are "ineffective" and lack a sense that they can control their destiny (Valentine, 1968, pp. 88–89). In the literature on the culture of poverty generally, there was a set of assumptions about character reminiscent of Spencer:

> Personal identity, character, and world view are weak, disorganized, and restricted: On the level of the individual, major characteristics are a strong feeling of marginality, of helplessness, of dependency and of inferiority . . . weak ego structure, confusion of sexual identification, lack of impulse control . . . little ability to defer gratification and to plan for the future . . . resignation and fatalism . . . provincial and locally oriented . . . very little sense of history [Valentine, 1968, p. 133].

The emotional life of the poor was described along similar lines. The poor were said to be drawn into "the search for excitement or 'thrill' " . . . use of alcohol . . . gambling of all kinds . . . adventuring with sex and aggression, frequently leading to 'trouble.' . . . Many lower class individuals feel that their lives are subject to a set of forces over which they have relatively little control" (Valentine, 1968, p. 137).

Together, these traits produced a common set of economic behaviors among the poor. In Oscar Lewis's depiction, the poor had "strong present-time orientation; little ability to defer gratification and plan for the future; [a] sense of resignation and fatalism" (Leeds, 1971, p. 241). They exhibited "absence of savings, chronic shortage of cash, pawning, borrowing from usurers" (p. 247). For Lewis and other culture-of-poverty theorists, these traits were viewed as arising from the characteristics of individuals rather than from the constraints of economic structures.

There has been a trenchant anthropological critique of these assumptions, which I have drawn on for the examples above. Among other things, the critique calls for a more complex and less stereotypical concept of culture, a greater appreciation of the constraints poverty exerts as understood from the perspective of the poor instead from the perspective of the middle class, and more complex descriptions based on directly observed ethnographic data. Frustratingly, and frighteningly, however, this set of assumptions is still alive and well. Perhaps emboldened by the current Bush administration, right-wing spokesmen like David Brooks are

almost eager to articulate them once again. In an editorial in the
New York Times, Brooks derided liberal assumptions that more
money would reduce poverty rates as outmoded and wrong. Lib-
erals wrongly assume, he wrote, that "economic forces determine
culture and shape behavior." "In reality, culture shapes economics.
A person's behavior determines his or her economic destiny. If
people live in an environment that fosters industriousness, sobri-
ety, fidelity, punctuality and dependability, they will thrive. But the
Great Society welfare system encouraged or enabled bad behavior,
and popular culture glamorizes irresponsibility" (p. A23).

Like the culture-of-poverty theorists, Brooks places the blame
for poverty squarely on the character faults of those who are poor.
He ignores the powerful structural forces flowing from an economic system that requires a certain degree of unemployment and
systematically degrades the benefits of work. He ignores the effects
of persistent racist and sexist attitudes on the part of employers,
police, educators, and bureaucrats, among others. He callously
ignores the factors that weigh heavily against poor women and people of color: lack of universal health insurance, lack of a living
wage, lack of adequate child care, and lack of adequate elder care,
among other things. There is a certain fit between his claims and
the claim that those remaining on the welfare rolls may suffer from
depression. For Brooks, the cause of "bad behavior" is popular culture and the welfare system itself; for advocates of screening for
depression in Temporary Aid for Needy Families offices, the cause
is states of the brain. Both views fail to contend adequately with the
impact of poverty and its attendant constraints.

CULTURE AND MENTAL ILLNESS

To conclude, I return to the issues raised by Surgeon General
Satcher's supplement. Phillip Rack has written about diagnosis in
the African Caribbean case in ways that are illuminating here. Rack
(1982) describes a syndrome called "West Indian psychosis," said to
be found among people of African Caribbean descent and characterized by "excitement and over-activity, with pressure of thought
and speech . . . bizarre behaviour . . . violence . . . talk [which is]
fragmented or incoherent" (p. 113). This diagnosis is usually taken
to be an attack of an endogenous psychosis, but Rack argues that

"when an African, Afro-Caribbean, or Asian patient behaves in a manner that would, in a British patient, point to a diagnosis of mania, the practitioner should keep in mind the possibility that this is a stress reaction, and not an attack of an endogenous psychosis" (p. 115). Rack suggests it is perhaps hard for clinicians to see a stress reaction instead of an endogenous psychosis because of certain preconceptions. The stereotypes of the "wild West Indian" or "the image of the big wild, dangerous black man or woman" are deep in the minds of many white people, partly because some West Indian speech styles sound to English ears "sharp, intense, abrupt, and hard-edged, with sudden changes of pitch, coupled with an ebullience of manner that suggests intense emotion or extraversion. Also there is a great deal of genuine anger, frustration, and bitterness among certain sections of the Afro-Caribbean community in Britain, and it causes acts of violence that attract a great deal of media coverage" (p. 116). Rack's first point is that when angry outbursts are constructed as endogenous psychosis rather than reactions to particular social contexts and experiences, this is in keeping with the tendency to deny social inequalities. His second point is that clinicians may be more comfortable linking the cognitive disordering of schizophrenia with their cultural conceptions of "blackness" than with their cultural conceptions of "whiteness."

The dominant model operating in the surgeon general's supplement is that there is something concrete and real in the world (and increasingly in the brain) that corresponds one to one with the major psychiatric diagnoses. Identifying this real thing, in the brains, say, of patients, is the proper first step to getting them the proper treatment. Identifying observer bias and removing it will clear the way to more frequently correct diagnosis. But there are at least three troubling aspects of this view. First, what if the categories into which psychiatry divides disorders themselves already have cultural assumptions embedded in them, not fixed for all time, but, as I have sketched for mood disorders, changing with the times? Second, what if our only route to the real is always through linguistic categories that are necessarily saturated with culturally constituted sets of meanings? Third, what if the interests of product-centered pharmaceutical corporations dovetail with seeing psychological states as physical states, extricable from social context? If these are so, can a pharmacogenomics specific to race be far behind? If any of these conditions were to hold, the job of removing the effects of racialized perceptions becomes far more difficult.

My object in saying this is not to create a cloud of pessimism over the endeavor of the supplement. It is to ask whether the problem of differential treatment for mental illness by race can be addressed without going much further to eliminate the social factors the supplement identifies and then tries to correct: poverty and racist attitudes. The supplement uses its powerful epidemiological tools to uncover patterns flowing from poverty and racism that affect mental health diagnoses and their treatment. Future ethnographies we can envision would, I feel sure, reveal more than we now realize about the way preconceptions based on racial categories permeate psychiatric ideas and practices. I hope the strengths of both approaches will come together with enough vigor to prevent us from imagining too quickly that pharmacological means based on brain mechanisms will provide an answer. I hope we keep this question at the forefront: Will making more and better medicines available to African Americans who suffer more stress due to poverty and racism provide something we want to call a solution, let alone a cure?

Notes

Thanks to Leith Mullings, Amy Schulz, and the other members of the conference for many helpful suggestions.

1. See also Brown and Keith (2003); Minsky and others (2003); Neighbors, Trierweiler, Ford, and Muroff (2003); and Williams and Harris-Reid (1999) for more background on racial difference in mental health diagnosis.
2. The research was supported by the Spencer Foundation, the National Science Foundation, the Guggenheim Foundation, and Princeton University. I am responsible for what I have written here.
3. See Martin (1994, 1999) and Harvey (1989).
4. "Bipolar Expeditions: Toward an Anthropology of Moods," book manuscript under contract to Princeton University Press.
5. I am grateful to Leith Mullings for suggesting that I think about the culture of poverty literature in this light.

References

Alcott, L. M. *Moods.* Boston: Loring, 1864.

Ayd, F. J. (ed.). *Mood Disorders: The World's Major Public Health Problem.* Baltimore: Ayd Medical Communications, 1978.

Brooks, D. "More Than Money. " *New York Times,* Mar. 2, 2004, p. A23.

Brown, D. R., and Keith, V. M. "The Epidemiology of Mental Disorders and Mental Health Among African American Women." In D. R. Brown and V. M. Keith (eds.), *In and Out of Our Right Minds: The Mental Health of African American Women.* New York: Columbia University Press, 2003.

Cardinal, M. *The Words to Say It.* Cambridge, Mass.: Van Vactor and Goodheart, 1983.

Corrigan, J. *Business of the Heart: Religion and Emotion in the Nineteenth Century.* Berkeley: University of California Press, 2002.

"Depressed and on Welfare." *60 Minutes,* Nov. 10, 2002. CBS-TV.

Gibbons, K. *Sights Unseen.* New York: Putnam, 1995.

Goodwin, F. K., and Jamison, K. R. *Manic-Depressive Illness.* New York: Oxford University Press, 1990.

Harvey, D. *The Condition of Postmodernity: An Enquiry into the Origins of Social Change.* Oxford: Basil Blackwell, 1989.

Healy, D. *The Antidepressant Era.* Cambridge, Mass.: Harvard University Press, 1997.

Jamison, K. R. *An Unquiet Mind.* New York: Knopf, 1995.

Leeds, A. "The Concept of the 'Culture of Poverty': Conceptual, Logical and Empirical Problems, with Perspectives from Brazil and Peru." In E. B. Leacock (ed.), *The Culture of Poverty: A Critique.* New York: Simon & Schuster, 1971.

Lunbeck, E. *The Psychiatric Persuasion: Knowledge, Gender, and Power in Modern America.* Princeton, N.J.: Princeton University Press, 1994.

MacLennan, R. "The Global CNS Therapeutics Markets: An Overview." May 29, 2002. www.frost.com/prod/serviet/market-insight.pag?docid=IKHA-5ALUC3&ctxht=FomCtx1&ctxixpLink=FomCtx2&ctxixpLabel+FomCtx3.

Martin, E. *Flexible Bodies: Tracking Immunity in America from the Days of Polio to the Age of AIDS.* Boston: Beacon Press, 1994.

Martin, E. "Flexible Survivors." *Anthropology Newsletter,* 1999, *40*(6), 5–7.

Minsky, S., and others. "Diagnostic Patterns in Latino, African American, and European American Psychiatric Patients." *Archives of General Psychiatry,* 2003, *60*(6), 637–644.

Mondimore, F. M. *Bipolar Disorder: A Guide for Patients and Families.* Baltimore: Johns Hopkins University Press, 1999.

Morrison, T. *Playing in the Dark: Whiteness and the Literary Imagination.* New York: Random House, 1993.

Neighbors, H. W., Trierweiler, S. J., Ford, B. C., and Muroff, J. R. "Racial Differences in DSM Diagnosis Using a Semi-Structured Instrument: The Importance of Clinical Judgment in the Diagnosis of African Americans." *Journal of Health and Social Behavior,* 2003, *44*(3), 237–256.

Padgett, A. *A Child of Silence*. New York: Mysterious Press, 1993.

Pfister, J. "Glamorizing the Psychological: The Politics of the Performances of Modern Psychological Identities." In J. Pfister and N. Schnog (eds.), *Inventing the Psychological: Toward a Cultural History of Emotional Life in America*. New Haven, Conn.: Yale University Press, 1997.

Rack, P. *Race, Culture, and Mental Disorder*. London: Tavistock, 1982.

Sartorius, N. "Depressive Disorders, a Major Public Health Problem." In F. J. Ayd (ed.), *Mood Disorders: The World's Major Public Health Problem*. Baltimore: Ayd Medical Communications, 1978.

Schnog, N. "Changing Emotions: Moods and the Nineteenth-Century American Woman Writer." In J. Pfister and N. Schnog (eds.), *Inventing the Psychological: Toward a Cultural History of Emotional Life in America*. New Haven, Conn.: Yale University Press, 1997.

SerVaas, C. "The Post Investigates Manic-Depression." *Saturday Evening Post*, 1996, *268*(2), 46–52.

Stocking, G. W. *Victorian Anthropology*. New York: Free Press, 1987.

Turkle, S. *Life on the Screen: Identity in the Age of the Internet*. New York: Simon & Schuster, 1995.

U.S. Department of Health and Human Services. *Mental Health: Culture, Race and Ethnicity—A Supplement to Mental Health: A Report of the Surgeon General*. Rockville, Md.: U.S. Department of Health and Human Services, Substance Abuse and Mental Health Services Administration, Center for Mental Health Services, 2001.

Valentine, C. A. *Culture and Poverty: Critique and Counter-Proposals*. Chicago: University of Chicago Press, 1968.

Walser, R. "Deep Jazz: Notes on Interiority, Race, and Criticism." In J. Pfister and N. Schnog (eds.), *Inventing the Psychological: Toward a Cultural History of Emotional Life in America*. New Haven, Conn.: Yale University Press, 1997.

Willocks, T. *Green River Rising*. London: J. Cape, 1994.

Williams, D. R., and Harris-Reid, M. H. "Race and Mental Health: Emerging Patterns and Promising Approaches." In A. V. Horwitz and T. L. Scheid (eds.), *A Handbook for the Study of Mental Health*. Cambridge: Cambridge University Press, 1999.

Whybrow, P. *A Mood Apart: Depression, Mania, and Other Afflictions of the Self*. New York: Basic Books, 1997.

CHAPTER FOUR

CONSTRUCTING WHITENESS IN HEALTH DISPARITIES RESEARCH

Jessie Daniels, Amy J. Schulz

> *My project is an effort to avert the critical gaze from the racial object to the racial subject; from the described and imagined, to the describers and imaginers; from the serving to the served.*
> TONI MORRISON (1990)

Over the past two decades, the body of research documenting and examining racial differences in health has grown exponentially, from fewer than 20 publications between 1980 and 1989, to more than 130 between 1990 and 1999, and over 700 in the first four years of the new millennium.[1] This literature has documented racial disparities in a substantial range of health outcomes, often comparing the health of one or more racialized groups to the health of whites. In other words, the search for explanations regarding the cause of racial disparities in health—and indeed, often the definition of racial disparities itself—is largely framed in terms of explicit or implicit comparisons of racialized groups to the referent group of white.

Often unspoken and unexamined in these comparisons is the category of whiteness itself: what it contains or represents and just what a comparison to whites tells us. Scholars examining the question of whiteness have noted that in contrast to other racial groups, whiteness has often been defined by what it is not (Frankenberg, 1993; Fine, 1997)—not marked, not deficit, not raced.

As Toni Morrison suggests in the quotation that serves as the epigraph for this chapter, there is a long tradition within the United States of constructing whiteness (the racial subject) against racialized others (the racial object) and in the process displacing the focus of critical analysis. Here we turn our lens to the often invisible—or at least underinterrogated—concept of whiteness within the context of the literature on racial disparities in health. Specifically, we examine how whiteness is constructed in the active literature documenting and interpreting racial disparities in health and the implications of these constructions for efforts to eradicate inequalities in health. We draw on the concepts of racial formation and "racial projects" that emphasize the fluidity, mutability, and historically constructed nature of race, as well as the social and political processes through which racial categories are created and transformed (Nagel, 1996; Nobles, 2000; Omi and Winant, 2002; Stevens, 2003; Winant, 1997). A racial project is simultaneously an interpretation, representation, or explanation of racial dynamics. In particular, we apply Winant's concept (1997) of "racial projects" to examine the construction of whiteness in ongoing dialogues about race and racial disparities in health. We consider the ways that varying constructions of whiteness enter into, influence, and are influenced by discussions of racial disparities in health, and the role of those constructions in the reproduction or disruption of racial categories and the inequitable distribution of resources along racial lines.

Race and Racial Classification in Health

The problem of whiteness and what it means or represents reflects larger dilemmas related to historical as well as contemporary constructions of race. Questions regarding race as a scientific category transcend disciplinary boundaries (Freeman, 1998; American Anthropological Association, 1998; Duster, 2003b), reflecting the pervasive influence of racialized thinking in scientific endeavors. Although widely used as analytical categories, racial classification systems have been soundly critiqued as unscientific, poorly defined, and contingent on both historical and geographical context. Despite persistent associations between racial categories and health out-

comes, scholars both within and outside public health continue to
raise critical questions about the use of racial classifications as
analytical categories (Bhopal, 1998; Duster, 2003a; Epstein, Moreno,
and Bacchetti, 1997; Farley, Richards, and Bell, 1995; Hahn, 1999;
Hahn and Stroup, 1994; Hahn, Mulinare, and Teutsch, 1992; Hahn,
Mendlein, and Helgerson, 1993; Jackson, 1989; Kaufman, 1999;
Mullings, 2004; Nobles, 2000; Witzig, 1996; Williams, 1997), including questions about their relation to historical processes that created
contemporary inequalities, contemporary definitions, meanings, and
interpretations, and their limits in identifying etiological pathways
through which differential health outcomes are produced.

Critics point to the lack of a biological, genetic, or other "scientific" basis for racial classification systems and ensuing difficulties in creating clear and consistent definitions (Hahn, 1999;
Kaufman, 1999; Hahn, Mendlein, and Helgerson, 1993). Two illus-
trative examples involve classifications employed in census data
and birth certificates, both commonly used in health research in
the United States. In 1790, the U.S. Census had three categories:
Free Persons (white, and all other free persons except Indians not
taxed), slaves (counted as three-fifths of a person), and Indians living on reservations (not taxed). By 1850, categories had shifted to
more explicitly racial language, denoting simply white and free
person of color. By 1890, an expanded range of racial categories
included white; black (persons with three-quarters or more "black
blood"); mulatto (one-half black ancestry); quadroon (one-fourth
black ancestry); and octoroon (one-eighth black ancestry). By
1910, these categories had contracted to aggregate the previous
distinctions in percentage ancestry into just white, black, and
mulatto categories. In 1930 and 1940, census takers were instructed
to categorize individuals with white and American Indian ancestry
as "Indian," and those of African and American Indian ancestry as
"negroes" "unless the Indian ancestry 'very definitely predomi-
nates'" (Forbes, 1993, p. 91). In other words, any American Indian
ancestry overrode white ancestry to identify individuals as Indian
(not white), while African ancestry overrode American Indian
ancestry, except in cases where African ancestry was small. The U.S.
racial paradigm of hypodescent means that a small amount of
African ancestry overrides a much larger amount of European
ancestry. The 2000 Census reflected renewed expansion of racial

options, including five racial categories and two ethnic categories (Hispanic or Latino; and not Hispanic or Latino). Respondents were allowed to indicate both race and ethnicity (Office of Management and Budget, 1978), further expanding the range of ethnic options available. The historically contingent nature of these racial categories highlights their socially and politically constructed nature and belies any coherent biological basis or interpretation of contemporary racial groups (Nobles, 2000).

Similarly, racial classification systems used on birth records in the United States reflect changing gender as well as racial ideologies and practicalities. Prior to 1989, the race of infants indicated on birth certificates was derived using a complex algorithm. Specifically, infants' race was coded as paternal race regardless of maternal race, with two exceptions. In instances where the father's race was white and the mother's race was any other, maternal (rather than paternal) race was used to define the infant's race. In contrast, if either parent was Hawaiian, the infant's race was coded as Hawaiian on the birth certificate. In 1989, this system of racial classification was modified, in part due to increasing numbers of children born for whom the father was not present and therefore father's race was unknown. Both the previous and the current system systematically simplify hereditary complexities, although using different racial and gender heuristics to do so. The examples of the census and birth certificate racial categories highlight the historical, social, and political nature of racial classification systems and make clear their limitations as indicators of biological or genetic makeup (see Hahn, Mendlein, and Helgerson, 1993; Cooper and David, 1986; Cooper and Freeman, 1999; Kaufman, 1999; Watson and others, 1993 for more detailed discussions of the limitations of racial classification systems as indicators of biological or genetic composition).

These illustrations of the socially, historically, and politically contingent nature of race, combined with the persistent interpretation of racial categories that emerged out of the specific historical and political context of the United States as scientifically meaningful, have contributed to lively debate about how persistent racial differences in health outcomes are best understood and addressed. Even as race is increasingly recognized as a social construct and racial categories as problematic from an analytical perspective (Bhopal and Donaldson, 1998; Fullilove, 1998; Williams, 1997; Witzig, 1996), scholars differ as to how best to address this problem. Some have suggested that race should be abandoned entirely in public health research (Fullilove, 1998) and replaced by explicit attention to the political and social processes that it represents (for example, socioeconomic differences, racial discrimination). Others, who would concur that we must explicitly attend to the political and social processes that create racial disparities in health, argue that we must continue to use racial and ethnic categories to monitor progress toward elimination of racial disparities (Baker, 1998; Duster, 2003a; LaVeist, 1994; Mullings, 2004). In other words, racial categories reflect racialized social systems in the United States, and those systems have an impact on the health of groups defined by race differently. Attaining equitable health outcomes can be assessed only if we continue to monitor the health of racially defined groups, recognizing that these differences are produced through social and political processes.

Even as these discussions about how best to recognize the socially constructed nature of race have emerged, interpretations of race as reflecting immutable characteristics of individuals continue, with racial differences in health viewed as emerging from biological or genetic differences (Herrnstein and Murray, 1994; Last, 1995; Rushton, 1994; Snyderman and Rothman, 1988). Understanding this struggle over the very meaning of race is central to an analysis of the interplay of race, gender, and class in health, as well as to an understanding of whiteness within health and in U.S. social and political systems more broadly.

These debates about the validity and certainly the reliability of the construct of race as an analytical category have unfolded in the context of a virtual explosion of research drawing attention to racial differences in health and mortality over the past quarter-century. Within this literature, the most common referent group is white (or, more rarely, Caucasian, European, or Western; Bhopal, 1998). Despite critical examination of the homogenizing influence of racial or ethnic categories that collapse diverse national, linguistic, and other identity groups into a single category (for example, Gimenez, 1989; Williams, Lavizzo-Mourey, and Warren, 1994) and a trend toward increasing complexity of comparisons within various racialized groups (for example, disaggregating analyses of blacks into African Americans and African Caribbeans; disaggregating "Latinos" into Cuban, Puerto Rican, and Mexican American), there has been relatively little critique of the aggregation of multiple groups into the white racial category (Bhopal, 1998). Furthermore, there has been relatively little explicit examination in the public health literature of how some groups come to be defined as white and the subsequent implications for health. How is it that the category of white or whiteness is both pervasive as a comparison or referent group in the literature on racial disparities in health and at the same time its composition and the meaning or interpretation of comparisons to whites remain largely uninterrogated? And perhaps more important, what are the implications of this invisibility for understanding and addressing the inequalities in health with which this literature is concerned?

To begin to examine this question, we borrow the concept of racial projects. This concept emerged in an attempt to capture the active and dynamic efforts of social groups to organize the distribution of resources along racial lines (Omi and Winant, 2002). Conceptualizing whiteness, like other racial categories, as socially constructed allows whiteness to be examined as dynamic, as actively created and maintained, rather than as static, given, or immutable. Thought of in this way, whiteness is not genetically derived or granted but is accomplished through the active efforts of human beings who construct and maintain social boundaries—for example, defining who is white and who is not (see Buck, 2001; Daniels, 1997; Ignatiev, 1995). Creating and maintaining whiteness as a bounded category that is largely not visible or marked, and yet manages to retain privilege, is neither a modest nor a simple venture. A defining feature of whiteness, then, is the absence or unmarked invisibility of "white" as a racial category. As many scholars have noted, this invisible and absent quality of whiteness is itself a mechanism of privilege (Allen, 1993; Dyer, 1997; Feagin and Vera, 1994; Fine, Weis, Powell, and Wong, 1997; Frankenberg, 1993; Ignatiev, 1995; Kincheloe, Steinberg, Rodriguez, and Chenault, 1998; McIntosh, 1988; Roediger, 1991, 1998), deflecting attention from whiteness while simultaneously playing a role in the racialization of those groups that are defined as not white.

Winant (1997) suggests that "the problem of the meaning of whiteness appears as a direct consequence of the movement challenge posed in the 1960s to white supremacy" (pp. 48–49). As civil rights movements disrupted previously homogeneous notions of whiteness, whites and whiteness were no longer exempt from the complex racialization processes that are the hallmark of U.S. history. Rather, whiteness has become a more contested and visibly negotiated racial category. The disruption of the homogeneity of whiteness brought about by the civil rights movement opened up both the possibility of an interrogation of white privilege, as well as challenges to civil rights legislation such as affirmative action through newly galvanized whites who envisioned themselves as under attack. A series of recent scholarly works has examined in detail the intersections of race and gender, and in some cases class and religion, in negotiations that define who is white and who is not, as well as the meaning of inclusion in various racial categories (for example, Buck, 2001; Daniels, 1997; Chehade, 2001; Majaj, 2000; Ferber, 2004). The concept of "whiteness projects" encourages explicit analyses of active efforts to negotiate conceptualizations of whiteness that may serve to reproduce or to disrupt racial inequalities.

Winant (1997) has sketched several useful typologies for understanding contemporary "white racial projects": far right, new right, neoconservative, neoliberal, and new abolitionist. He describes the whiteness project of the far right as putting forward biological notions of race as part of a racialized ideology that views racial differences (racial hierarchies) as immutable and inherent, grounded in genetic or biological difference. Effectively, this conservative racial project seeks to maintain white privilege through the argument that whites are genetically or biologically distinct from and superior to other racial groups.

Winant (1997) describes new right racial projects as differing from those of the far right in their acceptance of participation by members of nonwhite racial groups, provided that such participation "is pursued on a 'color-blind' basis and adheres to the rest of the authoritarian, nationalist program" (p. 44; see also Mullings, forthcoming). Despite the appearance of inclusiveness of nonwhite racial groups, new right racial projects emphasize the maintenance of white racial privilege through cultural representations of race that play on racial fears and exacerbate divisions among racial groups—for example, through the 1988 Willie Horton campaign ads employed by George H. W. Bush (Winant, 1994). A more recent example comes from Wilton's case study (2002) of community opposition to the placement of special-needs housing in a San Pedro, California, neighborhood. Wilton demonstrates the ways opponents to the housing project galvanized a NIMBY ("not in my back yard") campaign that deployed a romanticized, European, and "whitened" construction of community that marked "special needs" as outsiders, unwelcome and unwanted in the community. Wilton's study provides an example of the ways in which the new right racial project of whiteness emphasizes the maintenance of white racial privilege through cultural representations of race that play on racial fears and exacerbate divisions among racial groups.

Neoconservative whiteness is similarly rooted in the politics of the right but seeks to preserve white advantage through denial of racial difference (Winant, 1997). Such efforts simultaneously valorize universalism and individualism, and in so doing they seek to obscure or deny differences that may emerge from social inequalities. For example, in *The End of Racism* (1995), D'Souza writes that "racism can be overcome" by "revising our most basic assumptions about race," including the notion that "Affirmative Action is a policy that assures equal opportunity for disadvantaged African Americans and other minorities" (pp. 2–3). D'Souza and other neoconservatives' opposition to affirmative action policies simultaneously appeals to universalism (job or academic performance standards) and individualism (achievement in meeting those standards). Thus, for neoconservatives, "the end of racism" comes with renewed focus on universal standards and individual achievement without regard to race. Yet the focus on universal, race-blind standards within a context in which race still matters (that is, in which whites are more likely to have access to the kinds of material and social resources that enable them to achieve those standards) is a strategy that reinforces and privileges whiteness. Advocates are actively working to make this "color-blind" racial project the underpinning of contemporary legal theory and social practices (Mullings, forthcoming).

In contrast to these projects, neoliberal whiteness "seeks to *limit* white advantage through denial of racial difference" (Winant, 1997, p. 45). Winant describes neoliberal whiteness projects as encompassing social democratic political perspectives that focus on social structure, as opposed to the cultural representations of race that are employed in the various right-wing racial projects. Within this whiteness project, inherent racial differences are negated, and any systematic racial inequality is attributed to structural, often economically rooted, phenomena. Neoliberal whiteness maintains that if structural disadvantages that disproportionately affect black, Hispanic, and Native American groups were equalized, then racial differences would disappear.

The final category in Winant's typology is new abolitionist racial projects. New abolitionist projects emphasize the historical development of whiteness and white privilege as central to the emergence of U.S. capitalism. These studies focus attention on the relations between historical formations of race and class in the United States and promote the deconstruction or repudiation of white racial privilege. Here we employ Winant's notions of various racial projects as a way of continuing the disruption of homogeneous whiteness as it is constructed in health disparities research. To do this, we examine the constructions of whiteness that emerge within the context of two literatures in public health: broadly, the literature on racial disparities in health that focuses on social structural explanations for those differences, and discussions of genetic explanations for racial health disparities that have emerged in the wake of the Human Genome Project.

Constructing Whiteness in the Context of Racial Disparities in Health

The literature on racial disparities in health by definition involves comparisons across groups defined by some racial classification system. Perhaps the most common of these comparisons take the form of the following general proposition: [Black/Hispanic/Native American] [children or adults] have higher rates of [the condition, disease, or "disability" under investigation] than whites, primarily because of [explanatory variable].

This proposition constructs whiteness in two ways. First, it establishes a comparison between whites as a referent group and some "other" group whose health is evaluated in comparison to that of whites. In an ideal world, such comparisons may demonstrate arenas in which health outcomes do not differ by race, challenging ideas of racial group difference. If, however, funders are less likely to support research in areas in which substantial racial differences are not apparent, or if publishers are less likely to publish articles that find no statistically significant differences (for discussions of publication bias, see Phillips, 2000; Scargle, 2000; Stern, 1997), the literature will reinforce racial health differences while minimizing similarities (Gould, 1996; Lewontin, Rose, and Kamin, 1984, Stevens, 2003, Tucker, 1996).

Equally important, however, are the theoretical or conceptual frameworks that underlie questions about racial disparities. Whether such theoretical frameworks are implicit or explicit, they guide the way that research questions are framed, as well as the interpretation of results. We have already noted the absence of a scientific foundation for racial categories or even a clear and shared definition of what race is across and, in some cases, within disciplinary boundaries. Precisely because of the socially constructed and situated nature of racial constructs, comparisons of racial groups "leave room for multiple interpretations, including biologic or cultural notions of race as an essential or unchanging constituent of a person" (Muntaner 1999, p. 122). In other words, the use of racial categories and comparisons with no consistent foundation for theorizing, understanding, or interpreting observed racial differences (or their absence) in health outcomes provides space for a wide range of potential explanations. Each of these "explanations" implicitly or explicitly constructs both race and whiteness.

For example, within the literature on racial disparities in cardiovascular disease, comparisons of black or Latino and Latina to white Americans show disparities not only in cardiovascular mortality rates (Cooper and others, 2000; Wong, Shapiro, Boscardin, and Ettner, 2002) but also in multiple risk factors, including high blood pressure (Cooper and Rotimi, 1997; National Heart Lung and Blood Institute, 2004; Crespo, Loria, and Burt, 1996), obesity (James, 1999; Kumanyika, 2001), physical activity (Brownson and others, 2001; Crespo Loria, and Burt, 1996), and intake of micronutrients and macronutrients associated with cardiovascular risk (Li and others, 2000). In the absence of an explicitly social theory of race, analyses explaining racial disparities in cardiovascular disease in terms of biological, "lifestyle," or "cultural" factors can reify racial differences and obscure connections to socially structured inequalities. In other words, explaining racial differences in health in terms of individual biology, genes, or behavior can locate health problems in the bodies of those most negatively affected by social inequalities. Such explanations fail to make explicit connections to histories of racism and the struggles against oppression by subordinated groups (Bonilla-Silva, 2003; Mullings, forthcoming). In the process, they also take out of the equation—and thus make invisible—the processes through which whites maintain positions of relative advantage or privilege within racial hierarchies. In this sense, such explanations are consistent with the "color-blind" strategies of neoconservative and neoliberal whiteness projects described above, in that they explain racial disparities in health in nonracial terms. The example of cardiovascular disease is one to which we will return in a moment. First, we want to place this discussion within a historical context.

The failure to make explicit connections between biological and behavioral factors and race as a socially constructed system of inequality can also reinforce racial inequalities by playing on racial fears to exacerbate divisions between groups. A historic example of this is offered by Shah (2001), who describes the explicit construction of Chinese immigrants living in cramped, substandard housing in San Francisco. The communicable diseases that were, not surprisingly, common under these conditions were constructed as a "pestilence" that posed a "danger to the white public" (p. 251). Here the disproportionate occurrence of communicable diseases among Chinese immigrants led to constructions that associated disease with the Chinese immigrants themselves rather than with their relative disadvantage within a racial system, which led to their disproportionate residence in substandard housing.

Even more extreme is the construction of "Negro diseases" such as drapetomania (running away from enslavement), which defined resistance to slavery as a mental illness (Williams and Harris-Reid, 1999). Samuel A. Cartwright, M.D., writing on this topic in the 1850s, said, "With the advantage of proper medical advice, strictly followed, this troublesome practice that many Negroes have of running away can be almost entirely prevented." The recommended treatment was whipping, as well as keeping slaves in a submissive state and treating them like children, with "care, kindness, attention to humanity to prevent and cure them from running away" (Cartwright, 1981, p. 71; Jackson, 2002; Wren, 1985).

Defining individual responses to enslavement as a mental illness requiring treatment provided a justification for continued enslavement, with treatment of the medical condition the responsibility of the slave owner (Szasz, 1971). Simultaneously, locating the "problem" within the bodies and minds of slaves shifted the lens away from the structured economic system of slavery and the white slaveholders whom it benefited. More recent examples can be found in the literature on HIV/AIDS, in which the identification of HIV/AIDS among Haitians and gay men contributed to stigmatization of affected communities and impeded effective response (Altman, 1986; Brandt, 1987; Cohen, 1996; Sontag, 1989).

In each of these examples, the identification of a particular group most negatively affected by a health or social condition, combined with cultural representations that play on racial fears and stereotypes, serves to define particular health concerns within those groups most harmed, contributes to their stigmatization, and obscures white privilege in a manner that is consistent with Winant's typology of new right whiteness projects.

Examples such as these demonstrate the processes through which the causes of racial disparities in health can be located within those groups most visibly affected, rather than in the social relations that systematically advantage whites in relation to other racial groups. What remains invisible is whiteness itself, as well as its role in the process of creating and sustaining racial disparities in health by contributing to unequal access to the resources necessary to maintain health. The failure to explicitly conceptualize race as a set of social relations leaves descriptions of racial differences in biological or behavioral factors associated with differential health outcomes open to interpretations as produced through biological, genetic, or culturally patterned lifestyle differences. In other words, they "explain racial inequality as the outcome of nonracial dynamics" (Bonilla-Silva, 2003, p. 2), a hallmark of "colorblind racism." Such studies can be interpreted in ways that foster neoliberal, neoconservative, or new right whiteness projects.

In an effort to move toward a more explicit analysis that links racial disparities in health to social contextual factors, a literature on social disparities in health has emerged. This literature attempts to address the discrepant "life chances" between poor or working-class and middle-class people and between whites and blacks, Hispanics, or other racialized groups. This body of research attempts to explain racial and class differences in health outcomes through the identification of unequal exposures to social conditions that influence health—for example, access to employment opportunities, exposure to unfair treatment, or exposure to noxious environments.

To return to our earlier example of racial differences in cardiovascular disease, research framed in terms of social determinants of health might attempt to explicitly link racial disparities in cardiovascular disease to differentials in access to the resources or environments necessary to maintain health. Studies in this vein examine, for example, racial or socioeconomic variations in access to healthy and affordable fruits and vegetables and their implications for dietary practices (Cheadle and others, 1991; Morland, Wing, Diez-Roux, and Poole, 2002; Nestle and Jacobson, 2000; Swinburn, Egger, and Raza, 1999; Travers, 1996; Zenk and others, 2005), access to educational and employment opportunities and their implications for socioeconomic status (Massey and Denton, 1993; Orfield, 1993, 2001; Wacquant and Wilson, 1989), the location of health care providers and pharmacies and their implications for access to health care (McLafferty, 1982; Whiteis, 1992), and neighborhood concentrations of poverty and wealth and implications for cardiovascular risks (Diez-Roux and others, 2001; Kaufman, Cooper, and McGee, 1997). This literature reflects a move toward a more explicit theoretical conceptualization of racial disparities in health as resulting from differential access to the resources necessary to maintain health (for example, education, income, access to nutritious foods), which, in turn, influence health-related behaviors and biological processes associated with cardiovascular disease.

How is whiteness constructed in this literature? Explanations of racial disparities in health that focus attention on differential access to resources to promote health (such as grocery stores) and differential exposure to environments that are not conducive to health (such as restricted employment opportunities) shift the explanatory lens from the biology and the behaviors of racialized groups to the contexts within which people reside. This explanatory shift, depending on the theoretical framework and the explanation for why there is differential distribution of resources conducive to health, may help disrupt racial categories.

Specifically, these analyses test the extent to which racial differences in health emerge from differences in social environments rather than from differences in inherent characteristics of racial groups. They seek to document the contributions of differential access to health-promoting resources and differential exposure to health risks. They essentially suggest that there are not inherent differences between racial groups but that differences in health emerge through differences in the social determinants of health. Extending the argument that race would not matter if exposures to x were more equitably distributed contributes to understanding how social conditions contribute to or create racial differences in health. However, without an explicit analysis of how risks come to be distributed differentially, such analyses stop short of making the theoretical or empirical link to the processes that create these unequal distributions of resources and risks. In other words, they fail to specifically theorize the ways that racial categories and racialized processes contribute to the accrual of advantage by whites and the extent to which those benefits accrue at the expense of nonwhite people's health. This leaves whiteness, and specifically the way whiteness is protective of health, unmarked, invisible, and unnoticed. Given that the research is ostensibly addressing the issue of race, and indeed disparities in health, the invisibility of whiteness in this context becomes all the more difficult to name.

Some of this literature, however, is more explicit in theorizing the processes through which whiteness accrues privilege while disadvantage accumulates among racially labeled groups. For example, an active body of research explicitly examines the ways that race-based residential segregation and urban renewal efforts have served to concentrate poverty and disadvantage in segregated black or Latino and Latina urban communities while concentrating wealth and advantage in segregated white communities, with subsequent implications for health (Acevedo-Garcia, Lochner, Osypuk, and Subramanian, 2003; Fullilove, 2004; Schulz, Williams, Israel, and Lempert, 2002; Williams and Collins, 2001). This work links processes of racialization and discrimination to the distribution of resources available to maintain health, probing the ways that whites accrue advantage and blacks, Latinos and Latinas, and other racialized groups accrue systematic disadvantage in terms of exposures to risks and access to protective factors. Similarly, analyses that probe the intersections of race and gender and class, including the racialized and gendered nature of the labor market, help to explicate the reciprocal nature of advantage and disadvantage and their role in producing racial disparities in health (Mullings and Wali, 2001; Chapter Twelve, this volume).

Finally, analyses that turn the lens on the cultural production of difference and differential access to the means of constructing cultural interpretations (see Geronimus and Thompson, 2004; Chapter Two, this volume) further interrogate the production of inequalities, including the role of whiteness in sustaining systems of racial inequality. Explicit examination of whiteness projects can make more visible the processes through which racial hierarchies are reproduced. Bringing such analyses to research on racial disparities in health moves us toward what Winant has termed "new abolitionist" whiteness projects—those that explicitly focus on deconstructing or decentering white racial privilege by analyzing the construction of whiteness. Placing whiteness under such a critical lens in future studies of racial disparities in health can contribute to an examination of the complex forms that whiteness projects take, ranging from those that reproduce racial hierarchies to those that may disrupt and potentially transform those hierarchies. Scholars have raised important concerns and caveats about contemporary investigations of whiteness (Arnesen, 2001; Fine, 1997; Stein, 2001; Winant, 1997) while encouraging continued critical attention to the contribution of whiteness in social, political, and cultural processes that perpetuate racial inequalities.

In the following section, we examine the emergence of various whiteness projects within the context of the Human Genome Project over the past decade or so. Building on our analysis of the absence of an explicit theory of race as a set of social relations, we examine how that absence enables the production of a variety of racial projects that construct whiteness while enabling it to remain relatively invisible. This invisibility facilitates whiteness projects that simultaneously perpetuate inequalities (and thus disparities in health) while undermining the potential for more transformational whiteness projects that could contribute to the disruption of racial hierarchies and the health disparities that they produce.

CONSTRUCTING WHITENESS THROUGH GENETIC EXPLANATIONS FOR RACIAL DISPARITIES

Writing in 1997, Winant asserted that the neoconservative racial project was "far more complicated now than ever before, largely due to the present unavailability of biologistic forms of racism as a convenient rationale for white supremacy" (p. 45). However, in the first years of the twenty-first century, there has been a dramatic resurgence in the availability of biology as an explanation for persistent racial differences. In fact, the interest among scholars, mainstream media, and the lay public in biological or genetic explanations for differences among racial groups has been so pronounced that Rothman describes this "genetic frame" as a new "way of thinking" (2001, p. 2). While not the equivalent of the biologistic racism of the far right racial project, the biologically based individualism of neoconservative whiteness constructs and reinforces notions of race as fixed, rooted in physical bodies rather than in social constructs, while it also seeks to abrogate racial disparities in health. The interplay of assumptions and constructions of race and the inevitably of whiteness are visible as discussions of genomic research, particularly aspects of genomic research concerned with racial disparities, unfold.

BACKGROUND TO HUMAN GENOME RESEARCH

Genomic research, and in particular the Human Genome Project (HGP), has substantially altered biomedical and health research in racial disparities, precipitating a move toward analysis of genomic characteristics of individuals or groups (Duster, 2003a, 2003b; Haraway, 1997; Katz Rothman, 1998, 2001; Stevens, 2002, 2003). Begun in 1990 and completed in 2003, the HGP was conducted by the International Human Genome Research Consortium.[2] Alongside this academic consortium, a number of privately owned biotechnology firms, such as Celera, began attempts to map the human genome, with an eye toward turning a profit from genetic knowledge, particularly in the field of health (Malakoff and Service, 2001). The goal of both the privately funded efforts and the academic HGP was to "analyze the structure of human DNA and to determine the location of an estimated 100,000 human genes" (Guyer and Collins, 1993, p. 1145). (The total number of human genes is now estimated to be much lower, around 25,000; Stein, 2004).[3] The completion of the HGP has made it possible to identify and isolate human genes, particularly those associated with disease (van Ommen, 2002). Completion of the project and mapping of the human genome single-nucleotide polymorphisms (SNPs) are widely regarded, by both genomic researchers and the lay public, as holding out great promise for the future of diagnostics, treatment, and prevention of disease (Chice, Cariou, and Mira, 2002; Wade, 2002b).

Frequently considered the medical equivalent of landing on the moon, the HGP seemed to offer improved opportunities for early diagnosis and treatment when, in 1994, two leading scientists wrote that "the ability to predict the development of disease makes possible early intervention to limit the severity of a disease or to use gene therapy to cure inherited disorders" (Gottesman and Collins, 1994, p. 591). While some have tempered their enthusiasm in the years since the start of the HGP, neither the unfulfilled goal of early diagnosis and intervention to limit the severity of disease nor the illusive promise of gene therapy to cure inherited disorders has deterred ardent proponents of the possibilities of genomic research for disease diagnosis, prevention, and treatment (Stevens, 2003).

The HGP, and genomic research more broadly, are having a ripple effect on public health research agendas having to do with disparities. Evidence of this ripple effect can be seen in the growing body of literature that addresses the implications of genomic research for health promotion and disease prevention (Austin, Peyser, and Khoury, 2000; Khoury, Burke, and Thomson, 2000; Beskow, Khoury, Baker, and Thrasher, 2001; Chadwick, 2004; Gerard, Hayes, and Rothstein, 2002; Wilkinson and Targonski, 2003). This emerging literature calls for a variety of responses to genomic research by those who work in public health, including "how to address barriers to widespread application" (Gerard, Hayes, and Rothstein, 2002, p. 173) and "the integration of genomic competencies among public health professionals" (Beskow, Khoury, Baker, and Thrasher, 2001, p. 2). At the same time, a more critical voice has emerged among scholars within public health, medicine, genetics research, and related disciplines calling for a more equivocal and nuanced response to the emergent emphasis on genetic solutions to public health concerns (Anderson and Nickerson, 2005; Bonham, Warshauer-Baker, and Collins, 2005), including a concern about overemphasizing genetic explanations for public health problems (Kaufman and Hall, 2003; Stevens, 2003).

Funded in the United States by the National Institutes of Health (NIH), the HGP had an annual budget of approximately $350 million, easily making it the largest recipient of NIH funds. Some have speculated that in the wake of NIH sponsorship of the HGP, it will be increasingly difficult to obtain NIH funds for public health research that does not address genomes, such as environmental and behavioral health research (Wilkinson and Targonski, 2003). We contend that this shift toward the genomic has profound implications for an understanding of racial disparities in health and, in particular, the reproduction of whiteness within public health research and practice that seeks to address racial disparities.

WHITENESS AND THE HUMAN GENOME

The director of the National Human Genome Research Institute (NHGRI) at the National Institutes of Health, Francis Collins, has stated that the HGP "helped to inform us about how remarkably similar all human beings are—99.9% at the DNA level. Those who wish to draw precise racial boundaries around certain groups will not be able to use science as a legitimate justification" (Collins and Mansoura, 2001, p. 221). Other scientists working in the area of population genetics often (though not universally) echo this disavowal of the existence of race: "One important conclusion of human population genetics is that races do not exist" (Cavalli-Sforza, 1997, pp. 52–53). As one researcher has noted, referring to Herrnstein and Murray's 1994 work, "This is not the sociobiology seen in *The Bell Curve,* in which genetically based intelligence differentials are asserted to characterize different races" (Dunklee, 2003, p. 154). Reframed within Winant's typology, this is not the essentialism of the far right whiteness project. Rather, the HGP resonates with neoconservative whiteness projects as it universalizes, emphasizing similarities in human genetic material across races, while it simultaneously elevates the individual. This is particularly evident in both the sampling for the HGP and the claims based on those samples.

Rarely mentioned in the literature, and even less often scrutinized, are the samples and the sampling strategy used in the HGP and the associated private ventures on which this claim of "shared humanity" is based. Scientists working on the HGP from both the academic consortium and the privately funded biotechnology firms originally proposed to include a "diverse" sample of DNA for mapping the human genome: that is, chromosomal samples taken from people of a variety of racial and ethnic backgrounds. For example, the Web site for the academic consortium responsible for the HGP in the United States indicates that "candidates were recruited from a diverse population" (http://www.genome.gov/11006943). The private effort to map the human genome, led by the biotech firm Celera, claimed to be using an even more deliberately diverse chromosomal sample. Venter and others (2001) write, "Celera and the IRB believed that the initial version of a completed human genome should be a composite derived from multiple donors of diverse ethnic backgrounds" (p. 1306). DNA samples were collected from twenty-one volunteer male and female donors who self-identified their racial/ethnic category. From those donors, DNA was selected from five subjects (one African American, one Asian Chinese, one Hispanic Mexican, and two Caucasians, two of whom were male and three female). The decision about whose DNA to sequence was based on "a complex mix of factors, including the goal of achieving diversity, as well as technical issues such as the quality of the DNA libraries and availability of immortalized cell lines" (p. 1307). Thus, both the academic consortium and the private firm involved in mapping the human genome originally sought to include DNA from people of diverse racial/ethnic backgrounds as well as gender. On completion of 90 percent of the mapping project, Collins of the NHGRI and Venter of Celera, former competitors in the race to map the human genome, held a joint press conference with President Clinton to announce the completion of a "rough draft of the human genome" (Wade, 2000), ostensibly on this diverse sample of DNA.

However, both the academic HGP and the privately funded mapping project have been criticized for not selecting a sample

that is diverse enough to serve as the map of the human genome
(Jackson, 1997). In fact, the chromosomal reference samples for
the academic HGP were taken from "sixty-seven northern American and northern European men" with a large portion oversam-
pled from Utah (Stevens, 2002, p. 110). As for the private venture
at Celera, after the project was completed, Celera's CEO, Craig
Venter, revealed the mapping that his firm had done had not been
on the diverse chromosomal sample of donated DNA but rather on
his (Venter's) own DNA (Wade, 2002a). Explaining the use of his
own DNA, Venter cited both "privacy concerns" for volunteers who
submitted DNA to the project and his curiosity about the uniqueness of his own DNA (Wade, 2002a).[4] The point of noting this discrepancy here between the claim of shared genetic universality and
the limited sampling diversity (to vastly understate the case) of
DNA actually used for mapping the human genome is to raise one
of the central dilemmas for those interested in critically engaging
the genomic literature and the construction of whiteness. On the
one hand, charging that the DNA sample was not "diverse enough"
across racial and ethnic groups presumes that there are significant
genetic racial differences between groups that should be studied.
Indeed, Fatimah Jackson (1997) argues forcefully against the
applicability of the heavily North American and northern European sample of the HGP to people who are descendants of African
ancestors. She calls for separate genetic studies of Africans directed
by Africans and African Americans.[5] But this critique of the limited genome sample, while powerful, does little to upend the
reliance on biologically based notions of racial taxonomies. More
to the point for our discussion here, this type of argument leaves
the normativity of whiteness unexamined by calling for further
mapping of ostensibly genetically distinct racial groupings rather
than interrogating the notion that whiteness is a homogeneous
and genetically discreet category. Yet accepting the use of a limited, and predominantly Caucasian, DNA sample as the map of all
humankind morphs whiteness into that which is universally human
and reifies race as a putatively scientific category (Duster, 2001,
2005). Returning again to Winant's typology, neoconservative
whiteness combines a dual assertion of the universal alongside the
assertion of the uniqueness of the individual. That Venter in his
private venture used only his (Caucasian, male) DNA for mapping

(Wade, 2002a) passed with little comment because of the assumption of universality of this genetic sample: any (white) North American or northern European man is just as human as the next. As it plays out in the HGP, the universal "shared inheritance of all humankind" is invoked by leaders of one faction of the HGP researchers, while another researcher asserts his individual curiosity about his own DNA. In a very real sense, then, the mapping of the human genome is both a universal appeal to humankind and based on the DNA of a putatively white genome. Yet this is rarely explicitly stated or called into question. Given the pervasiveness of whiteness as a racialized norm in the United States, it is not surprising that a map constructed from the DNA of northern Europeans and Americans is assumed to represent *"the human"* genome (Cross, 2001, p. 435).

Alongside and following shortly after the HGP began, genetic researchers, led by Luigi Luca Cavalli-Sforza of Stanford University, proposed the Human Genome Diversity Project (HGDP) in 1991. Its explicit purpose was to map the diversity of the 0.1 percent of variation in human genomes by extracting genetic samples from a variety of geographically distinct populations, with a particular focus on indigenous peoples around the world. These DNA samples were to be multiplied and stored for future research. The HGDP, unlike the HGP, has met with strenuous criticism (Dodson and Williamson, 1999; Greely, 2001; Katz Rothman, 2001; Reardon, 2001; Resnik, 1999). Although the project languished without funding for a number of years, due in no small measure to opposition by indigenous people (Cross, 2001; Greely, 2001), it was given new life in a formal working relationship with the HGP (Stevens, 2002, p. 110).[6] The goal of mapping genetic diversity is doubly ironic, given both the minute proportion of variation (0.1 percent) and Cavalli-Sforza's statement quoted above that "races do not exist" (Cavalli-Sforza, 1997). As Jacqueline Stevens notes, Cavalli-Sforza's statement that races do not exist is "overshadowed" by the HGDP, "for if they do not exist, then it makes no sense to study the small differences among them" (Stevens, 2002, p. 109). What is left unquestioned and unexamined here is the whiteness of the baseline of comparison. The variation of 0.1 percent is variation from some norm, and given the predominance of Caucasians in the sample establishing that norm, it is a putatively white genomic standard; mapping the variation from that norm is a project inherently concerned with mapping difference from whiteness.

Undaunted by the criticisms and initial failure of the HGDP, another group of genetic researchers has proposed the "HapMap" project (Couzin, 2002; Gottlieb, 2002). One of the discoveries of the HGP was that many genes, rather than being transmitted to new generations at random, are passed down in blocks known as haplotypes (Gabriel and others, 2002). These haplotypes remain largely unchanged through generations; therefore, genome researchers hypothesize that there may be only a handful of variations across the entire human population. Furthermore, some genetic researchers speculate that these small variations may play an important role in the development of diseases such as asthma, cancer, and diabetes (Collins, 1999). Several countries involved in the HGP have already signed on to the HapMap project, and $100 million in funding will be shared by researchers in the United States, Canada, Britain, China, and Japan (Couzin, 2002; Gottlieb, 2002). The research aim is to decode the genetic sources of disease by comparing the genomes of people in four ethnic groups: Japanese, Han Chinese, the Yoruba people of Nigeria, and Americans of northern and western European descent (Couzin, 2002).[7] Clearly, the HapMap (like the HGDP) project holds the potential for naturalizing racial categories and challenging claims about the social construction of race by asserting a biological essence of race (Dunklee, 2003; Duster, 2003a; Katz Rothman, 2001; Stevens, 2002, 2003).

The HapMap's quest to find genetic markers for fundamentally social racial and ethnic groups, like the goal of the HGDP, is a move away from the ostensibly universal notions of the HGP. Indeed, Charles Murray (coauthor of *The Bell Curve*) has been quoted as saying: "As the HapMap project gets underway, this would seem to be a good time to put bets on the table regarding how the results will affect the ongoing debate about whether race is a valid and/or useful construct. . . . The HapMap results will move the current consensus toward the traditional end. Race will regain credibility as a useful, albeit imprecise, way to categorize human beings" (quoted in Cohen and others, 2003).

Here, the promise of genomic research in any sense of the universal ("we are all one," "99.9% the same DNA") has disappeared. In its place is a move toward reconstructing "race"—and thus, inevitably whiteness—in a manner that reproduces racial difference as immutable genetic difference.

Many genomic researchers share an assumption that the goal of genetic research is to identify the specific genes and gene variants that influence the diagnosis, prevention, and treatment of disease, with little or no emphasis on race at a genomic level (Collins, Green, Guttmacher, and Guyer, 2003). However, a subset of researchers continues to use self-identified and inherently social racial categorizations as a means to identify populations for genetic study, arguing that it is more economical to categorize people based on phenotypically based notions of race rather than to look exclusively at individual genetic composition for prevention, diagnosis, and treatment of disease (Risch, Burchard, Ziv, and Tang, 2002). Risch, Burchard, Ziv, and Tang (2002) argue that "population genetic studies have recapitulated the classical definition of races based on continental ancestry—namely African, Caucasian (Europe and Middle East), Asian, Pacific Islander (for example, Australian, New Guinean, and Melanesian), and Native American" (p. 3). The continued use of "race" as a heuristic device for investigation at the genomic level is paradoxical, when on its face individualized genetic therapy would mean testing and categorization on the individual level. This return to the use of classical racial categories in population genetics studies despite empirical evidence documenting the clear limits of these categories as indicative of ancestry or heritage (such as the U.S. Census and birth record examples described earlier in this chapter) highlights the power of these socially constructed categories within science, as well as the role of scientific research in continuing to reproduce these categories. This reification of race in scientific research is, at times, rendered graphically (see Figure 4.1).

This is a particularly pernicious use of racial categories. While the evidence from genetic research confirms the similarities of human beings across racial categories, geneticists like Risch want to continue to use social categories as a "practical" matter to underwrite the enormous costs of authentically individualized genetic testing and screening.

As Bonham, Warshauer-Baker, and Collins (2005) point out, attributing racial variations in patterns of disease to the genetic composition of racial or ethnic groups is based on a series of imperfect

FIGURE 4.1. EVOLUTIONARY TREE OF HUMAN RACES

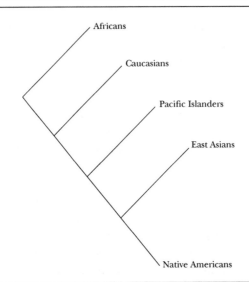

Note: This drawing originally appeared in the journal *Genome Biology* with the caption "Population genetic studies of world populations support the categorization into five major groups."

Source: Risch, Burchard, Ziv, and Tang (2002, Fig. 1).

assumptions. Specifically, "self-identified race is a surrogate for ancestral geographic origin, which is a surrogate for variation across the genome, which is a surrogate for variation in disease-relevant alleles, which is a surrogate for individual disease risk" (p. 13, citing Collins, 2004). With each imperfect assumption, the link between socially constructed racial categories and genetic sources of disease gets less clear, like a copy of a copy of a copy that continues to blur with each reproduction; yet the genetic frame, and the supposedly biological basis for whiteness, remains unchallenged. This reliance on race as a sorting mechanism of convenience in the face of genomic research that demonstrates this is a less than completely reliable proxy simultaneously naturalizes racial disparities while holding out the promise of eliminating racial disparities in health. And it leaves the whiteness within those disparities unexamined.

Furthermore, scholars have also pointed out the impulse to attach genetic conditions to labeled racial or ethnic groups, while those attached to "whites" remain invisible. For example, genetically linked conditions such as Tay-Sachs or sickle cell anemia have become labeled as "Jewish" and "black" diseases, respectively, because they are associated with people who are descendants of Ashkenazi Jews and African Americans. However, a disease such as cystic fibrosis, which is genetically linked to subgroups of the white population, does not get labeled as difference (Katz Rothman, 1998). The link, then, between genetic condition and whiteness is ephemeral, while the connection between genetic condition and members of (already) labeled racial and ethnic groups is intractable. Schwalbe and others (2000) have pointed to the process of identifying and labeling groups as crucial to the process of reproducing inequalities. Thus, the HapMap's explicit quest to locate difference at the genetic level contributes to a whiteness project that both reifies racial categories and contributes to the identification of disease risk as located within racialized groups.

Returning again to Winant's typology of different whiteness projects, the classical definition of races mentioned here seems to move away from the neoconservative whiteness project and toward the far right whiteness project of biological essentialism. Indeed, Risch's "evolutionary tree of human races" is actually quite close to de Gobineau's conceptualization in *Inequality of the Races* (1853), an essay widely regarded as crucial in the development of contemporary Western "racist culture" (Goldberg, 1993). Here we have moved fully from the neoconservative racial project on to the far right racial project in which race is seen as biologically based and whiteness morphs (Duster, 2001) into a discrete line, distinct from others and solidified. Thus, the explicit quest to locate difference at the genetic level contributes to a whiteness project that reifies racial categories and return to pre–civil rights movement constructions of race and whiteness as inherent, biological difference.

WHITENESS IN HEALTH DISPARITIES RESEARCH

Scholars both within and outside the field of public health have drawn attention to the limits of analyses and interventions that focus on biological or behavioral explanations for health and disease, without understanding the social contexts within which health and disease are produced (Geronimus, 2000; House and others, 1994; House and Williams, 2000; Link and Phelan, 1995; Lupton, 1995; Schulz, Williams, Israel, and Lempert, 2002; Williams and Collins, 2001). Specifically, they have argued that such a focus serves to locate the causes of poor health within the bodies of those individuals or groups who are most visibly affected by social, economic, and political powerlessness while drawing attention away from the broader social processes that influence opportunities for health as well as risk of disease (Lupton, 1995; Muntaner, 1999; Shah, 2001).

In this chapter, we have examined one aspect of this process: the ways that race and whiteness are constructed in the literature on racial disparities in health and the ways that this literature may contribute to the reification or reproduction of the racial categories that are fundamental to the production of racial inequalities (Schwalbe and others, 2000). We suggest that this challenge resurfaces particularly in the absence of a specifically social theory of race and of whiteness. Following Muntaner (1999), we argue that the absence of an explicitly social theory of race allows a wide range of interpretations of racial disparities in health to emerge, implicitly or explicitly locating the causes of health and disease within individuals, particular groups (such as Mexicans, Chinese Americans, or the poor), or social relations (such as hierarchies of race and class).

These interpretations, each of which can be linked to various whiteness or, more broadly, racial, projects, do not occur in isolation from the larger social and political context. Over the past several decades in the United States, neoliberal and neoconservative whiteness projects have been in constant flux. Recently, as the mainstream of U.S. politics has moved rightward, challenges have emerged to social and behavioral epidemiological research on health disparities (Zielhuis and Kiemeny, 2001), while biomedical and genomic research on racial disparities in health have reemerged.

Nelkin and Lindee (1995) suggested a decade ago that the power of genetic explanations for racial disparities in health may derive in part from the exoneration of the individual, "removing moral responsibility by providing a biological 'excuse.' Genes are the agents of destiny: We are the victims of a molecule, captives of our heredity" (p. 129). Yet as Kaufman and Hall (2003) point out more recently, "The myth of genetic determinism cuts both ways, however, for although it absolves the individual from responsibility, it also absolves the society at large. Deterministic biological explanations ('it's in my genes')—much like theological explanations ('the devil made me do it')—locate problems (and therefore solutions) within individuals" (p. 117). Genetic explanations for racial disparities in health ignore the historically situated and contextual nature of processes of racialization, shifting the lens away from the ways that those processes are linked to the social, political, and economic conditions that influence health. Instead, by locating the cause of health disparities within the genes—or haplotypes—of racialized groups, they suggest that there is "something innately pathologic" about that group, reinforcing their "essential physical inferiority in the modern world" (p. 117). Such interpretations obscure the social processes that create inequality, contribute to the stigmatization of racialized groups (and thus perpetuate inequalities), and allow whiteness to remain invisible and uninterrogated.

While we have focused particular attention on genetic research in the latter half of this chapter, this same process may play out with any research that does not put forward a specifically social theory of race. For example, research into the extent to which behaviors or cultural practices contribute to racial disparities in health, without explicit theoretical linkages to social and historical contexts, can reproduce ideas of immutable difference between racial groups. To the extent that culture, for example, comes to be perceived as an innate characteristic distinct to particular racial or ethnic groups, it "inherits the role of race . . . [and] becomes determinist and teleological," reproducing the idea of inherent differences between groups (Malik, 1996, p. 150).

Explicitly theorizing race as a social construct encourages us to examine how processes of racialization are linked to social, political, and economic conditions that influence health outcomes. By moving beyond the use of race as an atheoretical and ahistorical category and toward analysis of the processes through which racial constructs are produced and linked to differences in health, researchers can contribute to etiological research that identifies the underlying—or fundamental—causes of racial disparities in health. This includes an understanding of the ways that race is implicated in the construction of class, as well as the ways that class is implicated in the construction of race (Buck, 2001).

Even more so, it is imperative for those vested in understanding and addressing health disparities—whether population geneticists, social epidemiologists, or public health practitioners—to examine critically the assumptions and implicit as well as explicit theoretical frameworks that we bring to our work. Only in so doing can we begin to understand the ways that socially constructed racial categories permeate our own implicit assumptions and interpretations, as well as the ways that research on racial disparities in health may, purposefully or inadvertently, reproduce the racial categories that are themselves fundamental to the processes of inequality. Scholars who make explicit connections between social conditions and the historical and locally contingent production of whiteness and its connections to relative advantage in the distribution of material, political, and cultural resources begin to disrupt the invisibility of whiteness and offer the potential for transformational racial projects to emerge.

Notes
We thank Dana M. Britton, Troy Duster, Michelle Fine, Martine Hackett, Lora Lempert, Leith Mullings, Julie Netherland, and Barbara Katz Rothman for their thoughtful comments on earlier versions of this chapter.
1. PubMed search conducted February 2005 using the search term *racial disparities*.
2. The International Human Genome Sequencing Consortium includes: the Whitehead Institute/MIT Center for Genome Research, Cambridge, Mass.; Wellcome Trust Sanger Institute, Wellcome Trust Genome Campus, Hinxton, Cambridgeshire, U.K.; Washington University School of Medicine Genome Sequencing Center, St. Louis, Mo.; U.S. Department of Energy Joint Genome Institute, Walnut Creek, Calif.; Baylor College of Medicine Human Genome Sequencing Center, Department of Molecular and Human Genetics, Houston, Tex.; RIKEN Genomic Sciences Center, Yokohama, Japan; Genoscope and CNRS UMR-8030, Evry, France; GTC Sequencing Center, Genome Therapeutics Corporation, Waltham, Mass.; Department of Genome Analysis, Institute of Molecular Biotechnology, Jena, Germany; Beijing Genomics Institute/Human Genome Center, Institute of Genetics, Chinese Academy of Sciences, Beijing, China; Multimegabase Sequencing Center, Institute for Systems Biology, Seattle, Wash.; Stanford Genome Technology Center, Stanford, Calif.; Stanford Human Genome Center and Department of Genetics, Stanford University School of Medicine, Stanford, Calif.; University of Washington Genome Center,

Seattle, Wash.; Department of Molecular Biology, Keio University School of Medicine, Tokyo, Japan; University of Texas Southwestern Medical Center at Dallas, Dallas, Tex.; University of Oklahoma's Advanced Center for Genome Technology, Department of Chemistry and Biochemistry, University of Oklahoma, Norman, Okla.; Max Planck Institute for Molecular Genetics, Berlin, Germany; Cold Spring Harbor Laboratory, Lita Annenberg Hazen Genome Center, Cold Spring Harbor, N.Y.; and GBF—German Research Centre for Biotechnology, Braunschweig, Germany.

3. We thank Troy Duster for this point.

4. Since he had his DNA sequenced, Venter has been following an individually tailored regime for a condition that is known to be a precursor to Alzheimer's (Wade, 2002a). Most of the genetic research community involved in mapping the human genome found Venter's announcement less than noteworthy. Collins of the NHGRI, who shared the joint press conference with Venter, declined to comment on the revelation (Wade, 2002a).

5. And, indeed, a project known as G-RAP, Genomic Research in African-American Pedigree, is under way at Howard University, based precisely on the notion of understanding "gene-based differences."

6. In April 2005, National Geographic and IBM partnered with population geneticists to form the Genographic Project. The project's aim, strikingly similar to the HDGP, is to collect DNA from hundreds of thousands of people around the world over the next five years, including indigenous peoples. Again, we thank Troy Duster for this point.

7. According to a News Advisory titled "Background on Ethical and Sampling Issues Raised by the International HapMap Project," the NHGRI's Web site describes the rationale for selecting these groups in these terms: "These four populations were selected to include people with ancestry from widely separate geographic regions. Researchers have found that most human populations share the common haplotype patterns. Research already suggests that the overall organization of genetic variation is similar in all four populations, but that there will be enough differences in haplotype frequencies to justify genome-wide studies of samples from these populations." http://genome.gov/10005337.

References

Acevedo-Garcia, D., Lochner, K. A., Osypuk, T. L., and Subramanian, S. V. "Future Directions in Residential Segregation and Health Research: A Multilevel Approach." *American Journal of Public Health*, 2003, *93*(2), 215–221.

Allen, T. *The Invention of the White Race: Racial Oppression and Social Control.* New York: Verso, 1993.

Altman D. *AIDS in the Mind of America.* New York: Doubleday, 1986.

American Anthropological Association. "Statement on 'Race.' " 1998. http://www.aaanet.org/stmts/racepp.htm.

Anderson, N. B., and Nickerson, K. J. "Genes, Race and Psychology in the Genome Era: An Introduction." *American Psychologist,* 2005, *60*(1), 5–8.

Arnesen, E. "Whiteness and the Historian's Imagination." *International Labor and Working-Class History, 60,* 2001, 3–32.

Austin, M. A., Peyser, P. A., and Khoury, M. J. "The Interface of Genetics and Public Health: Research and Educational Challenges." *Annual Review of Public Health,* 2000, *21,* 81–99.

Baker, L. *From Savage to Negro: Anthropology and the Construction of Race, 1896–1954.* Berkeley: University of California Press, 1998.

Beskow, L. M., Khoury, M. J., Baker, T. G., and Thrasher, J. F. "The Integration of Genomics into Public Health Research, Policy and Practice in the United States." *Community Genetics,* 2001, *4*(1), 2–11.

Bhopal, R. "Spectre of Racism in Health and Health Care: Lessons from History and the United States." *British Medical Journal,* June 27, 1998, p. 316.

Bhopal, R., and Donaldson, L. "White, European, Western, Caucasian or What? Inappropriate Labeling in Research on Race, Ethnicity, and Health." *American Journal of Public Health,* 1998, *88*(9), 1303–1307.

Bonham, V. L., Warshauer-Baker, E., and Collins, F. S. "Race and Ethnicity in the Genome Era: The Complexity of the Constructs." *American Psychologist,* 2005, *60*(1), 9–15.

Bonilla-Silva, E. *Racism Without Racists: Color-Blind Racism and the Persistence of Racial Inequality in the United States.* Lanham, Md.: Rowman & Littlefield, 2003.

Brandt, A. M. *No Magic Bullet: A Social History of Venereal Disease in the United States Since 1880.* New York: Oxford University Press, 1987.

Brownson, R. C., and others. "Environmental and Policy Determinants of Physical Activity in the United States." *American Journal of Public Health,* 2001, *91*(12), 1995–2003.

Buck, P. D. *Worked to the Bone: Race, Class, Power, and Privilege in Kentucky.* New York: Monthly Review Press, 2001.

Cartwright, S. A. "Report on the Diseases and Peculiarities of the Negro Race." In A. L. Caplan, H. T. Englehardt, and J. J. McCartney (eds.), *Concepts of Health and Disease: Interdisciplinary Perspectives.* Reading, Mass.: Addison-Wesley, 1981.

Cavalli-Sforza, L. L. "Race Differences: Genetic Evidence." In E. Smith and W. Sapp (eds.), *Plain Talk About the Human Genome Project.* Tuskegee, Ala.: Tuskegee University, 1997.

Chadwick, R. "Nutrigenomics, Individualism and Public Health." *Nutrition*, 2004, *63*(1), 161–166.

Cheadle, A., and others. "Community-Level Comparisons Between the Grocery Store Environment and Individual Dietary Practices." *Preventive Medicine*, 1991, *20*(2), 250–261.

Chehade, C. *Big Little White Lies.* Kearney, Neb.: Morris Publishing, 2001.

Chice, J. D., Cariou, A., and Mira, J. P. "Bench-to-Bedside Review: Fulfilling Promises of the Human Genome Project." *Critical Care*, 2002, *6*(3), 211–215.

Cohen, C. "Contested Membership: Black Gay Identities and the Politics of AIDS." In S. Seidman (ed.), *Queer Theory: Sociology*. Oxford: Blackwell, 1996.

Cohen, E., and others. "HapMap: Revolution or Hype?" *New Atlantis*, 2003, *1*, 129–130.

Collins, F. S. "The Human Genome and the Future of Medicine." *Annals of the New York Academy of Sciences,* June 30, 1999, pp. 42–55.

Collins, F. S. "What We Do and Don't Know About 'Race,' 'Ethnicity,' Genetics and Health at the Dawn of the Genome Era." *Nature Genetics*, 2004, *36*(11 suppl.), S13–S15.

Collins, F. S., Green, E. D., Guttmacher, A. E., and Guyer, M. S. "A Vision for the Future of Genomics Research." *Nature*, Apr. 24, 2003, pp. 835–847.

Collins, F. S., and Mansoura, M. K. "The Human Genome Project: Revealing the Shared Inheritance of All Humankind." *Cancer*, 2001, *91*(1 suppl.), 221–225.

Cooper, R., and David, R. "The Biological Concept of Race and Its Application to Public Health and Epidemiology." *Journal of Health Politics, Policy and Law*, 1986, *11*(1), 97–116.

Cooper, R. S., and Freeman, V. L. "Limitations in the Use of Race in the Study of Disease Causation." *Journal of the National Medical Association*, 1999, *91*(7), 379–383.

Cooper, R., and Rotimi, C. "Hypertension in Blacks." *American Journal of Hypertension*, 1997, *10*, 804–812.

Cooper, R., and others. "Trends and Disparities in Coronary Heart Disease, Stroke and Other Cardiovascular Diseases in the United States: Findings of the National Conference on Cardiovascular Disease Prevention." *Circulation*, 2000, *102*(25), 3137–3147.

Couzin, J. "HUMAN GENOME: HapMap Launched with Pledges of $100 Million." *Science*, 2002, *298*, 941–942.

Crespo, C. J., Loria, C. M., and Burt, V. L. "Hypertension and Other Cardiovascular Disease Risk Factors Among Mexican Americans, Cuban Americans, and Puerto Ricans from the Hispanic Health and Nutrition Examination Survey." *Public Health Report*, 1996, *111*(suppl. 2), 7–10.

Cross, K. "Framing Whiteness: The Human Genome Diversity Project (As Seen on TV)." *Science as Culture,* 2001, *10*(3), 411–438.

Daniels, J. *White Lies: Race, Class, Gender and Sexuality in White Supremacist Discourse.* New York: Routledge, 1997.

Diez-Roux, A. V., and others. "Neighborhood of Residence and Incidence of Coronary Heart Disease." *New England Journal of Medicine,* 2001, *345*(2), 99–106.

Dodson, M., and Williamson, R. "Indigenous Peoples and the Morality of the Human Genome Diversity Project." *Journal of Medical Ethics,* 1999, *25*(2), 204–212.

D'Souza, D. *The End of Racism: Principles for a Multicultural Society.* New York: Free Press, 1995.

Dunklee, B. "Sequencing the Trellis: The Production of Race in the New Human Genomics." Unpublished doctoral dissertation, Brown University, 2003.

Duster, T. "The Morphing Properties of Whiteness." In B. Rasmussen, E. Klinenberg, I. Nexica, and M. Wray (eds.), *The Making and Unmaking of Whiteness,* Durham, N.C.: Duke University Press, 2001.

Duster, T. *Backdoor to Eugenics.* (2nd ed.) New York: Routledge, 2003a.

Duster, T. "Buried Alive: The Concept of Race in Science." In A. H. Goodman, D. Heath, and H. S. Lindee (eds.), *Genetic Nature/Culture: Anthropology and Science Beyond the Two-Culture Divide.* Berkeley: University of California Press, 2003b.

Duster, T. "Race and Reification in Science." *Science,* Feb. 18, 2005, pp. 1050–1051.

Dyer, R. *White.* New York: Routledge, 1997.

Epstein, M., Moreno, R., and Bacchetti, P. "The Underreporting of Deaths of American Indian Children in California, 1979 Through 1993." *American Journal of Public Health,* 1997, *87*(8), 1363–1366.

Farley, D. O., Richards, T., and Bell, R. M. "Effects of Reporting Methods on Infant Mortality Rate Estimates for Racial and Ethnic Subgroup." *Journal of Health Care for the Poor and Underserved,* 1995, *6*(1), 60–75.

Feagin, J., and Vera, H. *White Racism: The Basics.* New York: Routledge, 1994.

Ferber, A. L. (ed.). *Home-Grown Hate: Gender and Organized Racism.* New York: Routledge, 2004.

Fine, M. "Witnessing Whiteness. In M. Fine, L. Weis, L. C. Powell, and L. M. Wong (eds.), *Off White: Readings on Race, Power and Society.* New York: Routledge, 1997.

Fine, M., Weis, L., Powell, L. C., and Wong, L .M. (eds.). *Off White: Readings on Race, Power and Society.* New York: Routledge, 1997.

Forbes, J. D. *Africans and Native Americans: The Language of Race and the Evolution of Red-Black Peoples.* Urbana: University of Illinois Press, 1993.

Frankenberg, R. *White Women, Race Matters: The Social Construction of Whiteness.* Minneapolis: University of Minnesota Press, 1993.

Freeman, H. P. "The Meaning of Race in Science—Considerations for Cancer Research: Concerns of Special Populations in the National Cancer Program." *Cancer,* 1998, *82*(1), 219–225.

Fullilove, M. T. "Comment: Abandoning 'Race' as a Variable in Public Health Research—an Idea Whose Time Has Come." *American Journal of Public Health,* 1998, *88*(9), 1297–1298.

Fullilove, M. T. *Root Shock: How Tearing Up City Neighborhoods Hurts America, and What We Can Do About It.* New York: Random House, 2004.

Gabriel, S. B., and others. "The Structure of Haplotype Blocks in the Human Genome." *Science,* 2002, *296,* 2225–2229.

Gerard, S., Hayes, M., and Rothstein, M. A. "On the Edge of Tomorrow: Fitting Genomics into Public Health Policy." *Journal of Law and Medical Ethics,* 2002, *30*(3 suppl.), 173–176.

Geronimus, A. T. "To Mitigate, Resist or Undo: Addressing Structural Influences on the Health of Urban Populations." *American Journal of Public Health,* 2000, *90*(6), 867–872.

Geronimus, A. T., and Thompson, J. P. "To Denigrate, Ignore or Disrupt: Racial Inequality in Health and the Impact of Policy-Induced Breakdown of African American Communities." *DuBois Review,* 2004, *1*(2), 247–279.

Gimenez, M. E. "Latino/Hispanic?—Who Needs a Name? The Case Against Standardized Terminology." *International Journal of Health Services,* 1989, *19*(3), 557–571.

Gobineau, A. *Essai sur l'inegalité des races humaines/The Inequality of Human Races* (A. Collins, trans.). New York: H. Fertig, 1967. (Originally published 1853.)

Goldberg, D. T. *Racist Culture.* Malden, Mass.: Blackwell, 1993.

Gottesman, M. M., and Collins, F. S. "The Role of the Human Genome Project in Disease Prevention." *Preventive Medicine,* 1994, *23*(5), 591–594.

Gottlieb, S. "Scientists Unveil the Next Step in the Human Genome Project." *British Medical Journal,* Nov. 9, 2002, p. 1056.

Gould, S. J. *The Mismeasure of Man.* New York: Norton, 1996.

Greely, H. T. "Human Genome Diversity: What About the Other Human Genome Project?" *Nature Reviews Genetics,* 2001, *2*(3), 222–227.

Guyer, M. S., and Collins, F. S. "The Human Genome Project and the Future of Medicine." *Pediatrics and Adolescent Medicine,* 1993, *147*(11), 1145–1147.

Hahn, R. A. "Why Race Is Differentially Classified on U.S. Birth and Infant Death Certificates: An Examination of Two Hypotheses." *Epidemiology,* 1999, *10,* 108–111.

Hahn, R. A., Mendlein, J. M., and Helgerson, S. D. "Differential Classification of American Indian Race on Birth and Death Certificates, U.S. Reservation States, 1983–1985." *IHS Primary Care Provider,* 1993, *18,* 8–11.

Hahn, R. A., Mulinare, J., and Teutsch, S. M. "Inconsistencies in Coding of Race and Ethnicity Between Birth and Death in U.S. Infants." *Journal of the American Medical Association,* 1992, *267*(2), 259–263.

Hahn, R. A., and Stroup, D. F. "Race and Ethnicity in Public Health Surveillance: Criteria for the Scientific Use of Social Categories." *Public Health Reports,* 1994, *109*(1), 7–15.

Haraway, D. *Modest-Witness, Second-Millennium: Femaleman Meets Oncomouse: Feminism and Technoscience.* New York: Routledge, 1997.

Herrnstein, R. J., and Murray, C. *The Bell Curve: Intelligence and Class Structure in American Life.* New York: Free Press, 1994.

House, J. S., and Williams, D. R. "Understanding and Reducing Socioeconomic and Racial/Ethnic Disparities in Health." In B. D. Smedley and S. L. Syme (eds.), *Promoting Health: Intervention Strategies from Social and Behavioral Research.* Washington, D.C.: National Academy Press, 2000.

House, J. S., and others. "The Social Stratification of Aging and Health." *Journal of Health and Social Behavior,* 1994, *35*(3), 213–234.

Ignatiev, N. *How the Irish Became White.* New York: Routledge, 1995.

Jackson, F. "Assessing the Human Genome Project: An African American Bioanthropological Critique." In E. Smith and W. Sapp (eds.), *Plain Talk About the Human Genome Project.* Tuskegee, Ala.: Tuskegee University Press, 1997.

Jackson, F.L.C. "Race and Ethnicity as Biological Constructs." *Ethnicity and Disease,* 1989, *2,* 120–125.

Jackson, V. "In Our Own Voices: African American Stories of Oppression, Survival and Recovery in the Mental Health System." 2002. http://www.patdeegan.com/cp_socialjustice.html#africanamerican.

James, S. A. "Primordial Prevention of Cardiovascular Disease Among African Americans: A Social Epidemiological Perspective." *Preventive Medicine,* 1999, *29*(6 part 2), S84–S89.

Katz Rothman, B. *Genetic Maps and Human Imaginations: The Limits of Science in Understanding Who We Are.* New York: Norton, 1998.

Katz Rothman, B. *The Book of Life: A Personal and Ethical Guide to Race, Normality, and the Human Gene Study.* Boston: Beacon Press, 2001.

Kaufman, J. S. "How Inconsistencies in Racial Classification Demystify the Race Construct in Public Health Statistics." *Epidemiology,* 1999, *10*(2), 101–103.

Kaufman, J. S., Cooper, R. S., and McGee, D. L. "Socioeconomic Status and Health in Blacks and Whites: The Problem of Residual Confounding and the Resiliency of Race." *Epidemiology,* 1997, *8*(6), 621–628.

Kaufman J. S., and Hall, S. A. "The Slavery Hypertension Hypothesis: Dissemination and Appeal of a Modern Race Theory." *Epidemiology,* 2003, *14*(1), 111–118.

Khoury M. J., Burke, W., and Thomson, E. J. (eds.). *Genetics and Public Health in the Twenty-First Century: Using Genetic Information to Improve Health and Prevent Disease.* New York: Oxford University Press, 2000.

Kincheloe, J. L., Steinberg, S. R., Rodriguez, N. M., and Chenault, R. E. (eds.). *White Reign: Deploying Whiteness in America.* New York: St. Martin's Press, 1998.

Kumanyika, S. "Minisymposum on Obesity: Overview and Some Strategic Considerations." *Annual Review of Public Health,* 2001, *22,* 309–335.

Last, J. M. (ed.). *A Dictionary of Epidemiology.* (3rd ed.) New York: Oxford University Press, 1995.

LaVeist, T. A. "Beyond Dummy Variables and Sample Selection: What Health Services Researchers Ought to Know About Race as a Variable." *HSR: Health Services Research,* 1994, *29*(1), 1–16.

Lewontin, R., Rose, S., and Kamin, L. *Not in Our Genes: Biology, Ideology and Human Nature.* New York: Random House, 1984.

Li, R., and others. "Trends in Fruit and Vegetable Consumption Among Adults in 16 U.S. States: Behavioral Risk Factor Surveillance System, 1990–1996." *American Journal of Public Health,* 2000, *90,* 777–781.

Link, B. G., and Phelan, J. "Social Conditions as Fundamental Causes of Disease." *Journal of Health and Social Behavior,* 1995, *36* (special issue), 80–94.

Lupton, D. *The Imperative of Health: Public Health and the Regulated Body.* Thousand Oaks, Calif.: Sage, 1995.

Majaj, L. S. "Arab Americans and the Meanings of Race." In A. Singh and P. Schmidt (eds.), *Postcolonial Theory and the United States.* Oxford: University Press of Mississippi, 2000.

Malakoff, D., and Service, R. F. "Genomania Meets the Bottom Line." *Science,* Feb. 16, 2001, pp. 1193–1203.

Malik, K. *The Meaning of Race: Race, History and Culture in Western Society.* New York: New York University Press, 1996.

Massey, D., and Denton, N. *American Apartheid: Segregation and the Making of the Underclass.* Cambridge, Mass.: Harvard University Press, 1993.

McIntosh, P. *White Privilege and Male Privilege: A Personal Account of Coming to See Correspondences Through Work in Women's Studies.* Wellesley, Mass.: Wellesley College Center for Research on Women, 1988.

McLafferty, S. "Neighborhood Characteristics and Hospital Closures: A Comparison of the Public, Private, and Voluntary Hospital Systems." *Social Science and Medicine,* 1982, *16*(19), 1667–1674.

Morland, K., Wing, S., Diez-Roux, A., and Poole, C. "Neighborhood Characteristics Associated with the Location of Food Stores and Food Service Places." *American Journal of Preventive Medicine,* 2002, *22*(1), 23–29.

Morrison, T. *Playing in the Dark: Whiteness and the Literary Imagination.* New York: Vintage Books, 1990.

Mullings, L. "Race and Globalization: Racialization from Below." *Souls: A Critical Journal of Black Politics, Culture and Society,* 2004, *6*(2), 1–9.

Mullings, L. "Interrogating Racism: Toward an Anti-Racist Anthropology." *Annual Review of Anthropology,* forthcoming.

Mullings, L., and Wali, A. *Stress and Resilience: The Social Context of Reproduction in Central Harlem.* New York: Kluwer Academic/Plenum Publishers, 2001.

Muntaner, C. "Invited Commentary: Social Mechanisms, Race and Social Epidemiology." *American Journal of Epidemiology,* 1999, *150*(2), 121–126.

Nagel, J. *American Indian Ethnic Renewal: Red Power and the Resurgence of Identity and Power.* New York: Oxford University Press, 1996.

National Heart Lung and Blood Institute. *The Seventh Report of the Joint National Committee on Prevention, Detection, Evaluation and Treatment of High Blood Pressure.* Bethesda, Md.: U.S. Department of Health and Human Services, National Institutes of Health, Aug. 2004.

Nelkin, D., and Lindee, M. S. *The DNA Mystique: The Gene as a Cultural Icon.* New York: Freeman, 1995.

Nestle, M., and Jacobson, M. F. "Halting the Obesity Epidemic: A Public Health Policy Approach." *Public Health Reports,* 2000, *115*(1), 12–24.

Nobles, M. *Shades of Citizenship: Race and the Census in Modern Politics.* Palo Alto, Calif.: Stanford University Press, 2000.

Office of Management and Budget. *Race and Ethnic Standards for Federal Statistics and Administrative Reporting. Statistical Policy Handbook.* Washington, D.C.: Office of Federal Statistical Policy and Standards, 1978.

Omi, M., and Winant, H. "Racial Formation." In P. Essed and D. T. Goldberg (eds.), *Race Critical Theories.* Malden, Mass.: Blackwell, 2002.

Orfield, G. *The Growth of Segregation in American Schools: Changing Patterns of Separation and Poverty Since 1968.* Cambridge, Mass.: Harvard Project on School Desegregation, 1993.

Orfield, G. *Schools More Separate: Consequences of a Decade of Resegregation— New Research Findings from the Civil Rights Project at Harvard University.* Cambridge, Mass.: Harvard University Press, 2001.

Phillips, C. V. "Publication Bias in Situ." *BMC Medical Research Methodology*, 2000, *4*(20). http://www.biomedcentral.com/content/pdf/1471-2288-4-20.pdf.

Reardon, J. "The Human Genome Diversity Project: A Case Study in Coproduction." *Social Studies of Science*, 2001, *3*(3), 357–388.

Resnik D. B. "The Human Genome Diversity Project: Ethical Problems and Solutions." *Politics and the Life Sciences*, 1999, *18*(1), 15–23.

Risch, N., Burchard, E., Ziv, E., and Tang, H. "Categorization of Humans in Biomedical Research: Genes, Race, and Disease." *Genome Biology*, 2002, *3*(7), 1–12. http://genomebiology.com/2002/3/7/comment/2007.

Roediger, D. *The Wages of Whiteness: Race and the Making of the American Working Class.* New York: Verso, 1991.

Roediger, D. (ed.). *Black on White: Black Writers on What It Means to Be White.* New York: Schocken, 1998.

Rushton, J. P. *Race, Evolution and Behavior.* New Brunswick, N.J.: Transaction, 1994.

Scargle, J. D. "Publication Bias: The 'File Drawer' Problem in Scientific Inference." *Journal of Scientific Exploration*, 2000, *14*(1), 91–106.

Schulz, A. J., Williams, D. R., Israel, B. A., and Lempert, L. B. "Racial and Spatial Relations as Fundamental Determinants of Health in Detroit." *Milbank Quarterly*, 2002, *80*(4), 677–707.

Schwalbe, M., and others. "Generic Processes in the Reproduction of Inequality: An Interactionist Analysis." *Social Forces*, 2000, *79*(2), 419–452.

Shah, N. *Contagious Divides: Epidemics and Race in San Francisco's Chinatown.* Berkeley: University of California Press, 2001.

Snyderman, M., and Rothman, S. *The IQ Controversy: The Media and Public Policy.* New Brunswick, N.J.: Transaction, 1988.

Sontag, S. *AIDS and Its Metaphors.* New York: Farrar, Straus and Giroux, 1989.

Stein, J. "Whiteness and United States History: An Assessment." *International Labor and Working-Class History*, 2001, *60*, 1–2.

Stein, L. "Human Genome: End of the Beginning." *Nature*, Oct. 21, 2004, pp. 915–916.

Stern, J. "Publication Bias: Evidence of Delayed Publication in a Cohort Study of Clinical Research Projects." *British Medical Journal*, 1997, *315*, 640–645.

Stevens, J. "Symbolic Matter: DNA and Other Linguistic Stuff." *Social Text*, 2002, *20*(1), 105–136.

Stevens, J. "Racial Meanings and Scientific Methods: Changing Policies for NIH-Sponsored Publications Reporting Human Variation." *Journal of Health Politics, Policy and Law*, 2003, *28*(6), 1033–1087.

Swinburn, G., Egger, G., and Raza, F. "Dissecting Obesogenic Environments: The Development and Application of a Framework for Identifying and Prioritizing Environmental Interventions for Obesity." *Preventive Medicine,* 1999, *29*(6 part 1), 563–570.

Szasz, T. S. "The Sane Slave: An Historical Note on the Use of Medical Diagnosis as Justificatory Rhetoric." *American Journal of Psychotherapy,* 1971, *25*(2), 228–239.

Travers, K. D. "The Social Organization of Nutritional Inequities." *Social Science and Medicine,* 1996, *43*(4), 543–553.

Tucker, W. H. *The Science and Politics of Racial Research.* Urbana: University of Illinois Press, 1996.

van Ommen, G. J. "The Human Genome Project and the Future of Diagnostics, Treatment and Prevention." *Journal of Inherited and Metabolic Diseases,* 2002, *25*(3), 183–188.

Venter, J. C., and others. "The Sequence of the Human Genome." *Science,* Feb. 16, 2001, pp. 1304–1351.

Wacquant, L.J.D., and Wilson, W. J. "The Cost of Racial and Class Exclusion in the Inner City." *Annals of the American Academy of Political and Social Science,* 1989, *501,* 8–25.

Wade, N. "Reading the Book of Life: The Overview; Genetic Code of Human Life Is Cracked by Scientists." *New York Times,* June 27, 2000, p. A1.

Wade, N. "Scientist Reveals Secret of Genome: It's His." *New York Times,* Apr. 27, 2002a, p. A1.

Wade, N. "Genetic Decoding May Bring Advances in Worldwide Fight Against Malaria." *New York Times,* Oct. 3, 2002b, p. A1.

Watson, C. C., and others. "Classification of American Indian Race on Birth and Infant Death Certificates—California and Montana." *Morbidity and Mortality Weekly Report,* 1993, *42*(12), 220–223.

Whiteis, D. G. "Hospital and Community Characteristics in Closures of Urban Hospitals, 1980–87." *Public Health Reports,* 1992, *107*(4), 409–416.

Wilkinson, J. M., and Targonski, P. V. "Health Promotion in a Changing World: Preparing for the Genomics Revolution." *American Journal of Health Promotion,* 2003, *18*(2), 157–161.

Williams, D. R. "Race and Health: Basic Questions, Emerging Directions." *Annals of Epidemiology,* 1997, *7*(5), 322–333.

Williams, D. R., and Collins, C. "Racial Residential Segregation: A Fundamental Cause of Racial Disparities in Health." *Public Health Reports,* 2001, *116,* 404–416.

Williams, D. R., and Harris-Reid, M. "Race and Mental Health: Emerging Patterns and Promising Approaches." In A. V. Horwitz and T. L.

Scheid (eds.), *A Handbook for the Study of Mental Health: Social Contexts, Theories and Systems.* Cambridge: Cambridge University Press, 1999.

Williams, D. R., Lavizzo-Mourey, R., and Warren, R. C. "The Concept of Race and Health Status in America." *Public Health Reports,* 1994, *109*(1), 26–41.

Wilton, R. D. "Colouring Special Needs: Locating Whiteness in NIMBY Conflicts." *Social and Cultural Geography,* 2002, *3*(3), 303–321.

Winant, H. *Racial Conditions: Politics, Theory and Comparison.* Minneapolis: University of Minnesota Press, 1994.

Winant, H. "Behind Blue Eyes: Whiteness and Contemporary U.S. Racial Politics." In M. Fine, L. Weis, L. C. Powell, and L. M. Wong (eds.), *Off White: Readings on Race, Power and Society.* New York: Routledge, 1997.

Witzig, R. "The Medicalization of Race: Scientific Legitimization of a Flawed Social Construct." *Annals of Internal Medicine,* 1996, *125*(8), 675–679.

Wong, M. D., Shapiro, M. F., Boscardin, W. J., and Ettner, S. L. "Contribution of Major Diseases to Disparities in Mortality." *New England Journal of Medicine,* 2002, *347*(20), 1585–1592.

Wren, T. "A Two-Fold Character: The Slave as Person and Property in Virginia Court Cases, 1800–1860." *Southern Studies,* 1985, *24,* 417–431.

Zenk, S., and others. "Neighborhood Racial Composition, Neighborhood Poverty, and Supermarket Accessibility in Metropolitan Detroit." *American Journal of Public Health,* 2005, *95*(4), 660–667.

Zielhuis, G. A., and Kiemeney, L. A. "Social Epidemiology? No Way." *International Journal of Epidemiology,* 2001, *30*(1), 43–44.

PART THREE

THE SOCIAL CONTEXT OF HEALTH AND ILLNESS

CHAPTER FIVE

THE INTERSECTION OF RACE, GENDER, AND SES

Health Paradoxes

Pamela Braboy Jackson,
David R. Williams

Race/ethnicity, gender, and socioeconomic position are social status categories that predict the differential distribution of disease, disability, and death in society (Krieger and others, 1993). Prior research has attended to variations in health by each of these categories, considered separately, or by two of them in combination. But health researchers seldom consider how health is distributed when these three social status categories are considered simultaneously. In this chapter, we focus on social disparities in health and underscore the complex interactions among these social categories. We begin by briefly documenting that race, gender, and socioeconomic status (SES) each matters in predicting variations in health. We then consider the complex patterns that emerge when we consider race/ethnicity, SES, and gender together. In highlighting some of the paradoxes in the health literature, we draw particular attention to members of the black middle class. We conclude with directions for future research, describing the ways in which intersectionality theory (Mullings and Wali, 2001; Weber and Parra-Medina, 2003) can be used to further our understanding of persistent health inequalities.

RACIAL DIFFERENCES IN HEALTH

The United States routinely reports health statistics by race. However, members of the major racial/ethnic groups are divided over preferred terminology. For example, a large national study found that 62 percent of whites prefer "white" (17 percent prefer "Caucasian"), 58 percent of Hispanics prefer "Hispanic" (12 percent prefer "Latino"), 44 percent of blacks prefer "black" (28 percent prefer "African American"), and 50 percent of American Indians prefer "American Indian" (37 percent prefer "Native American") (Tucker and others, 1996). In an effort to recognize individual dignity, we use the preferred terms for each group interchangeably.

Table 5.1 illustrates the magnitude and pervasiveness of racial disparities in health across different diseases by considering the top fifteen causes of death in the United States (Hoyert and others, 2001). These data are officially reported only for blacks and whites. The first column shows the age-adjusted rates for white men and women, and the second presents the black-white ratios for each condition for men and women. (The last two columns focus on gender differences that we will return to shortly.) A ratio greater than 1.0 means that blacks have a higher mortality rate compared to whites. If the ratio is less than 1.0, then the mortality rate is higher for whites.

As shown in Table 5.1, heart disease, cancer, and stroke are the three leading causes of death in America. Compared to whites, black men and women have mortality rates that are at least 20 percent higher for each of these outcomes. A similar pattern can be seen for almost all diseases. Black men have higher death rates than whites for eleven of the fifteen leading causes of death, and black women have higher rates than their white counterparts for twelve of the fifteen leading killers. Compared to their white counterparts, the rates for black men and women are at least twice as high for five causes of death (diabetes, nephritis, septicemia, hypertension, and homicide). Black men and women have lower rates than their white peers for pulmonary disease, suicide, and Alzheimer's disease.

TABLE 5.1. AGE-ADJUSTED DEATH RATES FOR WHITE MEN AND WOMEN FOR THE FIFTEEN LEADING CAUSES OF DEATH AND THE RACIAL AND GENDER DIFFERENCES IN THE UNITED STATES, 1999

Cause of Death	Whites		Racial Differences, Black/White Ratios		Gender Differences, Male/Female Ratios	
	Men	Women	Men	Women	Blacks	Whites
1. Heart disease	324.7	215.5	1.23	1.35	1.37	1.51
2. Cancer	246.5	168.6	1.38	1.19	1.70	1.46
3. Cerebrovascular disease (stroke)	60.0	58.7	1.46	1.33	1.12	1.02
4. Pulmonary disease	59.6	40.2	0.84	0.59	2.10	1.48
5. Accidents	50.0	22.7	1.24	1.04	2.62	2.20
6. Diabetes mellitus	25.8	20.5	1.88	2.46	0.96	1.26
7. Pneumonia and influenza	27.7	20.8	1.17	1.02	1.52	1.33
8. Alzheimer's disease	14.7	18.4	0.66	0.66	0.80	0.80
9. Nephritis	14.8	9.7	2.22	2.68	1.27	1.53
10. Septicemia	11.0	9.4	2.56	2.39	1.25	1.17
11. Suicide	19.4	4.4	0.54	0.36	6.50	4.41
12. Liver disease and cirrhosis	13.7	6.1	1.10	1.05	2.36	2.25
13. Hypertension	5.1	5.3	3.31	2.91	1.10	0.96
14. Homicide	5.5	2.2	6.35	3.41	4.65	2.50
15. Aortic aneurysm and dissection	9.0	3.8	0.70	1.05	1.58	2.37

Source: National Vital Statistics Reports (2001), per 100,000 population.

MAKING SENSE OF RACIAL DISPARITIES IN HEALTH

The first U.S. Census, conducted in 1790, enumerated whites, blacks (as three-fifths of a person), and civilized Indians (those who paid taxes). This was done to comply with Article One of the U.S. Constitution. Over time, racial categories have been added and altered to keep track of new immigrants. The U.S. racial groupings do not capture race in a biological sense but are socially constructed (American Association of Physical Anthropology, 1996; Williams, 1997). Historically and currently, these social categories have reflected differential access to power and resources in society.

There are large racial differences in SES. For example, compared to whites, African Americans, Hispanics, American Indians, and some Asian groups have higher rates of poverty and unemployment and lower levels of median family income, educational attainment, and wealth (Williams, forthcoming). Adjusting racial differences for indicators of SES typically reduces the size of these differences substantially but does not completely eliminate them. That is, there appears to be an additional effect of racial/ethnic status even after SES is controlled. There is growing recognition among health researchers that there may be other factors shaping racial differences in health in addition to SES (LaVeist, 2002).

GENDER DIFFERENCES IN HEALTH

Like race/ethnicity, gender is a highly visible characteristic. Similar to race/ethnicity, SES is patterned by gender, with men having higher levels of SES than women (Andes, 1992; Grodsky and Pager, 2001; Tienda and Lii, 1987). Accordingly, we might have expected that women, an economically disadvantaged group compared to men, would fare worse than men in terms of health. The last two columns of Table 5.1 show, surprisingly, that across a broad range of disease conditions, men have higher death rates than women. Ratios greater than 1.0 reflect higher mortality rates for men compared to women, while ratios less than 1.0 mean that women have higher death rates than men. For both African Americans and whites, the two racial groups for which these data are available, men show higher death rates than women for thirteen of the fifteen leading causes of death. Moreover, men have death rates that are at least twice as high as those of women for accidents, suicide, cirrhosis of the liver, and homicide.

Making these gender comparisons in health is in no way intended to deny or minimize the historic and ongoing systems of exploitation that have adversely affected women in general, and women of color in particular, in the United States (Krieger and others, 1993; Sanchez-Hucles, 1997) or the pressing need to reduce health and other inequalities for women. Women continue to be disadvantaged on multiple social dimensions, and women of color continue to experience disparities for many indicators of health (Lillie-Blanton, Martinez, Taylor, and Robinson, 1993; Williams, 2002). Nonetheless, gender disparities in health dramatically illustrate that factors other than economic status can powerfully shape the distribution of health.

MAKING SENSE OF GENDER DIFFERENCES IN HEALTH

In most Western societies, men claim more power, prestige, and property than women. In general, these resources are linked to positive health outcomes (Reynolds and Ross, 1998). However, gender as a socially constructed category often produces unexpected health risks due to social roles and expectations that can be linked to gender role occupancy. For example, deeply held cultural views about maleness and masculinity can shape men's beliefs in ways that can lead to increased health risks for some men. Research indicates that beliefs about masculinity and manhood that are deeply rooted in culture and supported by social institutions play a role in shaping the behavioral patterns of men in ways that have adverse consequences for health (Williams, 2003). Compared to women, for example, men are more likely to smoke cigarettes and twice as likely to consume five or more drinks of alcohol in a single day (Eberhardt and others, 2001). Importantly, engaging in high-risk behaviors, refraining from engaging in health-promoting activities, and claiming that risky behaviors such as alcohol drinking will not negatively affect performance (for example, driving) are often demonstrations of the norms of masculinity in the larger culture and strategies that men use to construct and reinforce their masculinity (Courtenay, 2000).

Health care institutions and practitioners also respond differently to men and women. For example, in the emergency room, men with depressive symptoms (inconsistent with gender norms) are more likely to be hospitalized than women with the same symptoms, and women with antisocial behavior or substance use problems are more likely to be hospitalized than men with those presenting symptoms (Rosenfield, 1999). There are also large gender differences in the typical medical encounter. Compared to women, health care providers spend less time with men; provide them with fewer services, less health information, and less advice; and are less likely to talk about the need to change behaviors to improve health (Courtenay, 2000). Men also tend to have lower levels of adherence to medical regimens than women (Rose, Kim, Dennison, and Hill, 2000).

INTERSECTIONS OF RACE/ETHNICITY, SES, AND GENDER

Socioeconomic status is a term conventionally used to refer to an individual's or group's location in the structure of society, which determines differential access to power, privilege, and desirable resources. It is typically assessed by education, income, or occupational status. SES is one of the strongest known determinants of variations in health (Adler and others, 1993; Williams and Collins, 1995). Table 5.2 illustrates the power of SES by presenting the percentage of persons reporting fair or poor health by income for black, white, and Hispanic men and women in the United States. These data reveal that there are large differences in health by income for blacks, whites, and Hispanics. Moreover, while the largest effects of SES are at the lowest categories of income, there is a stepwise progression of risk in the relationship between SES and health status, with each higher level of income associated with better health status for both men and women in each racial group. At the same time, some racial/ethnic and gender differences remain evident when groups are compared at similar levels of SES.

Clearly, the associations among race/ethnicity, gender, SES, and health are complex. National data reveal that the patterns

TABLE 5.2. PERCENTAGE OF MEN AND WOMEN REPORTING
FAIR OR POOR HEALTH BY RACE AND INCOME, 1995

	Men			Women		
Income	*White*	*Black*	*Hispanic*	*White*	*Black*	*Hispanic*
Poor	30.5	37.4	26.9	30.2	38.2	30.4
Near poor	21.3	22.6	19.2	17.9	26.1	24.3
Middle income	9.3	13.1	11.9	9.2	14.6	13.5
High income	4.2	4.8	5.8	9.2	7.0	

Note: Poor = below federal poverty level; near poor = less than twice the poverty
level; middle income = more than twice poverty level but less than $50,000;
high income = $50,000 or more.

Source: Pamuk and others (1998).

appear to vary depending on the specific group and specific indicator of health status under consideration (Pamuk and others,
1998). For example, it is frequently observed, for multiple indicators of health status, that differences between socioeconomic categories within each racial group are larger than differences
between races (Navarro, 1989; Williams, 1999). Moreover, numerous paradoxes are evident when race, ethnicity, gender, and SES are
simultaneously considered. Observed patterns of association among
race/ethnicity, gender, and SES may reflect complex interactions
among these social factors and the long-term effects of exposure to
social and economic adversity during childhood, cultural practices
and beliefs, nativity differences, migration history, acculturation
processes, individual and institutional discrimination, and the non-
comparability of SES indicators across race/ethnic populations
(Kaufman, Cooper, and McGee, 1997; Williams, 1997).

Elucidating all of these processes is beyond the scope of this
chapter. We illustrate the kind of research that is needed by focusing in detail on a largely unrecognized and high-risk pattern in the
minority health literature. While the "epidemiological paradox" surrounding the health achievements of some Latino and Asian groups
(in the light of their socioeconomic, migration, or discriminatory
histories) has been given much attention (Franzini, Ribble, and Keddie, 2001), another is also evident. We refer to this paradox as the

intersectionality paradox because it captures the recurring dilemma of certain health problems faced at the intersection of race, SES, and gender by members of the black middle class. In some instances, African American women are at risk, and in other instances their male counterparts seem to be particularly vulnerable. We now turn our attention to this oft-ignored segment of the population.

The Intersectionality Paradox: The Black Middle Class

The definition and composition of the black middle class has changed over time. DuBois (1996) initially characterized it as consisting of married households where the husband engaged in a professional job and the unemployed wife maintained the home. Frazier (1997), however, identified the black middle class only in terms of personal occupation, including professional and technical workers; managers, officials, and proprietors; clerical and sales workers; artisans; and supervisors. More recently, Wilson (1987) defined the black middle class as those who occupy white-collar jobs (professional, managerial, and clerical workers). Oliver and Shapiro (1995) augmented Wilson's definition, identifying the black middle class along the dimensions of education (college educated), occupation (white-collar workers), household income (ranging between $25,000 and $50,000), and wealth (for example, home ownership). And still others focus specifically on white-collar workers who work in or live in predominantly white settings (Hochschild, 1993). In many communities, prestige is afforded to those who have symbolic power beyond objective characteristics such as income. Political, religious, and military officials such as civil servants or clergy, for example, are included in this category (Cayton and Mitchell, 1970). These individuals have played a long-standing role in serving the psychological needs of the black community, primarily through affirmation of black identity.

The black middle class emerged during the pre-Reconstruction era (Cayton and Mitchell, 1970). Although this group was relatively small, there is some evidence that following Reconstruction, many cities had an active black professional class (Gatewood, 2000). The amount of political power afforded this group was very restricted, but they furnished the growing black working class with professional and business services. During the industrial era, the black middle class developed further. Descendants of the older bourgeoisie were soon joined by the new industrial class, who took advantage of the educational and employment opportunities afforded them during the early decades of the twentieth century (Gatewood, 2000). The mass migration from southern farms to northern cities between 1910 and 1950 and the increase in the number of black businesses during that time helped solidify the existence of the black middle class (Franklin, 1974). It was during this era that the black middle class expanded to include church, civic, political, and labor group leaders (Cayton and Mitchell, 1970; Gatewood, 2000).

The 1960s and 1970s witnessed a growing number of African Americans entering a wide range of occupations. Blacks became more visible as chief executives of many cities, especially as city mayors in the late 1960s (Biles, 1992). Following government intervention policies, minority representation in state and bureaucratic jobs increased substantially (Collins, 1993). Some minorities were able to take full advantage of affirmative action efforts that helped to increase black representation in professional and managerial positions (Allen and Farley, 1986), resulting in increasing class differentiation (Wilson, 1987).

A constant feature of black life in America that has transcended the changing occupational opportunity structure is residential segregation (Alba, Logan, and Stults, 2000; Massey and Denton, 1993). The hypersegregation of middle-class African Americans significantly reduces the returns typically associated with home ownership, limits educational opportunities for African American children, and is related to racial disparities in health (Williams and Collins, 2001). Research further indicates that successful blacks receive fewer returns on their education and possess much less wealth than their white counterparts (Oliver and Shapiro, 1995). These statistics shed light on the racialized structure underlying American meritocracy and the tenuous position of the black middle class. Furthermore, they allude to a set of race-related stressors that all black Americans experience.

In the following section, we argue that at the intersection of race, class, and gender, new experiences emerge that undermine the benefits of being a member of the black middle class. In fact, Willie (1979) forewarns of this dilemma when he describes how the black middle class "who, because of school desegregation and affirmative action and other integration programs, are coming into direct contact with whites for the first time for extended interaction" (p. 157). Operating within the context of the historical legacy of racial discrimination, African Americans must combat a range of negative stereotypes that infiltrate their social interactions (Benjamin, 1991; Cose, 1993; Greenhaus, Parasuraman, and Wormley, 1990; Williams, Neighbors, and Jackson, 2003). The "race work" that has to be done is even more extensive among those who reside in predominantly white neighborhoods, which helps explain why many middle-class African Americans return to predominantly black neighborhoods (Taylor, 2002). Even this strategy, however, may have negative repercussions, as we discuss later.

The long-standing body of social science research on racial stereotypes has shown that whites' attitudes toward African Americans have changed over the past four decades (Schuman, Steeh, and Bobo, 1985). Other work indicates the emergence of a subtler form of racism, with many whites believing that African Americans do not embrace the American values of hard work, self-reliance, and self-discipline (Kinder and Sears, 1981). These stereotypes are also gendered. For example, black women are often depicted as sexually promiscuous, single mothers, and welfare recipients (Collins, 1990; Guy-Sheftall, 1990; Marshall, 1996; Mullings, 1994). Black men are perceived as dishonest, dangerous, lazy, and involved with drugs (Hacker, 1995; Majors and Billson, 1992). These stereotypes confront African Americans every day regardless of their social class standing and have significant implications for many health outcomes. We focus on the case of infant mortality rates among women and homicide rates among men. These indicators of premature death reflect a paradox at the intersection of race, class, and gender that draws our attention to the unique status of the black middle class.

MIDDLE-CLASS BLACK WOMEN

Affirmative action programs have provided many opportunities for qualified women to gain access to professional fields they would otherwise have been denied. For example, IBM's affirmative action program resulted in an increase in the proportion of female executives from 1.8 percent in 1980 to 13.3 percent in 1994 (Pathways and Progress, 1996). Similarly, the total number of African American women on public Fortune 1000 corporate boards increased from 223 in 1992 to 342 by 1996 (Norment, 2002). Nonetheless, many professional occupations remain male-dominated fields. In 2002, for example, women were only 10.8 percent of all engineers, 30.7 percent of all doctors, and 29.2 percent of all lawyers (U.S. Department of Labor, 2003).

Among middle-class black women who are employed in managerial and professional occupations, the majority work in industries dominated by government and nonprofit employment: health, social services, and education (Council of Economic Advisers, 1998). Black women are the most underrepresented subgroup in private-sector professional jobs. As such, African American women are likely to be a minority in professional workplace settings.

Work groups have been characterized as uniform (that is, homogeneous), skewed, tilted, or balanced in proportional representation (Kanter, 1977). Tokens—minority group members who work in skewed work settings—are identified by ascribed characteristics (gender, race, ethnicity), attached to which are sets of assumptions about the culture, competence, and behavior of the status occupant. Kanter (1977) argues that women who occupy token positions in their organizational settings experience performance pressures (added pressure to perform well), boundary heightening (feeling socially isolated), and role entrapment (typecasting by dominants). Thus, black women must not only contend with the cultural stereotypes of "black" and "female" but must also combat stereotypes of "black women" as matriarch. Some argue that "once in the labor market . . . all women are treated as mothers—former, actual, or potential" (Sokoloff, 1980, p. 216; Kennelly, 1999), but black women are also accused of spending "too much time away from home" working (Collins, 1990, p. 72).

Other evidence suggests that African American women face additional hostility in corporate workplaces from African American men, with whom they are often competing (Bell and Nkomo, 2001). One of the ways in which workers confront work problems is by seeking social support (Loscocco and Spitze, 1990). In a sample of black professionals, however, Jackson and Saunders (forthcoming) find that 71 percent of men but only 59 percent of women turn to family members or colleagues for advice about dealing with work problems. These professional black women are much more likely than their male peers to try to handle work problems on their own. Furthermore, Bailey, Wolfe, and Wolfe (1996) report that the support of supervisors and coworkers does not reduce levels of depression among the black professional women in their study. Thus, professional African American women may actually be disadvantaged in regard to the important resource of social support (Gray and Keith, 2003).

While it is useful to examine the relationship between individual social characteristics and health outcomes, we also believe that differences in social class intersect with race and gender to account for the paradox facing some African American women (Martin, 1994). African American middle-class women are disadvantaged on a variety of health outcomes. In national data, the highest SES group of African American women has equivalent or higher rates of infant mortality, low birth weight, hypertension, and excess weight than the lowest SES group of white women (Pamuk and others, 1998). Of these health outcomes, we discuss infant mortality, an often-used indicator of the general well-being of a population. African American women are more than twice as likely to suffer the loss of an infant than their non-Hispanic white counterparts. Moreover, the black-white differential in infant mortality becomes larger as maternal education increases.

As shown in Table 5.3, infant mortality rates are strongly patterned by educational level for both black and white women, with increasing years of education predicting lower levels of infant mortality. Among whites, women who did not complete high school have an infant mortality rate that is 2.4 times the rate of women who graduated from college. Similarly, among African Americans, women with less than twelve years of education have an infant mortality rate that is 1.5 times as high as that of college graduates.

Racial differences at every level of education are striking. Infants born to black women in the lowest education category are 1.7 times as likely to die before their first birthday as are infants born to similarly educated white females. At every other level of education, the black-white ratio is greater than two. In fact, there is an even greater gap between the infant mortality rates of non-Hispanic white and African American mothers who have sixteen

TABLE 5.3. INFANT MORTALITY RATES, MOTHERS
AGED TWENTY YEARS AND OLDER, 1995

Maternal Education	White	Black	Black-to-White Ratio
Less than 12 years	9.9	17.3	1.74
12 years	6.5	14.8	2.28
13–15 years	5.1	12.3	2.41
16 years or more	4.2	11.4	2.71

Source: Pamuk and others (1998).

or more years of schooling than between those with less than twelve years of education (Pamuk and others, 1998).

The black-white difference in infant mortality has been linked to a complex web of biological (for example, genetic heritage), socioeconomic (for example, access to neonatal technology), and behavioral factors (for example, diet). A more recent emphasis has been placed on the role played by psychosocial stressors (James, 1993; McLean, Hatfield-Timajchy, Wingo, and Floyd, 1993; Mullings and Wali, 2001; Rini, Wadhwa, and Sandman, 1999) and a lack of support systems available to middle-class African American women (Hogan and others, 2000). These concerns are crystallized when we consider how race/ethnicity, gender, and SES converge to create the paradox facing those interested in the alarming rate of black infant mortality: highly educated African American women have a higher infant mortality rate than less educated non-Hispanic white women.

Intersectionality theory provides a useful lens through which such health disparities may be more clearly viewed because of the attention paid to resources that are available to actors as a result of the amount of power afforded to a group (Weber and Parra-Medina, 2003). In terms of infant mortality, we highlight the fact that African American professional women must navigate within the confines of organizations that are structured by both racial and gender divisions. Patterns of dominance and deference also intersect with these master status characteristics. More specifically, we argue that middle-class status is experienced in a less profound and beneficial way for these women than for any other group because they are not in a position to mobilize all of the resources that should be at their disposal given their social class standing.

First, African American women earn lower wages at each education level and realize less of a payoff for additional education than otherwise similar nonblack women and especially men (Bradbury, 2002). Income provides the means to pay the bills, feed the children, and obtain shelter and medical care for members of the household. It is the most soluble dimension of social class position. When it is scarce, people become vulnerable to negative events and psychological distress (Thoits, 1995).

The figures in Table 5.4 represent the median family incomes reported in 1996. The data clearly indicate that median family income rises with each higher level of education regardless of gender and race/ethnicity. Several patterns are noteworthy. First, at all levels of education, black and Hispanic men and women tend to reside in households with lower levels of income than their white counterparts. Other data reveal that individual earnings at every level of education are markedly greater for whites compared to their black and Hispanic peers, but only for men (Williams and Collins, 1995). However, at the level of household economic resources, both black and Hispanic men and women are disadvantaged. The lower levels of household income for black than for Hispanic women reflect the reality that African American women are more likely than their Latino peers to be the primary wage earner in the household. At every level of education, Asian households report the highest levels of income. However, whites have higher per capita income than Asians, and the higher median income for Asian households reflects the fact that they are more likely than white households to have multiple wage earners (DeNavas-Walt and Cleveland, 2002).

Women of all racial/ethnic groups earn considerably less income at every educational level compared to men. A striking pattern in Table 5.4 is the female disadvantage in household economic resources for many U.S. women at every level of education. This pattern is largest and most pronounced for African American women and persists for them at every level of education.

Second, the benefits of receiving social support may not outweigh the costs of providing social support. Social support is generally given or received, but upwardly mobile African American

TABLE 5.4. MEDIAN FAMILY INCOME AMONG ADULTS
TWENTY-FIVE YEARS OF AGE AND OVER, 1996

Sex, Race, and Hispanic Origin	Education			
	Less Than 12 Years	*12 Years*	*13–15 Years*	*16 or More Years*
Men				
White, non-Hispanic	$25,274	$41,200	$49,000	$67,952
Asian or Pacific Islander	$34,146	$44,612	$55,392	$68,327
Black, non-Hispanic	$19,957	$36,020	$42,500	$54,500
Hispanic	$24,000	$35,000	$43,734	$58,079
Women				
White, non-Hispanic	$18,471	$37,000	$45,510	$64,007
Asian or Pacific Islander	$37,420	$42,658	$57,300	$65,675
Black, non-Hispanic	$13,100	$23,556	$33,162	$47,100
Hispanic	$19,310	$32,000	$38,000	$56,765

Source: Pamuk and others (1998).

women are twice as likely as their white counterparts to give support resources to family and friends than they are to receive support from these sources (Higganbotham and Weber, 1992). As a result, African American women may feel overwhelmed by support requests. Perceived social support is associated with high depressive symptoms among black middle-class women (Warren, 1997).

Marriage is an important venue for social support and predictor of health across racial groups in the United States. On average, married persons live longer and enjoy better health than those who are nonmarried, especially the formerly married. Differential rates of marriage across race may also be a contributor to the elevated health risks of African American women. Blacks have lower rates of marriage and higher rates of marital dissolution than whites (Tucker, 2000). These differences appear to be driven not by cultural preferences but by the social and economic conditions that African Americans face. For both blacks and whites in the United States, rates of marriage are positively related to average male earnings and inversely to male unemployment rates (Bishop, 1980). Thus, African American women face real challenges finding mates given the high rates of unemployment, underemployment, and incarceration among black men.

National data reveal that men have higher levels of college completion than women. This pattern does not hold true for the black population. Accordingly, many professional African American women marry mates who are lower in educational and occupational status than themselves. Thus, on average, white women receive larger economic benefits from marriage than black women. Research needs to systematically assess the extent to which the actual costs and benefits of marriage may vary across race, class, and gender. Given their hypersegregation and low marriage rates, black professional women may lack the network ties that would enable them to compensate for the support resources they give to others. This added burden may very well be linked to poor health habits, less attention to personal health and well-being, and subsequent physical health problems, including those linked to birth outcomes.

MIDDLE-CLASS BLACK MEN

Middle-class African American men may be an understudied group of vulnerable men. Middle-class status does not provide African American men with the normally expected reductions for at least some health risks. For both African Americans and whites, rates of suicide are much higher for males than females. Over the past two decades, the suicide rate has remained relatively stable for white men but has increased for young black men (McLoyd and Lozoff, 2001). Several studies have found that while SES is inversely related to the suicide rate for whites, it is positively related to the suicide rate for African American males (Williams, 2003).

Three factors may contribute to higher level of stress and subsequent adverse consequences on middle-class African American men. First, the personal experience of discrimination based on race is an added burden that all African Americans face but may seem especially egregious to the black middle class because they feel that their socioeconomic success has earned them the right not to have to deal with such indignities. Again, a growing body of research reveals that these perceptions of discrimination are stressors that can adversely affect physical and mental health (Jackson, Thoits, and Taylor, 1995; Krieger, 1999; Williams, Neighbors, and Jackson, 2003). There is a positive association between perceptions of discrimination and education among African Americans, and African American men report higher levels of chronic and acute discrimination than African American women (Forman, Williams, and Jackson, 1997).

Second, middle-class status is often recent, tenuous, and marginal for African Americans (Collins, 1993, 1997). College-educated African Americans are more likely than whites to experience unemployment (Wilhelm, 1987; Council of Economic Advisers 1998). Middle-class African Americans have markedly lower levels of wealth than whites of similar income (Davern and Fisher, 1995). They are also less likely than whites of similar income to translate their higher economic status into desirable housing and neighborhood conditions (Alba, Logan, and Stults, 2000).

Third, unfulfilled expectations because black men's investment in education has not provided comparable gains in income may be a unique and additional source of stress and alienation for African American men (Anderson, 1999). Educational attainment is an important indicator of lifetime economic opportunities, with higher levels of education being associated with higher wages, higher family income, and lower unemployment (Council of Economic Advisers, 1998). Over the past several decades, the gap has narrowed between African American males and other Americans in the number of years of formal education. Although racial disparities in education still exist, there is only a narrow gap in educational attainment between African American and white men aged twenty-five to twenty-nine (Council of Economic Advisers, 1998). However, for African American men, higher education has not translated into additional income. At every level of education, minority men earn lower levels of income than whites, and differences in pay between whites on the one hand and African Americans and Hispanics on the other are larger for men than for women (Council of Economic Advisers, 1998). One of the ways in which these problems may become manifest is in homicide rates.

Table 5.5 presents the homicide rates for men and women stratified by race and education. Regardless of racial status, the homicide rate varies markedly by SES. Among adults aged twenty-five to forty-four, homicide rates are strongly patterned by education levels for both blacks and whites, males and females (Pamuk and others, 1998). The homicide rate for black males who have not completed high school is more than five times that of black males with some college education or more. Similarly, there is a ninefold difference for black females and a sixfold difference for white females by level of education. At the same time, elevated rates of homicide for African Americans compared with whites exist at all levels of individual SES, with striking racial differences in homicide even when blacks and whites are compared at similar levels of education. For example, the homicide death rate for African American men with some college education is eleven times that of their similarly educated white peers. Strikingly, the homicide rate of black males in the highest education category exceeds that of white males in the lowest education group!

Residential segregation plays a major role in racial differences in homicide. Sampson's empirical research (1987) has traced the pathways that lead from residential segregation to elevated homicide risk for African American males. Segregation creates restricted educational and employment opportunities for many poor black communities. These conditions produce a diminished pool of employable or stably employed males.

TABLE 5.5. HOMICIDE RATES AMONG ADULTS TWENTY-FIVE TO FORTY-FOUR YEARS OF AGE, BY EDUCATIONAL ATTAINMENT, SEX, AND RACE, 1994–1995

Education (in years)	Males		Females	
	White	Black	White	Black
All (data for 1995)	11.0	77.9	3.3	17.4
Less than 12 years	25.0	163.3	10.2	38.2
12 years	10.6	110.7	4.7	22.0
13 or more years	2.9	32.4	1.6	9.4

Source: Pamuk and others (1998).

Lack of access to jobs creates high rates of male unemployment and underemployment, which in turn generates the high rates of out-of-wedlock births, female-headed households, the "feminization of poverty," and the extreme concentration of poverty in many black communities (Testa, Astone, Krogh, and Neckerman, 1993; Wilson, 1996). For both blacks and whites, male employment and earnings are positively related to entry into marriage, and economic instability is positively related to marital dissolution (Bishop, 1980; Wilson, 1996). Single-parent households are associated with lower levels of social control and supervision of young males, which lead to elevated rates of violent behavior among males (Sampson, 1987). Research documents that the neighborhood characteristics associated with residential segregation and household characteristics that result from the concentration of poverty account for racial differences in violent behavior and homicide (Sampson and Wilson, 1995).

Importantly, these family and neighborhood factors that predict increased risk of violent crime and homicide are identical for blacks and whites (Sampson, 1987). However, because of residential segregation, blacks are more likely to be exposed to these conditions than members of other racial groups. For example, in not even one of the 171 largest cities in the United States do whites live in comparable conditions to blacks in terms of poverty rates or rates of single-parent households. Sampson and Wilson (1995, p. 41) concluded that "the sources of violent crime appear to be remarkably invariant across race and rooted instead in the structural differences among communities, cities, and states in economic and family organization." Thus, the elevated rates of violent crime and homicide for African Americans are determined by their greater exposure to poverty and lack of jobs created by segregation and by the family structures and processes that result from these economic conditions.

This leaves unanswered why middle-class black males have such an elevated risk of homicide. Again, segregation appears to provide the answer. African Americans in general, and middle-class African Americans in particular, are unique in the United States in terms of the experience of high levels of segregation (Massey, 2004). All other racial/ethnic minority groups in the United States have markedly lower levels of segregation than African Americans (Massey, 2004). Moreover, while the level of residential segregation varies by income for Latinos and Asians, the segregation of African Americans is high at all levels of income. In fact, the most affluent African Americans (annual income over $50,000) experience higher levels of residential segregation than the poorest Latinos and Asians (income under $15,000) (Massey, 2004).

These data also highlight that middle-class blacks are less able than their white counterparts to translate their higher economic status into desirable residential conditions. Research reveals that middle-class suburban African Americans reside in neighborhoods that are less segregated than those of poor central city blacks (Alba, Logan, and Stults, 2000). However, compared to their white counterparts, middle-class blacks live in poorer-quality neighborhoods, with white neighbors who are less affluent than they are. An analysis of 1990 census data revealed that suburban residence does not buy better housing conditions for blacks, with the suburban locations where African Americans reside being equivalent or inferior to those of blacks in central cities (Harris, 1999). Segregation is thus a neglected but powerful example of institutional racism in the United States that continues to have pervasive adverse consequences on SES and health.

Instructively, the high levels of segregation of blacks do not reflect their residential preferences. Of all the major racial/ethnic groups, blacks reveal the highest preference for residing in integrated areas (Massey, 2004). Thus, regardless of individual or household SES, black and white neighborhoods differ dramatically in the availability of jobs, family structure, opportunities for marriage, and exposure to conventional role models (Sampson and Wilson, 1995). This highlights the importance of future research that pays attention to social and economic characteristics of areas that may capture important aspects of the social context over and above individual or household characteristics.

Intersectionality theory paints an even more complex picture of the lives of socially mobile African American men. Leadership "schemas" in the United States include "male" as a critical attribute (Nye and Simonetta, 1996), thereby reducing the extent to which black men have to evoke justifications for their high-status job positions. Black professional men must overcome the cultural stereotypes that challenge their abilities. Based on personal interviews with a sample of African American professional workers, Cose (1993) finds that blacks often face a "dozen demons" that haunt them as they interact with colleagues within their organization. Some of these demons include under- or overidentifying with other African Americans and feeling that they constantly have to prove they are worthy of respect. Even here, being male does not guarantee that one will be afforded the symbolic resources of deference and respect. Rather, the cumulative effect of everyday racism (Essed, 1991) and structural discrimination reduces the life chances of African American men.

In particular, residential segregation may contribute to many professional black men finding themselves in a no-win situation. Those who reside in predominantly white neighborhoods must confront racial stereotypes at work and at home. For many, home is no longer a refuge from the racist world. They have to ruminate on unfriendly neighbors and the extent to which they are simply unfriendly people or pose a potential danger to self and family (Green, Strolovitch, and Wong, 1998). They may even have to worry that any need for assistance could be met with indifference. Consequently, some find themselves returning to predominantly black neighborhoods even though their social class position could buy them more elaborate housing in a predominantly white suburb (Taylor, 2002). Those who elect to live in the city, then, increase their probability of being the victim of a crime (Sampson, 1987). Even those who live in low-stress, low-crime areas (predominantly black suburbs, for example) expose themselves to other neighborhood conditions when visiting with family members. Blacks have larger families than whites (Jackson, 2000), and many middle-class blacks have large family networks, many residing in high-stress, low-SES contexts. Research reveals that the costs of caring for a large extended social network can adversely affect an individual's health (Kessler, Price, and Wortman, 1985). We contend that there is a similar fatal cost associated with caring for and about those who live in unstable neighborhoods.

CONCLUSION

Despite the gains made in the past decade toward improved health outcomes across America's racial/ethnic groups, there are still large disparities in health. This chapter emphasized the unique status and vulnerabilities faced by members of the black middle class. We

believe more systematic research is needed on the unique problems of these African American professionals (Jackson and Stewart, 2003). In particular, more attention should be paid to the
tokenism processes that African Americans in high-ranking positions experience (Yoder, 1994). Perhaps there exists an intricate
interplay among such factors as visibility (that is, feeling that your
work is always being noticed and scrutinized), colleagueship
(encouragement, feeling accepted as a colleague), and social atmos-
phere (sharing social time) rather than any single issue that characterizes work lives. These may be exacerbated by other aspects of
work and non-work-related stress.

Work-family research provides some insight into these issues
(Lundberg and Frankenhaeuser, 1999). For example, African
American women are more likely than white women to be simultaneously employed and caring for young children (Seltzer, 1994),
thus resulting in greater work-family strain. There is also some evidence that African American husbands report lower levels of marital well-being when their wives describe themselves as career women
rather than wage earners or housewives (Orbuch and Custer, 1995).
Thus, professional blacks (specifically those who are married) may
experience family-work conflict that often goes unnoticed in most
research studies.

Future research applying the intersectionality paradigm to
African American health should attend to how context affects family relationships. There are intriguing research findings on the ways
in which the social and economic circumstances of one spouse
affect the economic and health status of the other. For example,
U.S. data reveal that a woman's employment outside the home
benefits her mental health but adversely affects the psychological
well-being of her spouse (Rosenfield, 1992). Similarly, national
mortality data reveal that while a woman's earnings are positively
related to her longevity, they are inversely related to that of her
husband (McDonough, Williams, House, and Duncan, 1999). In
addition, at least five major epidemiological studies in the United
States, including the Framingham Heart Study, have found an
adverse effect of being married to well-educated women on men's
heart disease risk (Matthews, 2002).

At the same time, other research documents the positive effects
of women's employment on men and the family. Ono's work

(1998) indicates that in households with working wives, men's difficulties as providers have become less devastating for marital instability. Similarly, increasing economic resources for women in countries like the United States and Sweden, where dual-earning couples have become the norm, strengthen the institution of marriage, while the opposite occurs in more strongly gendered societies like Japan (Ono, 2003). Importantly, all of these findings come from studies of white populations or studies in which racial differences were not tested. We do not understand how the economic situations of socially advantaged men and women affect each other's health and the extent to which these patterns vary by race. African American women have been working outside the household in large numbers much longer than white women (Jackson, 2000), and this could lead to variations in some of these processes. What is needed is research that seeks to identify under what conditions a spouse's social circumstances can have positive or negative effects on health (see Orbuch and Custer, 1995). More generally, the available evidence clearly indicates that the impact of social structure and context on black husbands' and wives' social circumstances and health should be estimated jointly.

Lifestyle factors are also implicated in the epidemic of black infant mortality and homicide rates. For example, when compared to native black women, foreign-born blacks have a lower incidence of low-birth-weight babies (Hummer, Rogers, Nam, and LeClere, 1999), and certain health behaviors may play a role in these differences. Compared to foreign-born black women, native-born black women are four times more likely to smoke and nearly eight times as likely to use illegal drugs during pregnancy (Cabral and others, 1990). Researchers often view variations in health practices and beliefs as driven by individual differences in values and attitudes, but it is important to balance such views by attending to the ways in which health-related factors measured at the individual level are constrained by larger social structures and processes (Williams, 1998). For example, there are more retail outlets for the sale of alcohol in disadvantaged neighborhoods, and both the alcohol and tobacco industries heavily market their products to blacks and Hispanics.

Similarly, among men, certain lifestyle factors may be consequential for their health status. Men are socialized to project strength, autonomy, dominance, stoicism, and physical aggression and to avoid any expression of emotion or vulnerability that could be construed as weakness (Courtenay, 2000; Davis, Matthews, and Twamley, 1999). These beliefs about masculinity and manhood can lead men to take actions that harm their health, as well as to avoid engaging in health-protective behaviors. A comprehensive review of research on gender differences in health practices shows that women are more likely to engage in a broad range of preventive and health-promoting behaviors than men, while men are more likely than women to engage in more than thirty behaviors that increase their risk of morbidity, injury, and mortality (Courtenay, 2000).

This chapter emphasized that while SES might afford adults the wherewithal to engage in preventive health care, not feeling accepted by society (or one's professional peers) or confronting multiple sources of strain can undermine the potential benefits of material resources (Jackson, 1997). The examples we used of the types of health problems that some members of the black middle class face highlight this complexity. The growing evidence of the emotional and physical health consequences of perceived discrimination among African Americans implies the need to address more systemic problems in society. The challenge is how to characterize multiple adversities and resources over the life course and understand their health consequences. In essence, a variety of situational constraints can very well undermine the benefits associated with one's socioeconomic status (Bailey, Wolfe, and Wolfe, 1996).

Intersectionality theory sensitizes us to the complexity of health disparities as well as some of the health paradoxes permeating the health literature (Mullings and Wali, 2001; Weber and Parra-Medina, 2003). Moving beyond a "double-jeopardy" or "triple-jeopardy" paradigm, this perspective suggests that new identities (and therefore new challenges or new sets of stressors) are formed when multiple minority statuses (linked to limited resources and a different set of relationships) converge. For example, problems faced by many black professional women are also faced by other ethnic minority women within workplace settings dominated by white men (Yoder, 1994). However, men who find themselves in token positions (working in female-dominated work settings) do not experience gender discrimination (Williams, 1992), suggesting that dominant groups will use their power to maintain their privileged position (Reskin, 1988).

This chapter has focused heavily on the African American experience. Future research is needed to explore intersectionality paradoxes that might exist for other racial/ethnic populations. There is no generic minority health model that applies equally to all racial/ethnic groups. In fact, there is growing attention to the considerable diversity that exists within each of the broad racial/ethnic categories. The intersections of racial, gender, and socioeconomic factors as they influence health for each population group and subgroup need to be understood within their historical and social contexts.

References

Adler, N. E., and others. "Socioeconomic Inequalities in Health: No Easy Solution." *Journal of the American Medical Association,* 1993, *269,* 3140–3145.

Alba, R. D., Logan, J. R., and Stults, B. J. "How Segregated Are Middle-Class African Americans?" *Social Problems,* 2000, *47,* 543–558.

Allen, W. R., and Farley, R. "The Shifting Social and Economic Tides of Black America, 1950–1980." *Annual Review of Sociology,* 1986, *12,* 277–306.

American Association of Physical Anthropology. "AAPA Statement on Biological Aspects of Race." *American Journal of Physical Anthropology,* 1996, *101,* 569–570.

Anderson, E. "The Social Situation of the Black Executive: Black and White Identities in the Corporate World." In M. Lamont (ed.), *The Cultural Territories of Race: Black and White Boundaries.* Chicago: University of Chicago Press, 1999.

Andes, N. "Social Class and Gender: An Empirical Evaluation of Occupational Stratification." *Gender and Society,* 1992, *6,* 231–251.

Bailey, D., Wolfe, D., and Wolfe, C. R. "The Contextual Impact of Social Support Across Race and Gender: Implications for African American Women in the Workplace." *Journal of Black Studies,* 1996, *26,* 287–307.

Bell, E., and Nkomo, S. *Our Separate Ways.* Cambridge, Mass.: Harvard Business School Press, 2001.

Benjamin, L. *The Black Elite: Facing the Color Line in the Twilight of the Twentieth Century.* Chicago: Nelson-Hall, 1991.

Biles, R. "Black Mayors: A Historical Assessment." *Journal of Negro History,* 1992, *77,* 109–125.

Bishop, J. H. "Jobs, Cash Transfers, and Marital Instability: A Review of the Evidence." *Journal of Human Resources*, 1980, *15*, 301–334.

Bradbury, K. "Education and Wages in the 1980s and 1990s: Are All Groups Moving Up Together?" *New England Economic Journal*, Oct. 2002, pp. 19–46.

Cabral, H., and others. "Foreign-Born and U.S. Born Black Women: Differences in Health Behaviors and Birth Outcomes." *American Journal of Public Health*, 1990, *80*(1), 70–72.

Cayton, H. R., and Mitchell, G. S. *Black Workers and the New Unions.* Chapel Hill: University of North Carolina Press, 1970.

Collins, P. H. *Black Feminist Thought: Knowledge, Consciousness, and the Politics of Empowerment.* New York: Routledge, 1990.

Collins, S. M. "Blacks on the Bubble: The Vulnerability of Black Executives in White Corporations." *Sociological Quarterly*, 1993, *34*(3), 429–447.

Collins, S. M. "Black Mobility in White Corporations: Up the Corporate Ladder But Out on a Limb." *Social Problems*, 1997, *44*(1), 55–67.

Cose, E. *The Rage of a Privileged Class.* New York: HarperCollins, 1993.

Council of Economic Advisers for the President's Initiative on Race. *Changing America: Indicators of Social and Economic Well-Being by Race and Hispanic Origin.* Washington, D.C.: U.S. Government Printing Office, 1998.

Courtenay, W. "Constructions of Masculinity and Their Influence on Men's Well-Being: A Theory of Gender and Health." *Social Science and Medicine*, 2000, *50*, 1385–1401.

Davern, M. E., and Fisher, P. J. *Household Net Worth and Asset Ownership: 1995.* Washington, D.C.: U.S. Government Printing Office, 1995.

Davis, M., Matthews, K., and Twamley, E. W. "Is Life More Difficult on Mars or Venus? A Meta-Analytic Review of Sex Differences in Major and Minor Life Events." *Annals of Behavioral Medicine*, 1999, *21*, 83–97.

DeNavas-Walt, C., and Cleveland, R. W. *Money Income in the United States: 2000.* Washington, D.C.: U.S. Government Printing Office, 2002.

DuBois, W.E.B. *The Philadelphia Negro.* Philadelphia: University of Pennsylvania Press, 1996. (Originally published 1899.)

Eberhardt, M. S., and others. *Health, United States, 2001: With Urban and Rural Health Chartbook.* Hyattsville, Md.: National Center for Health Statistics, 2001.

Essed, P. *Understanding Everyday Racism: An Interdisciplinary Theory.* Thousand Oaks, Calif.: Sage, 1991.

Forman, T. A., Williams, D. R., and Jackson, J. S. "Race, Place, and Discrimination." In C. Gardner (ed.), *Perspectives on Social Problems.* Greenwich, Conn.: JAI Press, 1997.

Franklin, J. H. *From Slavery to Freedom.* New York: Knopf, 1974.

Franzini, L., Ribble, J. C., and Keddie, A. M. "Understanding the Hispanic Paradox." *Ethnicity and Disease,* 2001, *11*(3), 496–518.

Frazier, E. F. *Black Bourgeoisie: The Rise of a New Middle Class.* New York: Free Press, 1997. (Originally published 1957.)

Gatewood, W. *Aristocrats of Color: The Black Elite, 1880–1920.* Fayetteville: University of Arkansas Press, 2000.

Gray, B., and Keith, V. "The Benefits and Costs of Social Support for African American Women." In D. Brown and V. Keith (eds.), *In and Out of Our Right Minds: The Mental Health of African American Women.* New York: Columbia University Press, 2003.

Green, D. P., Strolovitch, D. Z., and Wong, J. S. "Defended Neighborhoods, Integration, and Racially Motivated Crime." *American Journal of Sociology,* 1998, *104,* 372–403.

Greenhaus, J. H., Parasuraman, S., and Wormley, W. M. "Effects of Race on Organizational Experiences, Job Performance Evaluations, and Career Outcomes." *Academy of Management Journal,* 1990, *33,* 64–86.

Grodsky, E., and Pager, D. "The Structure of Disadvantage: Individual and Occupational Determinants of the Black-White Wage Gap." *American Sociological Review,* 2001, *66,* 542–567.

Guy-Sheftall, B. *Daughters of Sorrow: Attitudes Toward Black Women, 1880–1920.* Brooklyn, N.Y.: Carlson, 1990.

Hacker, A. *Two Nations: Black and White, Separate, Hostile, Unequal.* New York: Ballantine, 1995.

Harris, D. R. *All Suburbs Are Not Created Equal: A New Look at Racial Differences in Suburban Locations.* Ann Arbor: Population Studies Center, University of Michigan, 1999.

Higganbotham, E., and Weber, L. "Moving Up with Kin and Community: Upward Social Mobility for Black and White Women." *Gender and Society,* 1992, *6,* 416–440.

Hochschild, A. "Middle-Class Blacks and the Ambiguities of Success." In P. M. Sniderman, P. E. Tetlock, and E. G. Carmines (eds.), *Prejudice, Politics, and the American Dilemma.* Stanford, Calif.: Stanford University Press, 1993.

Hogan, V. K., and others. "A Public Health Framework for Addressing Black and White Disparities in Preterm Delivery." *Journal of the American Medical Women's Association,* 2000, *56,* 12–80.

Hoyert, D. L., and others. *Deaths: Final Data for 1999.* Hyattsville, Md.: National Center for Health Statistics, 2001.

Hummer, R. A., Rogers, R. G., Nam, C. B., and LeClere, F. B. "Race/Ethnicity, Nativity, and U.S. Adult Mortality." *Social Science Quarterly,* 1999, *80,* 136–153.

Jackson, J. S. (ed.). *New Directions: African Americans in a Diversifying Nation.* Washington, D.C.: National Policy Association, 2000.

Jackson, P. B. "Role Occupancy and Minority Mental Health." *Journal of Health and Social Behavior,* 1997, *38,* 237–255.

Jackson, P. B., and Saunders, T. "Work Stress, Coping Resources, and Mental Health: A Study of America's Black Elite." *Research in Occupational Stress and Well Being.* Greenwich, Conn.: JAI Press/Elsevier, forthcoming.

Jackson, P. B., and Stewart, Q. T. "A Research Agenda for the Black Middle Class: Work Stress, Survival Strategies, and Mental Health." *Journal of Health and Social Behavior,* 2003, *44*(3), 442–455.

Jackson, P. B., Thoits, P., and Taylor, H. "Composition of the Workplace and Psychological Well-Being: The Effects of Tokenism on America's Black Elite." *Social Forces,* 1995, *74,* 543–557.

James, S. A. "Racial and Ethnic Differences in Infant Mortality and Low Birth Weight: A Psychosocial Critique." *Annals of Epidemiology,* 1993, *3*(2), 131–136.

Kanter, R. M. *Men and Women of the Corporation.* New York: Basic Books, 1977.

Kaufman, J. S., Cooper, R. S., and McGee, D. L. "Socioeconomic Status and Health in Blacks and Whites: The Problem of Residual Confounding and the Resiliency of Race." *Epidemiology,* 1997, *8,* 621–628.

Kennelly, I. "That Single-Mother Element: How White Employers Typify Black Women." *Gender and Society,* 1999, *13*(2), 168–192.

Kessler, R. C., Price, R. H., and Wortman, C. B. "Social Factors in Psychopathology: Stress, Social Support, and Coping Processes." *Annual Review of Psychology,* 1985, *36,* 531–572.

Kinder, D., and Sears, D. "Symbolic Racism versus Racial Threats to the Good Life." *Journal of Personality and Social Psychology,* 1981, *46,* 414–431.

Krieger, N. "Embodying Inequality: A Review of Concepts, Measures, and Methods for Studying Health Consequences of Discrimination." *International Journal of Health Services,* 1999, *29*(2), 295–352.

Krieger, N., and others. "Racism, Sexism, and Social Class: Implications for Studies of Health, Disease, and Well-Being." *American Journal of Preventive Medicine,* 1993, *9*(6 suppl.), 82–122.

LaVeist, T. A. (ed.). *Race, Ethnicity, and Health.* San Francisco: Jossey-Bass, 2002.

Lillie-Blanton, M., Martinez, R. M., Taylor, A. K., and Robinson, B. G. "Latina and African American Women: Continuing Disparities in Health." *International Journal of Health Services,* 1993, *23,* 555–584.

Loscocco, K., and Spitze, G. "Working Conditions, Social Support, and the Well-Being of Female and Male Factory Workers." *Journal of Health and Social Behavior,* 1990, *31,* 313–327.

Lundberg, U., and Frankenhaeuser, M. "Stress and Workload of Men and Women in High-Ranking Positions." *Journal of Occupational and Health Psychology,* 1999, *4*(2), 142–151.

Majors, R., and Billson, J. M. *Cool Pose: The Dilemmas of Black Manhood in America.* New York: Touchstone, 1992.

Marshall, A. "From Sexual Denigration to Self-Respect: Resisting Images of Black Female Sexuality." In D. Jarrett-Macauley (ed.), *Reconstructing Womanhood, Reconstructing Feminism: Writings on Black Women.* London: Routledge, 1996.

Martin, S. "Outsider Within the Station House: The Impact of Race and Gender on Black Women Police." *Social Problems,* 1994, *41,* 383–400.

Massey, D. "Segregation and Stratification: A Biosocial Perspective." *DuBois Review,* 2004, *1,* 7–25.

Massey, D., and Denton, N. *American Apartheid: Segregation and the Making of the Underclass.* Cambridge, Mass.: Harvard University Press, 1993.

Matthews, K. A. "Commentary: Is an Educated Wife Hazardous to Her Husband's Heart? Never, Always, or Sometimes?" *International Journal of Epidemiology,* 2002, *31,* 806–807.

McDonough, P., Williams, D. R., House, J., and Duncan, G. J. "Gender and the Socioeconomic Gradient in Mortality." *Journal of Health and Social Behavior,* 1999, *40,* 17–31.

McLean, D., Hatfield-Timajchy, K., Wingo, I., and Floyd, R. "Psychosocial Measurements: Implications for the Study of Preterm Delivery in Black Women." *American Journal of Preventive Medicine,* 1993, *9,* 39–81.

McLoyd, V. C., and Lozoff, B. "Racial and Ethnic Trends in Children's and Adolescents' Behavior and Development." In N. J. Smelser, W. J. Wilson, and F. Mitchell (eds.), *America Becoming: Racial Trends and Their Consequences.* Washington, D.C.: National Academy Press, 2001.

Mullings, L. "Images, Ideology, and Women of Color." In M. B. Zinn and B. T. Dill (eds.), *Women of Color in U.S. Society.* Philadelphia: Temple University Press, 1994.

Mullings, L., and Wali, A. *Stress and Resilience: The Social Context of Reproduction in Central Harlem.* Norwell, Mass.: Kluwer, 2001.

Navarro, V. "Race or Class, or Race and Class." *International Journal of Health Services,* 1989, *19,* 311–314.

Norment, L. "Black Women on Corporate Boards." *Ebony,* Mar. 2002, pp. 42–48.

Nye, J. L., and Simonetta, L. G. "Followers' Perceptions of Group Leaders: The Impact of Recognition-Based and Inference-Based Processes." In J. L. Nye and A. M. Brower (eds.), *What's Social About Social Cognition.* Thousand Oaks, Calif.: Sage, 1996.

Oliver, M. L., and Shapiro, T. M. *Black Wealth/White Wealth: A New Perspective on Racial Inequality.* New York: Routledge, 1995.

Ono, H. "Husbands' and Wives' Resources and Marital Dissolution." *Journal of Marriage and the Family,* 1998, *60,* 674–689.

Ono, H. "Women's Economic Standing, Marriage Timing, and Cross-National Contexts of Gender." *Journal of Marriage and Family,* 2003, *65,* 275–286.

Orbuch, T. L., and Custer, L. "The Social Context of Married Women's Work and Its Impact on Black Husbands and White Husbands." *Journal of Marriage and the Family,* 1995, *57,* 333–345.

Pamuk, E., and others. *Socioeconomic Status and Health Chartbook. Health, United States, 1998.* Hyattsville, Md.: National Center for Health Statistics, 1998.

Pathways and Progress. *Corporate Best Practices to Shatter the Glass Ceiling.* Chicago: Chicago Area Partnerships, 1996.

Reskin, B. "Bringing Men Back in: Sex Differentiation and the Devaluation of Women's Work." *Gender and Society,* 1988, *2,* 58–81.

Reynolds, J. R., and Ross, C. E. "Social Stratification and Health: Education's Benefit Beyond Economic Status and Social Origins." *Social Problems,* 1998, *45,* 221–247.

Rini, C., Wadhwa, P., and Sandman, C. "Psychological Adaptation and Birth Outcomes: The Role of Personal Resources, Stress, and Sociocultural Context in Pregnancy." *Health Psychology,* 1999, *18,* 333–345.

Rose, L., Kim, M., Dennison, C., and Hill, M. "The Contexts of Adherence for African Americans with High Blood Pressure." *Journal of Advanced Nursing,* 2000, *32*(3), 587–594.

Rosenfield, S. "The Costs of Sharing: Wives' Employment and Husbands' Mental Health." *Journal of Health and Social Behavior,* 1992, *33*(3), 213–225.

Rosenfield, S. "Gender and Mental Health: Do Women Have More Psychopathology, Men More, or Both the Same (and Why)?" In A. Horowitz and T. Scheid (eds.), *A Handbook for the Study of Mental Health: Social Contexts, Theories, and Systems.* Cambridge: Cambridge University Press, 1999.

Sampson, R. J. "Urban Black Violence: The Effect of Male Joblessness and Family Disruption." *American Journal of Sociology,* 1987, *93,* 348–382.

Sampson, R. J., and Wilson, W. "Toward a Theory of Race, Crime, and Urban Inequality." In J. Hagan and R. D. Peterson (eds.), *Crime and Inequality.* Stanford, Calif.: Stanford University Press, 1995.

Sanchez-Hucles, J. "Jeopardy Not Bonus Status for African American Women in the Work Force: Why Does the Myth of Advantage Persist?" *American Journal of Community Psychology,* 1997, *25,* 565–580.

Schuman, H., Steeh, C., and Bobo, L. *Racial Attitudes in America.* Cambridge, Mass.: Harvard University Press, 1985.

Seltzer, J. A. "Consequences of Marital Dissolution for Children." *Annual Review of Sociology,* 1994, *20,* 235–266.

Sokoloff, N. J. *Between Money and Love: The Dialectics of Women's Home and Market Work.* New York: Praeger, 1980.

Taylor, M. *Harlem: Between Heaven and Hell.* Minneapolis: University of Minnesota Press, 2002.

Testa, M., Astone, N. M., Krogh, M., and Neckerman, K. M. "Employment and Marriage Among Inner-City Fathers." In W. J. Wilson (ed.), *The Ghetto Underclass.* Thousand Oaks, Calif.: Sage, 1993.

Thoits, P. A. "Stress, Coping, and Social Support Processes: Where Are We? What Next?" *Journal of Health and Social Behavior,* 1995, *45*(extra issue), 53–79.

Tienda, M., and Lii, D.-T. "Minority Concentration and Earnings Inequality: Blacks, Hispanics, and Asians Compared." *American Journal of Sociology,* 1987, *93,* 141–165.

Tucker, C., and others. "Testing Methods of Collecting Racial and Ethnic Information: Results of the Current Population Survey Supplement on Race and Ethnicity." *Bureau of Labor Statistical Notes,* 1996, *40,* 1–149.

Tucker, M. *Considerations in the Development of Family Policy for African Americans.* Washington, D.C.: National Policy Association, 2000.

U.S. Bureau of the Census. *Current Population Survey.*

U.S. Department of Labor, Bureau of Labor Statistics. *Employment and Earnings.* Washington, D.C.: U.S. Government Printing Office, Jan. 2003.

Warren, B. J. "Depression, Stressful Life Events, Social Support, and Self-Esteem in Middle Class African American Women." *Archives of Psychiatric Nursing,* 1997, *11*(3), 107–117.

Weber, L., and Parra-Medina, D. "Intersectionality and Women's Health: Charting a Path to Eliminating Health Disparities." *Advances in Gender Research,* 2003, *7,* 181–230.

Wilhelm, S. M. "Economic Demise of Blacks in America: A Prelude to Genocide?" *Journal of Black Studies,* 1987, *17,* 201–254.

Williams, C. "The Glass Escalator: Hidden Advantages for Men in the Female Professions." *Social Problems*, 1992, *39*, 253–267.

Williams, D. R. "Race and Health: Basic Questions, Emerging Directions." *Annals of Epidemiology*, 1997, 7(5), 322–333.

Williams, D. R. "African-American Health: The Role of the Social Environment." *Journal of Urban Health*, 1998, 75(2), 300–321.

Williams, D. R. "Race, SES, and Health: The Added Effects of Racism and Discrimination." *Annals of the New York Academy of Sciences*, 1999, *896*, 173–188.

Williams, D. R. "Racial/Ethnic Variations in Women's Health: The Social Embeddedness of Health." *American Journal of Public Health*, 2002, 92(4), 588–597.

Williams, D. R. "The Health of Men: Structured Inequalities and Opportunities." *American Journal of Public Health*, 2003, 93(5), 724–731.

Williams, D. R. "The Health of U.S. Racial and Ethnic Populations." *Journal of Gerontology: Social Sciences*, forthcoming.

Williams, D. R., and Collins, C. "U.S. Socioeconomic and Racial Differences in Health." *Annual Review of Sociology*, 1995, *21*, 349–386.

Williams, D. R., and Collins, C. "Racial Residential Segregation: A Fundamental Cause of Racial Disparities in Health." *Public Health Reports*, 2001, *116*, 404–415.

Williams, D. R., Neighbors, H. W., and Jackson, J. S. "Racial/Ethnic Discrimination and Health: Findings from Community Studies." *American Journal of Public Health*, 2003, 93(2), 200–208.

Willie, C. V. *Caste and Class Controversy.* Bayside, N.Y.: General Hall, 1979.

Wilson, W. J. *The Truly Disadvantaged.* Chicago: University of Chicago Press, 1987.

Wilson, W. J. *When Work Disappears: The World of the New Urban Poor.* New York: Knopf, 1996.

Yoder, J. D. "Looking Beyond Numbers: The Effects of Gender Status, Job Prestige, and Occupational Gender-Typing on Tokenism Processes." *Social Psychology Quarterly*, 1994, *57*, 150–159.

Chapter Six

Identity Development, Discrimination, and Psychological Well-Being Among African American and Caribbean Black Adolescents

Cleopatra Howard Caldwell,
Barbara J. Guthrie, James S. Jackson

Much of the work on race, gender, class, and health has focused on adult populations, with little attention to youth from different ethnic backgrounds or gender groups (Guthrie, Caldwell, and Hunter, 1997). Male and female adolescents who are experiencing developmental transitions may cope with racialized and gendered experiences in different ways. In this chapter, we use an intersectionality framework to highlight the importance of considering the integral influences of race and gender on identity development, experiences with discrimination, and psychological well-being in ethnically diverse black adolescents. We use the term *black* to include the numerous distinct cultures that people of African ancestry who settled in the United States represent; however, it is most often used to refer jointly to the African Americans and Caribbean blacks (people from the Caribbean Islands who are of African descent) discussed in this chapter.

Our goal is to examine whether historical experiences and current social contexts of African Americans and Caribbean blacks within the United States offer potential explanations for different racial identity attitudes, experiences with discrimination, and psychological well-being among adolescents who participated in the recently completed National Survey of American Life (Jackson and others, 2004). By highlighting structural conditions that can impinge on the well-being of black youth, we hope to avoid the tendency to attribute problems in psychological functioning to inherent predispositions of adolescents. We also demonstrate the significance of using theoretical and analytical approaches that do not obscure the relevance of the joint influences of race and gender when empirically examining adolescent well-being.

INTERSECTIONALITY AS A THEORETICAL FRAMEWORK

Treating race, gender, and class solely as demographic variables excludes the cumulative, interlocking, and historically embedded influences that they can have in shaping the lives, adaptation, and social identities of racial groups in this country. One theoretical perspective that considers the effects of multiple influences and social identities is the intersectionality framework (Collins, 1991). Intersectionality refers to the fluid processes inherent in holding two or more social identities that are situated within a historical context (Collins, 1991; Crenshaw, 1995). Social identities such as race, gender, and class are defined as attributes that societies use to stratify or place individuals in a social hierarchy that can lead to the creation of different meanings for life experiences (Harding, 2004). An intersectional perspective may provide a more holistic lens to gain insights into health disparities and ultimately guide the development of more racially, gender-, and class-responsive health services, policies, and prevention interventions. In addition, it supports social action as a strategy for change that moves beyond an individual focus to societal interventions that have the potential to ensure more universal and equitable access to resources.

UNDERSTANDING ETHNIC AND GENDER DIFFERENCES IN BLACK YOUTHS' IDENTITY DEVELOPMENT

The intersectionality framework is especially useful for conceptualizing the multiple social identities that ethnic minority adolescents must navigate to reach adulthood in America (Garcia Coll, 2000). Adolescence represents a critical developmental period that can be visualized metaphorically as a bridge that connects childhood with adulthood (Guthrie and Low, 2005). One of the many developmental tasks (such as balancing autonomy and attachment and developing intimate relationships) associated with the successful transition into adulthood is identity achievement. Psychosocial identity must be constructed and is influenced by a number of structural determinants. Race, gender, class, family characteristics, community of residence, and societal values are a few determinants that may effectively facilitate or limit the range of opportunities available to youth as they construct social identities. According to Erikson (1968), identity achievement involves commitments to a career and a number of ideologies (political and religious, for example); however, ascribed characteristics, such as race and gender, are integrally involved in the identity development process.

For African American and Caribbean black youth, searching for an identity involves developing multiple identities that include an awareness of the need to function in their own and in mainstream cultural worlds as a male or female. Most black adolescents explore and come to terms with who they are after considering stereotypical social perceptions of their racial, gender, class, and age groups. Caribbean black adolescents, as part of immigrant families, face the additional task of negotiating identities that include the cultural duality of American society for African Americans and the culture of the country in which their parents or grandparents were raised (Waters, 1996). The historical experiences of both groups provide important contexts for understanding variations that may exist both within and across groups when considering racial and gender identity development, experiences with discrimination, and psychological well-being. We explore these issues in order to understand correlates of well-being among ethnically diverse black youth living in the United States.

Identity Development and African American Youth

The legacy of slavery continues to shape the experiences of African American people despite advances made since the civil rights movement. The traditions of oppression and racism persistently exert negative influences on the lives of many African Americans, resulting in more chronic economic disadvantage, less educational attainment, fewer career advancements, and poorer health outcomes than white Americans. The historical experiences of African Americans as a subgroup in American society provide a foundation for beginning to understand the significance of different developmental pathways to achieving multiple social identities among African American youth. As Burt and Halpin (1998, p. 15) note:

> While African American culture is woven within the fabric of the American experience, the collective history of African Americans in the United Sates is one of many contradictions. It is a history of struggle and triumph, of exclusion and inclusion, and of humility and pride, as well as denial and recognition. It is the purpose of research somehow to gain a better understanding of human lives; however, we cannot hypothesize African American identity without having a clear understanding of the identities of Americans. African Americans have shared challenging history; however, they have also demonstrated a remarkable collective resilience and fortitude. To understand and assess the identity development of African Americans accurately in this present day (or in the future), we must acknowledge and understand the history of the African American experience because according to this old Jabo (Liberian) proverb, "The fruit must have a stem before it grows."

This quotation suggests that African Americans have had many different experiences in America, with both negative and positive consequences for identity formation and psychological well-being. As members of a historically marginalized group, African American adolescents are especially challenged in developing social identities that include a positive sense of self as well as positive attitudes about black people as a group. Consequently, over the past two decades, a substantial body of research has emerged that examines different ways racial or ethnic identity can develop among African American youth.

Racial identity has been defined as a psychological attachment to a group or a collective identity based on race and a shared history rooted in racial oppression and discrimination (Thompson, 2001). The two most commonly used approaches to examining a racial or ethnic identity among African Americans involve stage models, in which a person is expected to progress from a more diffused identity to a more actualized identity, and multidimensional models of identity that consider the content and meaning of different aspects of a person's racial identity. Although stage models have been helpful in using a developmental approach to understanding racial identity and in conceptualizing multiple dimensions of racial identity, they have been criticized for positing each stage as a unitary concept with distinct developmental periods (Demo and Hughes, 1990; Thompson, 2001). Nevertheless, earlier efforts to conceptualize and measure racial identity relied on the stage model approach.

Grounded in the historical experiences of African Americans, Cross's model of Nigrescence is the most widely used stage model of African American racial identity development (Cross, 1971, 1991). The Nigrescence model consists of five stages of racial identity development that African Americans experience as they construct a psychologically healthy black identity. In the first stage, pre-encounter, individuals do not believe that race is an important component of their identity. This stage may involve an idealization of the dominant white society or simple placement of more emphasis on another identity component, such as gender or religion. In the second stage, encounter, individuals are faced with a profound experience or a collection of events directly linked to their race. This experience encourages them to reexamine their current identity and find or further develop their black identity. This experience can be positive or negative (Cross, 1991). The third stage, immersion/ emersion, is described as being extremely problack and antiwhite. Externally, individuals are obsessed with identifying with black culture, but internally they have not made the commitment to endorse all values and traditions associated with being black. The fourth stage, internalization, is characterized by having a feeling of inner security and satisfaction about being black. Moreover, individuals at this stage tend to have a less idealized view regarding the meaning of race. They are able to see both the positive and negative elements of being black or white. Internalization-commitment, the final stage, represents individuals who translate their internalized identities into action. Although some of Cross's original assumptions have been revised, this basic conceptual framework guides much of the current racial identity research on African Americans.

Subsequent models of ethnic identity development have used the original identity status work of Erikson (1968) and Marcia (1980) to articulate stages of ethnic identity development applicable to multiple groups of ethnic youth that deemphasize unique historical experiences and highlight similarities across groups as a way of describing universal experiences in ethnic identity development (for example, Phinney, 1990). Continued criticism of stage model approaches as being limited in focus propelled new efforts that expand Cross's original work to move beyond general processes and structures of group identity to include the significance and meaning of being black, which represents another approach to studying racial identity development. Sellers and others (1998) provide an excellent historical assessment of the racial identity literature, including its Afrocentric origins in W.E.B. Dubois's classic work (1903) on the double consciousness of Negroes in America delineated in *The Souls of Black Folk,* and attempts to stretch the U.S. Constitution to limit social contact between African Americans and whites prior to and after slavery. They offer an integrated conceptual framework called the Multidimensional Model of Racial Identity (MMRI). This model incorporates aspects of the historically embedded models of racial identity development and the more universal approaches in an effort to comprehensively address the construction of multiple racial identities that build on historical and cultural experiences that contribute to a unique group identity orientation for black people (Sellers and others, 1998).

The MMRI has four assumptions: (1) identities can be stable characteristics of the individual, and they can be influenced by specific situations; (2) individuals have multiple identities that are hierarchically ordered, and race can be viewed within the context of other identities; (3) individuals must construct their own identities; and (4) the significance and meanings assigned to race at a particular point in time matter more than a particular stage of development because they are likely to change across the life span due to life experiences (Sellers and others, 1998). Sellers and others (1997) further articulate multiple dimensions of racial identity that reflect beliefs and ideologies, including beliefs about black people as a group and beliefs about being black. Three beliefs that are especially critical during adolescence are beliefs about private regard, public regard, and racial centrality. Private regard is the individual's positive or negative evaluation of black people and his or her membership in that racial group, and public regard is the individual's evaluation of how positively or negatively other racial groups view black people as a group. Racial centrality refers to the extent to which an individual normatively defines himself or herself in terms of being black. This multidimensional approach incorporates psychological, sociological, and cultural dimensions, and it is sensitive to the fact that racial identities are not constructed in isolation; rather, they are often formed within the context of families, communities, and broader societal values that can reflect racism, sexism, and classism.

Because African American adolescents must make sense out of both their internal and external worlds to function effectively, it is critical to link different racial identity attitudes to external factors that have implications for their well-being. Discrimination based on institutional policies or interpersonal practices that consider attributes such as race or gender in efforts to control or limit power are examples of external factors that can influence racial identity development among African American youth. Recent research suggests that components of racial identity are associated with reported experiences with racial discrimination and psychological well-being in different ways. In a sample of 578 African American high school students, Sellers, Caldwell, Schmeelk-Cone, and Zimmerman (2003) found that experiences with racial discrimination were associated with lower levels of psychological distress for students for whom race was more central to their identity. Others have found that having a more central racial identity was related to more perceived stress (Caldwell and others, 2002) but also positive self-esteem (Rowley, Sellers, Chavous, and Smith, 1998) among African American adolescents.

Ogbu's theory of oppositional identities among African Americans (1990) is an important conceptual orientation to consider when examining the links among racial identity, racial discrimination, and the well-being of black youth because it focuses on the role of structural limitations and group identities. Essentially, it suggests that involuntary minorities (those who came to the United States through involuntary means, such as African Americans) assume an oppositional identity (one that rejects the behavior and symbols of the dominant group), which can result in an enhanced sense of self-worth because of the sense of a collective group identity. Thus, as a way of coping with discrimination and prejudice, African Americans assume a strong sense of solidarity with other blacks while challenging the rules of the dominant society to overcome the blocked opportunity structure.

Fordham and Ogbu (1986) suggest that structural and educational barriers in American society have led to oppositional identities in African American youth related to academic achievement. The controversial example that they provide is the peer rejection some youth fear because of getting good grades, which is symbolic of what it means to be white in that peer group. Those who oppose the "acting white" hypothesis suggest that it ignores the presence of individual and environmental protective factors that mitigate the impact of discriminatory experiences on youth outcomes. Spencer, Noll, Stoltzfus, and Harpalani (2001), for example, have argued that not considering cultural contexts results in misinterpretations of the behaviors and development of black youth as "pathological products of oppression." These brief examples make clear that the construction of racial identities is complex and influenced by a number of factors rooted in individual and group experiences that can be positive or negative during adolescence.

Gender identity development in African American youth has received far less attention than racial identity development. As Cole and Guy-Sheftall (2003, p. xxiv) so elegantly state:

> Rarely, except among a small group of feminist and other gender-progressives, is there serious consideration of the importance of moving beyond a race-only analysis in understanding the complexities of African American communities and the challenges they face. While we are certain that institutionalized racism and the

persistence of economic injustices are responsible for our contemporary plight as second-class citizens, we boldly assert that *gender* matters too. When we use the term *gender,* we are referring not solely to women or sexism, but also to the experiences of men, cultural definitions of womanhood and manhood, and the interconnections between race, gender, sexual orientations, age, class, and other oppressions. . . . How patriarchy is manifested within African American communities and how we define appropriate roles for black women and men—helps illuminate the status of black America in the twenty-first century.

Consequently, gender identity is dynamically embedded in and very critical to racial identity for black Americans. Gender identity development intensifies during adolescence and is malleable in the same way as racial identity. As the previous quotation suggests, consideration of gender identity is often secondary to racial identity development for African Americans because racial issues are viewed as being more attached to survival than gender (Fujino and King, 1994). Nevertheless, the experiences of African Americans in the United States based on gender can be very different. Scholars of African American female identity development note that their relational orientation (for example, connection, affiliation, and empathy) is consistent with the African American cultural perspective of communalism and collectivism (Collins, 1998; Stevens, 1997). As the first socializing agent, African American families play a key role in orienting their youth not only to an extended definition of self as "we" but also to the existing social environment in which they must function. The extended definition of self refers to the importance of maintaining immediate and extended family connectedness, and African American females are socialized to this orientation early in life.

There is a noticeable gap in the literature on the scholarship of African American males' identity development. Nevertheless, a few works suggest the precarious position of some African American males as they experience adolescence. In their assessment of challenges in raising African American adolescent males, Boyd-Franklin and Franklin (2000) assert that their life chances are affected by how they are viewed by others. In their search for identities as men, many African American males adopt what Majors and

Billson (1993) call a "cool pose," or a way to act calm when confronted with personal assaults. This protective posture allows them to cope with challenges to their manhood, including experiences such as being the victims of racial profiling or avoiding the label of "acting white" through poor school performance based on the belief that education will lead to little social mobility due to discrimination against black people (Fordham and Ogbu, 1986). For some young African American males, assuming a protective posture in response to such assaults is expressed as anger, violence, and mistrust toward white people (Boyd-Franklin and Franklin, 2000). For others, family socialization efforts effectively counterbalance external pressures, encouraging more adaptive responses to unsupportive environmental influences (Spencer, Noll, Stoltzfus, and Harpalani, 2001).

In general, social institutions and cultural environments promote the development of independence and autonomy in males and interdependence and relatedness in females (Maccoby, 1998). Thoughts and feeling about how to be male or female in American society and male or female as an African American may be in direct conflict with each other (Ward, 1996; Tolman, 1999). For example, African American families typically promote more gender role flexibility than what is expected in mainstream society, often because of the historical labor force participation of African American women. Based on data from the National Survey of Black Americans, Hunter and Sellers (1998) found that African Americans, regardless of gender, believed that housework and paid employment should be shared equally. They suggested that egalitarian gender roles may reflect the belief that African American men and women must do what is necessary and work together for their very survival. Gender equality tends to be the goal in childhood socialization for most African American parents, although successfully achieving this goal can vary by social class. Nevertheless, when evaluating the psychological well-being of African American adolescents, it is important to consider how the paradox of independence and interdependence in males and autonomy and attachment in females can couple with the struggle for positive racial identities to manifest in enhanced or compromised psychological functioning.

IDENTITY DEVELOPMENT AND CARIBBEAN BLACK YOUTH

The Caribbean black population from English-speaking islands grew substantially in the United States throughout the twentieth century, especially after the McCarran-Walter Act of 1952 and the Immigration Act of 1965 ended the quota systems that previously limited the levels of immigration to the United States from non-European countries. More Caribbean immigrants arrived in the United States from Jamaica, Trinidad and Tobago, Guyana, and Barbados during the ten years after the enactment of the 1965 Immigration Act than had come in the previous seventy years (Jacobson, 1998). In 1990, three-quarters of all Caribbean immigrants lived in one of six states: California, New York, New Jersey, Florida, Texas, or Illinois (Rong and Preissle, 1998), with the vast majority settling in predominantly black neighborhoods (Waters, 1999). The Caribbean youth population, or second-generation immigrants, has grown exponentially in the past few years as well. In 1998, for example, 50 percent of all the immigrants from Jamaica were under the age of twenty (Jacobson, 1998).

A major challenge facing all immigrants is the process of identity formation in a new country (Obeler, 1999). Few Caribbean black immigrants think of their homeland as one unified place of origin in any way except geographically. For this reason, many immigrants reject blanket terms created to describe them. Caribbean people adopt distinctive ethnic identities in order to distinguish themselves from one another. A Taino identity, for example, which recalls the culture and language of tribes indigenous to the Caribbean area that thrived before the arrival of colonial powers, was promoted in the Dominican Republic in order to separate them from their Haitian neighbors (Haslip-Viera, 2001). Emphasizing ethnic diversity may be a more natural approach to identity development among Caribbean people than the melting pot philosophy that commonly characterizes the labeling of ethnic groups in American society.

Constructing an identity is even more complicated for second-generation immigrants in the United States because of conflicting socialization messages from family members, peer groups, and society. Multiple identity options are available to these youth. Based on her study of 212 teenagers of Caribbean ancestry in New York City, Waters (1996) outlines three possible identity paths the youth followed in forming their ethnic identity: an American identity (42 percent), which is characterized by downplaying their ethnic background in an effort to be only American; an ethnic identity (30 percent), in which youth distanced themselves from African Americans and stressed the ethnic identity of their homeland; and an immigrant identity (28 percent), which reflected a strong attachment to their parents' national origins but did not reject African Americans. These identities represent a sense of self that incorporates the pressures of being an immigrant, a minority, and an adolescent in American society.

While many Caribbean black youth are aware of the different ethnic identities available to them, they also experience tremendous pressure to conform to broad ethnic labels standardized in American culture. Caribbean black youth face pressures from peers and pressures from within (a developmental need to fit in) to reject their ethnic identities and identify only as black or African American. Much of the pressure targeted toward the ethnic homogenization of Caribbean black immigrants also comes from the media, public schools, or governmental sources such as the Bureau of the Census. These pressures increase with every subsequent generation born in the United States, but this assimilation process can be resisted. Portes and Zhou (1993) offer the segmented assimilation process to account for different outcomes for second-generation immigrants adapting to American society. Although their thesis is not without its critics, they propose three pathways to integration into American society:[1] (1) assimilation into the mainstream, with access to upward mobility; (2) becoming part of the urban underclass, destined to downward mobility because of low parental or community resources; and (3) establishing ethnic enclaves or residential concentrations of their own ethnic group. Waters (1996, p. 70) summarizes Portes and Zhou's conclusions as follows: "For immigrants who come with strong ethnic networks, access to capital, and fewer ties to minorities in the United States, the second generation is more likely to resist acculturation and maintain strong ethnic ties to the parental generation. But for immigrants who face extreme discrimination in the

United States and who reside in proximity to American minorities, the second generation is likely to develop an 'adversarial stance' toward the dominant white society. This adversarial stance stresses that discrimination in the United States is very strong and devalues education as a vehicle of advancement."

Caribbean black adolescents living in close proximity to African Americans may be less ethnically identified than those who live in ethnic enclaves. In some instances, there are advantages to a Caribbean, rather than black or African American, identity. Rong and Preissle (1998) found that youth who identified themselves as Caribbean black did better in school, worked longer hours, and stayed in school longer than those who identified themselves as unhyphenated African American. These findings are consistent with the view that Caribbean blacks surpass African Americans in academic achievement and employment (Waters, 1999). This assessment ignores the voluntary versus involuntary entry into this country by these groups (Ogbu, 1990). It also ignores the influence of policies, such as the 1990 amendments to the Immigration and Nationality Act, that increased admission quotas to the United States for highly skilled workers from the Caribbean for selected undersupplied occupations (Conway, 2003). Such policies created opportunities for Caribbean black immigrant families to be more economically viable than many resident African American families. It also ignores what it means to be descendants of African slaves in America.

Mistrust of the dominant white society by African Americans is common, rooted in a long history of mistreatment and discriminatory practices (Terrell and Terrell, 1981). Schools are environments in which black adolescents can be exposed to racial discrimination that could foster this type of cultural mistrust with deleterious consequences. Biafora and others (1993) examined cultural mistrust and delinquent behavior among African American and Caribbean black adolescent males. They found that mistrust of white teachers and whites in general was related to delinquency for all youth, regardless of ethnic background. Interestingly, they also found that Caribbean black males, other than Haitians, reported lower levels of mistrust of whites than African American males. Others have found that African Americans and Caribbean blacks perceive racial discrimination fundamentally differently because most Caribbean blacks emigrate from countries where social class matters more than race (Rong and Preissle, 1998). In her qualitative study of Caribbean immigrants in New York, however, Waters (1999) found that the second generation's persistent experiences with racism and discrimination influenced their life chances and made them less optimistic about race relations and their chances for achieving success by hard work. Their beliefs were often in direct contrast to their parents' beliefs about how to succeed in American society.

As generation after generation of Caribbean black youth becomes more deeply immersed in American society, racial discrimination against blacks in general may influence their psychological functioning. Rumbaut (1994), for example, found that anticipated racial discrimination was related to more depressive symptoms and low self-esteem, while actual experiences with racial discrimination resulted in higher depressive symptoms among immigrant youth. Thus, African American and Caribbean black adolescents share a large part of the negative experiences of being black in America. Examining discrimination and multiple racial identity attitudes in Caribbean black youth with regard to how positive or negative they are about black people, how they believe other racial groups view black people, how central being black is to their own identity, and how any of these racial identity attitudes relate to their psychological well-being is an important next step in identity development work with this population. They are not immune to the discrimination that African Americans face, but the impact and meanings of such experiences may differ, especially by gender.

Similar to African American youth, gender identity formation among Caribbean black youth has not been the focus of much research, in either the Caribbean or in the United States, yet gender role distinctions are evident in the family life of blacks of Caribbean ancestry. After the end of the quota system in 1965, Caribbean black women immigrated to the United States in large numbers. During the 1970s, for example, Jamaican women were more than twice as likely to immigrate to the United States as men (Obeler, 1999). One role of Caribbean black women in families is to ensure that the cultural traditions of their homeland are passed on to their children. Parental discipline is viewed as critical to raising children correctly (Waters, 1999). An important family value passed on to females is that they must be self-reliant. They are taught autonomy from an early age; however, the idea of autonomy from a cultural perspective implies interdependence, involving the formation of reciprocal obligatory relationships within often female-centered social networks that can be relied on to respond in times of need (Bolles, 2003). Education, rather than depending on men, is a critical strategy for advancement and self-sufficiency for Caribbean black women.

A Test of the Intersection of Race and Gender

Racial and gender identity development among African American and Caribbean black youth living in the United States is shaped by a number of external forces, including family socialization practices, neighborhood and community resources, media messages, and societal factors such as immigration laws, educational and employment opportunities, prejudice, and institutional discrimination, to name a few. Examining the influences of specific racial identity attitudes and experiences with discrimination on adolescent well-being using an intersectionality approach can provide direction for how external forces can better support identity development and protect the well-being of diverse groups of black adolescents in American society.

Several empirical studies have found that a more fully developed racial identity is associated with less depressive symptoms (Arroyo and Zigler, 1995; Martinez and Dukes, 1997; Phinney, Lochner, and Murphy, 1990) and higher self-esteem (Munford, 1994; Phinney and Alipuria, 1990; Martinez and Dukes, 1997; Smith and others, 1999; Roberts and others, 1999) and that racial discrimination is associated with more psychological distress among youth (Sellers and others, 2003). Most of these studies are concerned only with African American youth, with little regard for possible ethnic or gender variations among black youth. In this chapter, we summarize preliminary findings from an empirical study that we conducted (Caldwell, Guthrie, and Jackson, 2005) using an intersectionality framework to analyze data obtained from the National Survey of American Life (Jackson and others, 2004). We used descriptive statistics and a series of multiple regression analyses to examine these issues for African American and Caribbean black male and female adolescents, ascertaining the combined influences of race and gender. Our goal is to interpret the findings within broader historical contexts associated with identity development and experiences with discrimination as they relate to the psychological well-being of diverse groups of black youth. Thus, we are able to consider structural factors that may account for differences found that are beyond the scope of the original study.

OVERVIEW OF THE NATIONAL SURVEY OF AMERICAN LIFE

The National Survey of American Life (NSAL) is the most comprehensive and detailed study of mental disorders and the mental health of black Americans ever conducted in the contiguous United States (Jackson and others, 2004). It is designed to explore intra- and intergroup racial and ethnic differences in mental disorders, psychological distress, and informal and formal service use as they are manifested in the context of a variety of stressors, risk and resilient factors, and coping resources among different ethnic groups. The adult samples include blacks of African descent (African Americans) ($N = 3,570$), the first-ever national probability sample of blacks of Caribbean descent (Caribbean blacks) ($N = 1,621$), and non-Hispanic whites (Americans largely of European descent) ($N = 891$) for a total sample of 6,082 individuals aged eighteen and over. Supplementary interviews were conducted with 1,193 African American and Caribbean black adolescents thirteen to nineteen years of age who were attached to the NSAL adult households (Jackson and others, 2004). The results reported in this chapter are based on the 1,170 adolescents who were thirteen to seventeen years old at the time of the interview. The eighteen- and nineteen-year-olds who screened into the study at age seventeen but did not complete their interview until after their eighteenth birthday were eliminated from these analyses ($N = 23$). The sample was weighted to adjust for unequal probabilities of selection, nonresponse, and poststratification to match the 2000 Census distribution of the African American and Caribbean black populations on several geographical and sociodemographic variables. The adolescent sample also was weighted to adjust for differential probability of selection of more than one adolescent per household based on gender. The overall sample response rate for African American and Caribbean black adolescents was 80.6 percent. The SAS Version 9.1 software package was used for data analysis.

The final sample consists of 810 African American youth and 360 youth from Caribbean black households with family members who emigrated from English-speaking islands in the Caribbean. The majority of Caribbean black youth are from households with family members from Jamaica, Haiti, or Trinidad and Tobago. Both groups were almost equally divided by gender (African American— 50 percent males, 50 percent females; Caribbean black—44 percent males and 56 percent females). The average age of the overall sample was fifteen years old, with an average of about a tenth-grade education. The median family income was $28,000.

RACIAL IDENTITY ATTITUDES

Black youth are similar to one another with regard to their racial identity attitudes. In general, all youth had very positive feelings about black people as a group (*Mean* = 3.66–3.81 on a 4.0 private regard scale as measured by the Multidimensional Inventory of Black Identity) (Sellers and others, 1997). African American males, however, had even higher private regard than African American females and Caribbean black males. There were no gender differences in how Caribbean black youth felt about black people. It is noteworthy that the overwhelming majority of black adolescents were able to form positive opinions about black people despite the negative stereotypes that are pervasive throughout society.

Families are often credited with providing protective influences to negate harmful stereotyping that can have deleterious consequences for identity development. Racial socialization is a specific practice used in black families to provide children and adolescents with knowledge and skills necessary to resist the internalization of prevailing negative images and messages about black people (Thornton, Chatters, Taylor, and Allen, 1990). Race-related socialization to existing social environments involves cultural and political interpretations and assumptions derived from a family's lived experiences of being black in America. Clearly, ethnic pride has been communicated to these youth, regardless of ethnic background. This suggests that differences that may exist between first-generation Caribbean blacks and African Americans regarding their place in American society may not be emphasized when pride in the social identity of blacks as a group is conveyed to contemporary black youth. Additional research is necessary to determine how interacting with other social institutions, such as black churches, civil rights groups, or ethnically oriented community organizations, also may contribute to the race-related socialization of black youth.

Caribbean black females' beliefs about how other racial groups feel about black people, or public regard attitudes, differed most from those of the other three groups. Specifically, Caribbean black females (*Mean* = 2.74 on a 4.0 scale) were least likely to say that other racial groups felt favorably toward black people when compared to Caribbean black males (*Mean* = 2.95), African American females (*Mean* = 2.86), and African American males (*Mean* = 2.99). These differences were not statistically different. Overall, most adolescents felt that other racial groups were generally positive about black people (*Mean* = 2.89). These findings indicate that contemporary black youth appear to have optimistic views about how other racial groups perceive black people in American society. Brown, Wallace, and Williams (2001) suggest that the inconsistencies found in reports of race relations between adults and adolescents may reflect developmental differences. They assert that "youth may not have lived long enough to accurately appraise the meaning and significance of race in the United States" (p. 100); therefore, adolescents' reports of optimistic assessments of race relations may be more grounded in idealism than in reality or may be influenced by the positive regard their parents have helped to foster.

Interestingly, there were no gender differences in the levels of racial centrality within racial groups; however, African American males (*Mean* = 3.42 on a 4.0 scale) reported slightly higher levels of racial centrality than Caribbean black males (*Mean* = 3.34), and African American females (*Mean* = 3.39) reported higher levels of racial centrality than Caribbean black females (*Mean* = 3.18). In considering the historical background of immigrant youth, Biafora and others (1993) concluded that Caribbean black adolescents may perceive less racial exclusion in American society than African American youth; therefore, race may be less central in their definitions of who they are. In addition, Rong and Preissle (1998) suggested that social class may be more important than race for Caribbean black identity given the significance of the class structure in the West Indies. That is, for people who come from a predominantly black country, class differences are apparent, while race is not. Thus, confronting racial hierarchies in America becomes the impetus for thinking about race. At first glance, historical context could perhaps explain the slight differences in racial centrality noted above; however, being black appears to be a highly central part of racial identity for both African American and Caribbean black youth. This finding reinforces the significance of race as a critical component of identity development for black youth in America regardless of their ethnic background.

Experiences with Discrimination

From a historical perspective, African American and Caribbean black adolescents' families came to America in different ways; nevertheless, their experiences with discrimination appear to be quite similar. When asked about different types of discrimination in their daily life—such as being treated with less courtesy than other people, being treated by teachers with less respect than other students or as if they are not smart, or being called names or insulted, to name a few encounters—youth in this study reported an average of five types of discriminatory encounters. Both African American (*Mean* = 5.40) and Caribbean black males (*Mean* = 6.1) reported experiencing more types of discrimination than their female counterparts (*Mean* = 4.83 and 4.25, respectively). The most frequent type of discrimination, encountered by 67 percent of the adolescents, was defined as "people acting as if they were better than you are." Discrimination most often was attributed to race or ancestry, regardless of ethnic/gender subgroup. Specifically, 48 percent of African American males, 43 percent of African American females, 49 percent of Caribbean black males, and 35 percent of Caribbean black females said that they thought the main reason that they had experienced any type of discrimination was their race/ancestry. Gender as an explanation for discrimination was offered by only 8 percent of African American males, 10 percent of African American females, 6 percent of Caribbean black males, and 7 percent of Caribbean black females. Age and physical appearance were identified as reasons for discrimination more frequently than gender but less frequently than race/ancestry.

While previous studies have found that African American youth report experiencing racial discrimination (Biafora and others, 1993; Brown and others, 2001), the Waters study (1999) is one of few that focuses on Caribbean black teenagers. The youth in this qualitative study reported that they constantly experienced being harassed by police and store owners, being turned down for jobs, and being attacked in white neighborhoods. The results of the current study also show that black youth appear to share a common fate when it comes to chronic, routine, and less overt experiences of unfair treatment or discrimination. The attribution of these experiences to race/ancestry is another indication of the vividness of race as a vital part of the life experiences of many black youth at this critical stage of development, especially for black males.

Although the measure of discrimination used in this study (Williams, Yu, Jackson, and Anderson, 1997) allowed unfair treatment to be attributed to several factors equally, gender was not a prominent selection. Adolescents may not be able to separate the influences of race and gender in their assessments of unfair treatment at this stage of development. But discrimination based on age and physical appearance may be easier to distinguish from discrimination based on race/ancestry when assessing unfair treatment. Perhaps because at this stage of development, adolescents are often preoccupied with how they dress as distinct from adults and are acutely aware that they are treated differently because of their age across an array of situations, attributing discriminatory episodes to these physical characteristics may be less ambiguous than those that can be attributed to gender bias. As these adolescents move into the world of employment, financial negotiations, or large-scale consumerisms, the vividness of gender bias may become clearer to them as a plausible explanation for their experiences with discrimination. While discriminatory episodes reported in this study were often not attributed to gender, we did find that males reported more discrimination than females. This suggests that gender and gender roles exert critical influences on experiences with discrimination.

RACIAL IDENTITY ATTITUDES, DISCRIMINATION, AND PSYCHOLOGICAL WELL-BEING

Correlates of self-esteem and depressive symptoms were revealed when these well-being indicators were regressed on different racial identity attitudes and experiences with discrimination by race and gender, while controlling for age and family income. The most consistent finding was that discriminatory experiences were associated with less self-esteem for all youth, an indication that discrimination is detrimental to the psychological well-being of black adolescents. Furthermore, African American and Caribbean black females who reported more experiences with discrimination also reported higher levels of depressive symptoms. Interestingly, this was not true for African American males, but this relationship did approach significance for Caribbean black males. The fact that African American and Caribbean black youth most often attributed their discriminatory experiences to race/ancestry underscores the reality that a sense of oppression remains an issue in the life experiences of many contemporary black youth. Future research must identify underlying mechanisms that can further elaborate the nature of these relationships. Other factors may mediate or moderate the conditions under which discriminatory experiences will influence psychological well-being, especially for African American males. For example, the combined influences of different racial identity attitudes and discrimination are promising future directions for research, with implications for intervention.

Our findings revealed varied relationships between different racial identity attitudes that youth hold on their psychological well-being, while controlling for discrimination. Specifically, we found that African American male and female youth with less positive feelings about black people (that is, private regard) had more depressive symptoms than those with more positive feelings about blacks. More private regard, however, was associated with more self-esteem for African American youth, regardless of gender. These findings are consistent with previous research indicating that a positive black identity among African American youth is associated with less depression and higher self-esteem (Arroyo and Zigler, 1995; Munford, 1994). They provide additional evidence that having positive attitudes about one's race among African American youth is protective against negative self-internalizations, perhaps because of a sense of connection to a larger group with similar historical experiences and a common fate (Cross, 1991; Sellers and others, 1997). What is interesting is that different racial identity attitudes were relevant for the psychological well-being of male and female Caribbean black youth.

Believing that other racial groups held less favorable views about black people (that is, public regard) was associated with more depressive symptoms for Caribbean black males. It is not clear from this research whether public regard is correlated with the amount of time Caribbean black males have been in the United States or whether they are currently living in Caribbean communities in America. This is important because males who have been in this country longer or those surrounded by other West Indians may have differential expectations regarding race relations (Rumbaut, 1994; Waters, 1999). These expectations could be based on their own experiences or on the values and beliefs of the first generation. We found that Caribbean black males reported more experience with discriminatory episodes than any other ethnic-gender subgroup. These negative encounters may have contributed to their assessment of less public regard for black people and feelings of depression. Or, highly identified West Indian males may believe that whites have valid reasons for treating African Americans in negative ways or holding negative views about them. Waters (1996) found that Caribbean black adolescents who distanced themselves from African Americans assumed that whites who held negative views about African Americans were justified. Consequently, the protections normally felt in the face of discrimination through group or collective identity as blacks in America may be weakened for highly identified Caribbean black males and may contribute to their experience of more depressive symptoms. Future research should explore both of these potential explanations for this finding using longitudinal data.

The fact that public regard was not associated with depressive symptoms for Caribbean black females or African American youth of either gender suggests that this finding cannot be easily explained by Ogbu's theory of oppositional identities in voluntary and involuntary immigrants (1990). It does provide support for Sellers and others' MMRI conceptualization (1998) of racial identities as being contextualized within other identities. That is, there is something unique about being Caribbean black and being Caribbean male that makes public regard critical for depression. Future research should pursue lines of inquiry aimed at elaborating Ogbu's oppositional identities orientation (1990) and other conceptualizations of identity development in black youth to incorporate a hierarchy between ethnicity and gender in different social contexts to assist in understanding these findings.

We also found that more racial centrality was associated with more depressive symptoms, but only for Caribbean black females. From a developmental perspective, adolescent girls grappling with the question of achieving a more general identity may take comfort in identifying with black people so that other worldviews that emphasize and value attributes that they may never achieve (being blond, blue-eyed, or very thin, for example) can be assessed more realistically. Racial centrality therefore should be critical to their psychological well-being. Because most Caribbean blacks emigrate from countries where social class matters more than race (Rong and Preissle, 1998), Caribbean black females may not be prepared to cope with persistent experiences with racism and discrimination that second-generation immigrants face in this country (Waters, 1999). This could expose them to what Spencer, Noll, Stoltzfus, and Harpalani (2001) describe as a "dissonance-producing environment" in which racial centrality could be associated with distress because of the constant exposure to discrimination. The fact that this finding was significant only for Caribbean black females again highlights the need to elaborate the interactive role of race and gender as integral to understanding adolescent well-being with an eye toward understanding the contributions of social context and social meanings. Clearly, determining whether race-related socialization messages that Caribbean black youth receive from parents or communities are gendered, especially with regard to coping with discrimination and depression, is a critical direction for future research.

CONCLUSIONS

In this chapter, we empirically demonstrated the significance of using an intersectionality framework for understanding nuanced differences in the relationship between experiences with discrimination, multiple racial identity attitudes, and psychological well-being among African American and Caribbean black male and female adolescents. We were interested in determining whether any of these differences might be understood by considering the historical experiences and current social contexts of the ethnic and gender group to which they belong. Such an approach has allowed us to consider the life experiences of black adolescents in a more contextualized way. Our findings show that African American and Caribbean black youth share a number of characteristics related to racial identity, discrimination, and well-being, regardless of gender, perhaps because of the strong ethnic homogenizing forces that are prevalent in American society. There were, however, unique findings that demonstrated the complexity of race and gender as embedded social identities that would have been missed if an intersectional approach had not been taken.

We found, for example, that racial centrality was negatively related to depressive symptoms for Caribbean black females, while public regard was negatively related to depressive symptoms for Caribbean black males. Less private regard was associated with more depressive symptoms for female youth regardless of ethnicity. Furthermore, African American and Caribbean black females who reported more experiences with discrimination also reported higher levels of depressive symptoms, while discriminatory experiences were associated with less self-esteem for all youth. This type of information is essential for developing gender-responsive health interventions for black youth for whom different racial identity attitudes could be incorporated to enhance their psychological well-being. Coping with discriminatory experiences should be incorporated into all interventions involving black youth, especially male youth, who reported that they experienced discriminatory events more frequently than females did. Framed with an intersectionality lens, such interventions must be developed in gender-responsive ways to reflect the life experiences of black males. Prior to developing any intervention program, we strongly suggest that focus groups be conducted with separate groups of male and female African American and Caribbean black adolescents to determine the meaning they attribute to these racial attitudes and experiences with discrimination so that effective intervention content can be developed.

As a society, we cannot afford to ignore how vital it is to understand the intersection of race, gender, and class as fundamental to the well-being of black youth if we are to create healthy environments that can facilitate their well-being as they navigate the challenges of adolescence. The ultimate implication is the reduction of health disparities as they transition into adulthood.

Notes

The National Survey of American Life was designed by James S. Jackson (principal investigator) and the staff of the Program for Research on Black Americans, Research Center for Group Dynamics, Institute for Social Research, University of Michigan. It was funded by the National Institute of Mental Health (U01-MH57716) with supplemental support from the Office of Behavioral and Social Science Research at the National Institutes of Health and the University of Michigan. We thank Elias Morrel-Samuels, who served as a research assistant for this project.

1. Portes and Zhou's segmented assimilation process (1993) proposed three paths to integration into American society: (1) assimilation into the mainstream, with access to upward mobility; (2) becoming part of the urban underclass, destined to downward mobility because of low parental or community resources; and (3) establishing ethnic enclaves or residential concentrations of one ethnic group. The last path has been criticized as being "anti-American," leading to a backdoor fragmentation of American society. The assimilation path assumes immigrants must purge themselves of their ethnic background to become American. It has been criticized and rejected in favor of other approaches for explaining adaptation among second-generation immigrants. These include the multiculturalists' perspective, which suggests that immigrants actively shape their own lives, and the structural perspective, which depicts American society as a stratified system of social inequality (Zhou, 1997). Each approach, however, acknowledges that variations in social and economic resources and opportunities, as well as experiences with discrimination, have implications for downward or upward mobility options for immigrant youth.

References

Arroyo, G., and Zigler, E. "Racial Identity, Academic Achievement, and the Psychological Well-Being of Economically Disadvantaged Adolescents." *Journal of Personality and Social Psychology,* 1995, *69,* 903–914.

Biafora, F. A., and others. "Cultural Mistrust and Racial Awareness Among Ethnically Diverse Black Adolescent Boys." *Journal of Black Psychology,* 1993, *19,* 266–281.

Bolles, A. L. "Women and Development." In R. S. Hillman and T. J. D'Agostino (eds.), *Understanding the Contemporary Caribbean*. Boulder, Colo.: Lynne Rienner, 2003.

Boyd-Franklin, N., and Franklin, A. J. *Boys into Men: Raising Our African American Teenage Sons*. New York: Penguin, 2000.

Brown, T. N., Wallace, J. M., and Williams, D. R. "Race-Related Correlates of Young Adults' Subjective Well-being." *Social Indicators Research*, 2001, *53*, 97–116.

Burt, J. M., and Halpin, G. "African American Identity Development: A Review of the Literature." Paper presented at the Annual Meeting of the Mid-South Educational Research Association, New Orleans, Nov. 4–6, 1998.

Caldwell, C. H., Guthrie, B. J., and Jackson, J. S. "Gender Differences in Perceived Discrimination, Racial Identity, and Psychological Well-Being Among African American and Caribbean Black Adolescents." Unpublished manuscript, 2005.

Caldwell, C. H., and others. "Racial Identity, Maternal Support, and Psychological Distress Among African American Adolescents." *Child Development*, 2002, *73*, 1322–1336.

Cole, J. B., and Guy-Sheftall, B. *Gender Talk: The Struggle for Women's Equality in African American Communities*. New York: Ballantine, 2003.

Collins, P. H. *Black Feminist Thought: Knowledge, Consciousness, and the Politics of Empowerment*. New York: Routledge, 1991.

Collins, P. H. *Fighting Words: Black Women and the Search for Justice*. Minneapolis: University of Minnesota Press, 1998.

Conway, D. "The Caribbean Diaspora." In R. S. Hillman and T. J. D'Agostino (eds.), *Understanding the Contemporary Caribbean*. Boulder, Colo.: Lynne Rienner, 2003.

Crenshaw, K. "Mapping the Margins: Intersectionality, Identity Politics, and Violence Against Women of Color." In K. Crenshaw, N. Gotanda, G. Peller, and K. Thomas (eds.), *Critical Race Theory*. New York: Free Press, 1995.

Cross, W. E., Jr. "The Negro-to-Black Conversion Experience." *Black World*, 1971, 13–27.

Cross, W. E., Jr. *Shades of Black: Diversity in African-American Identity*. Philadelphia: Temple University Press, 1991.

Demo, D., and Hughes, M. "Socialization and Racial Identity Among Black Americans." *Social Psychology Quarterly*, 1990, *53*, 364–374.

Dubois, W.E.B. *The Souls of Black Folk: Essays and Sketches*. Chicago: A. C. McClurg, 1903.

Erikson, E. *Identity, Youth, and Crisis*. New York: Norton, 1968.

Fordham, S., and Ogbu, J. "Black Students' School Success: Coping with the Burden of Acting White." *Urban Review*, 1986, *18*, 176–206.

Fujino, D. C., and King, K. R. "Toward a Model of Womanist Identity Development." Paper presented at the Annual Convention of the American Psychological Association, Los Angeles, 1994.

Garcia Coll, C. "Minorities in the United States: Sociocultural Context for Mental Health and Developmental Psychopathology." In A. J. Samoff, M. Lewis, and S. M. Miller (eds.), *Handbook of Developmental Psychopathology*. (2nd ed.) Norwell, Mass.: Kluwer, 2000.

Guthrie, B. J., Caldwell, C. H., and Hunter, A. G. "African American Adolescent Female Health: Strategies for the Next Millennium." In D. K. Wilson, J. R. Rodrigue, and W. C. Taylor (eds.), *Adolescent Health Promotion in Minority Populations*. Washington, D.C.: American Psychological Association, 1997.

Guthrie, B. J., and Low, L. K. "Adolescent Females' Health: Challenges and Opportunities." Unpublished manuscript, 2005.

Harding, S. (ed.). *The Feminist Standpoint Theory Reader.* New York: Routledge, 2004.

Haslip-Viera, G. *Taino Revival: Critical Perspectives on Puerto Rican Identity and Cultural Politics.* Princeton, N.J.: Markus Wiener, 2001.

Hunter, A. G., and Sellers, S. L. "Feminist Attitudes Among African American Women and Men." *Gender and Society*, 1998, *12*, 81–99.

Jackson, J. S., and others. "The National Survey of American Life: A Study of Racial, Ethnic and Cultural Influences on Mental Disorder and Mental Health." *International Journal of Methods in Psychiatric Research*, 2004, *13*, 196–207.

Jacobson, D. *The Immigration Reader: America in a Multidisciplinary Perspective.* Malden, Mass.: Blackwell, 1998.

Maccoby, E. *The Two Sexes: Growing Up Apart, Coming Together.* Cambridge, Mass.: Belknap Press, 1998.

Majors, R., and Billson, J. M. *Cool Pose.* New York: Touchstone, 1993.

Marcia, J. E. "Identity in Adolescence." In J. Adelson (ed.), *Handbook of Adolescent Psychology.* New Hoboken, N.J.: Wiley, 1980.

Martinez, R., and Dukes, R. "The Effects of Ethnic Identity, Ethnicity, and Gender on Adolescent Well-Being." *Journal of Youth and Adolescence*, 1997, *26*, 503–516.

Munford, M. "Relationship of Gender, Self-Esteem, Social Class, and Racial Identity in Depression Among Blacks." *Journal of Black Psychology*, 1994, *20*, 157–174.

Obeler, S. "Radicalizing Latinos in the United States: Towards a New Research Paradigm." In L. Goldin (ed.), *Identities on the Move: Transnational Processes in North America and the Caribbean Basin.* Austin: University of Texas Press, 1999.

Ogbu, J. "Minority Status and Literacy in Comparative Perspective." *Daedalus*, 1990, *119*, 141–168.

Phinney, J. S. "Ethnic Identity and Self-Esteem: A Review and Integration." *Hispanic Journal of Behavioral Sciences*, 1990, *13*, 193–208.

Phinney, J. S., and Alipuria, L. "Ethnic Identity in College Students from Four Ethnic Groups." *Journal of Adolescence*, 1990, *13*, 171–183.

Phinney, J. S., Lochner, B. T., and Murphy, R. "Ethnic Identity Development and Psychological Adjustment in Adolescence." In A. Stiffman and L. Davis (eds.), *Issues in Adolescent Mental Health*. Thousand Oaks, Calif.: Sage, 1990.

Portes, A., and Zhou, M. "The New Second Generation: Segmented Assimilation and Its Variants." *Annals of the American Academy of Political and Social Science*, 1993, *530*, 74–96.

Roberts, R., and others. "The Structure of Ethnic Identity of Young Adolescents from Diverse Ethnocultural Groups." *Journal of Early Adolescence*, 1999, *19*, 301–322.

Rong, X. L., and Preissle, J. *Educating Immigrant Students: What We Need to Know to Meet the Challenges*. Thousand Oaks, Calif.: Corwin Press, 1998.

Rowley, S. J., Sellers, R. M., Chavous, T. M., and Smith, M. A. "The Relationship Between Racial Identity and Self-Esteem in African American College and High School Students." *Journal of Personality and Social Psychology*, 1998, 74, 715–724.

Rumbaut, R. G. "The Crucible Within: Ethnic Identity, Self-Esteem, and Segmented Assimilation Among Children of Immigrants." *International Migration Review*, 1994, *28*, 748–794.

Sellers, R. M., Caldwell, C. H., Schmeelk-Cone, K. H., and Zimmerman, M. A. "The Role of Racial Identity and Racial Discrimination in the Mental Health of African American Young Adults." *Journal of Health and Social Behavior*, 2003, *44*, 302–317.

Sellers, R. M., and others. "Multidimensional Inventory of Black Identity: A Preliminary Investigation of Reliability and Construct Validity." *Journal of Personality and Social Psychology*, 1997, *73*, 805–815.

Sellers, R. M., and others. "Multidimensional Model of Racial Identity: A Reconceptualization of African American Racial Identity." *Personality and Social Psychology Review*, 1998, *2*, 18–39.

Smith, E. P., and others. "Ethnic Identity and Its Relationship to Self-Esteem, Perceived Efficacy and Prosocial Attitudes in Early Adolescence." *Journal of Adolescence*, 1999, *22*, 867–880.

Spencer, M. B., Noll, E., Stoltzfus, J., and Harpalani, V. "Identity and School Adjustment: Revisiting the 'Acting White' Assumption." *Educational Psychologist*, 2001, *36*, 21–30.

Stevens, J. W. "African American Female Adolescent Identity Development: A Three Dimensional Perspective." *Child Welfare*, 1997, *126*, 145–172.

Terrell, F., and Terrell, S. "An Inventory to Measure Cultural Mistrust Among Blacks." *Western Journal of Black Studies,* 1981, *5,* 180–185.

Thompson, V.L.S. "The Complexity of African American Racial Identification." *Journal of Black Studies,* 2001, *32,* 155–165.

Thornton, M., Chatters, L. M., Taylor, R. J., and Allen, W. A. "Socio-Demographic and Environmental Correlates of Racial Socialization by Black Parents." *Child Development,* 1990, *61,* 401–109.

Tolman, D. "Femininity as a Barrier to Positive Sexual Health for Adolescent Girls." *Journal of the American Medical Women's Association,* 1999, *54,* 133–138.

Ward, J. "Raising Resisters." In B. Leadbeater and N. Way (eds.), *Urban Girls: Resisting Stereotypes, Creating Identities.* New York: New York University Press, 1996.

Waters, M. C. "The Intersection of Gender, Race, and Ethnicity in Identity Development of Caribbean American Teens." In B. Leadbeater and N. Way (eds.), *Urban Girls: Resisting Stereotypes, Creating Identities.* New York: New York University Press, 1996.

Waters, M. C. *Black Identities: West Indian Immigrant Dreams and American Realities.* Cambridge, Mass.: Harvard University Press, 1999.

Williams, D., Yu, Y., Jackson, J., and Anderson, N. "Racial Differences in Physical and Mental Health: Socioeconomic Status, Stress, and Discrimination." *Journal of Health Psychology,* 1997, *2,* 335–351.

Zhou, M. "Segmented Assimilation: Issues, Controversies, and Recent Research on the New Second Generation." *International Migration Review,* 1997, *31,* 975–1008.

CHAPTER SEVEN

DISPARITIES IN LATINA HEALTH

An Intersectional Analysis

Ruth E. Zambrana, Bonnie Thornton Dill

Despite steady improvements in the overall health of the U.S. population, underserved racial and ethnic minorities, especially African American and Latino women, experience disproportionately higher rates of morbidity and mortality than nonminorities (National Center for Health Statistics, 2002; Office of Research on Women's Health, 2002; U.S. Department of Health and Human Services, 2000).[1]

Health disparities in populations where race, ethnicity, and gender intersect have been persistent and understudied. Latinas in particular have been systematically neglected in most research studies. Investigators have repeatedly documented that the intersection of factors such as socioeconomic differences, differential access to health care, quality of health care and services, and direct and indirect consequences of discrimination are all key determinants of Latinos' health disparities (Aguirre-Molina, Molina, and Zambrana, 2001; American College of Physicians, 2000; Commonwealth Fund, 2000; Smedley, Stith, and Nelson, 2003; Stryer, Clancy, and Simpson, 2002). However, few studies have examined the sociopolitical and structural factors that keep the above associations stable and in place. Since data are not situated in the political context of resource allocation as it affects employment and educational opportunities, in family and community contexts or in the context of the way low-income women of color are perceived and stereotyped, the reasons for these disparities in health outcomes remain poorly understood.

This chapter has three aims: (1) to provide an overview of the social, economic, and educational correlates associated with Latinas' health; (2) to present selected health behaviors and major chronic conditions that disproportionately burden Latinas in comparison to non-Latino black and white women;[2] and (3) to discuss innovative interventions and research directions to reduce health disparities among low-income Latino women. The Latina populations focused on in this chapter are Mexican American and Puerto Rican women, who represent the largest Latino subgroups and are also the most historically, economically, and socially disadvantaged groups in the United States. This chapter draws on available data to disentangle the politically constructed category of Latina in order to reveal how it is used to predicate ethnicity or culture as the sole determinant of health outcomes in spite of evidence to the contrary. Therefore, caution in the generalizability of data for all Latinas is warranted.

The conceptual lens that guides this discussion is an intersectional analysis, which helps to explain the persistence of patterns of inequality. This approach provides a more nuanced and complex understanding of Latina health and challenges researchers to pay more attention to the social production and maintenance of inequality as it is manifested in the intersection of adverse social conditions such as poverty and poor housing, access to health care, and the quality of health care received. Throughout this chapter, we simultaneously address inequity as the unequal distribution of social goods and resources that are associated with social conditions and experiences that affect health outcomes and the disparity in health outcomes that result from these interactions. (See Chapter Nine, this volume, and Carter-Pokras and Baquet, 2002, for discussion of differing definitions and [mis]understandings of these terms.)

THE INTERSECTIONAL LENS: THEORETICAL ASSUMPTIONS

Intersectional analyses provide an important lens for rethinking Latina health because they require that research findings be understood in relation to the distribution of power in the production of inequality. Thus, any examination of Latina health must explore and unpack relations of domination and subordination in the structural arrangements through which health services are delivered, in the political contexts that influence how and to whom resources are distributed, and in the stereotypes and representations that affect how patients are treated and what services are made available to them (Crenshaw, 1993). In addition, intersectional analysis requires the simultaneous examination of multiple dimensions of inequality and difference. It is not sufficient to focus solely on race/ethnicity, class, gender, nationality, or another dimension of difference and inequality. Intersectional analyses focus on the way these dimensions shape and influence one another. As a result, intersectional analysis requires us to think in complex and nuanced ways about identity and challenges us to look at both the points of cohesion and fracture within groups (Dill, 2002; Weber, 2001).

STRUCTURAL AND POLITICAL CONSIDERATIONS

Intersectional analyses challenge both the medical and public health models that place primary emphasis on individual attributes and self-responsibility as determinants of health; instead, they include a focus on the economic and social position of groups within the society and the associations among institutional practices, socioeconomic status, and health outcomes. For example, the location of health services in relation to low-income Latino communities structures access to health care and is a major factor affecting the health of Latina women, children, and families. The distribution of governmental resources, ranging from funding for research to the provision of public health services, is examined in terms of historical patterns and political considerations, which have led to a concentration of health resources in middle- and upper-income communities and the prioritization of research on diseases and illnesses that are more prevalent in those populations. An intersectional analysis therefore begins with several assumptions about the importance of social structure and its impact on Latino communities.

Such an approach recognizes that poverty is primarily the result of the unequal distribution of society's goods and resources (Adler and others, 1993). Examining the interaction of poverty with race/ethnicity and gender demonstrates that these factors, taken together, have a disproportionately negative effect on Latinas and result in detrimental health consequences. Mexican American and Puerto Rican women, historically underserved groups, experience poorer health status, suffer with undetected medical conditions longer, and die younger than the majority population (National Center for Health Statistics, 2002; Office of Research on Women's Health, 2002; U.S. Department of Health and Human Services, 2000; Aguirre-Molina and Pond, 2003; Stewart and Napoles-Springer, 2003). Intersectional analyses direct us to look at structural inequities by examining questions of social and economic justice, both to reveal the sources of these inequities and begin to redress them.

Race, ethnicity, and geography matter; they are all determinants of access to social capital or social resources. Social capital broadly refers to access to resources that improve educational, economic, and social position in society (Bourdieu, 1985; Ellen and Turner, 1997). Intersectional analysis draws attention to the policies, practices, and outcomes of institutional racism and discrimination, one result of which is the concentration of low-income Latinas in resource-poor neighborhoods with low-quality public systems such as schools and public health services. For example, access to quality education that provides the skill of literacy is essential to promoting and maintaining good health.

REPRESENTATIONAL CONSIDERATIONS

In addition to a focus on structural, political, historical, and locational factors, intersectional analyses emphasize the importance of the ways social groups and individuals are represented—the ways they are viewed and depicted in the society at large and the expectations associated with these depictions (hooks, 1992; Chin and Humikowski, 2002; Zambrana, Mogel, and Scrimshaw, 1987). Intersectional analyses challenge us to interrogate those representations— to locate and uncover their origins and multiple meanings and examine the reasons for their existence and persistence. The dominant representations of people of color build on and elaborate stereotypes that become the rationale for the differential treatment of groups and individuals (Arcia, Skinner, Bailey, and Correa, 2001;

Portes, 2000). In the case of Latinas, stereotypes that all Latinas are immigrants, do not speak English, cannot concisely articulate their symptoms, have too many children, and have come to the United States to get government handouts affect not only the ways dominant-culture providers treat their Latina patients but the kinds of public policies that are designed to determine their access to health care (Hernandez and Charney, 1998; Lillie-Blanton and Hudman, 2001; Perez, 2000; Reyes, 2001).[3] Language and culture are key aspects of representation. They intersect with socioeconomic status (SES), occupation, education, and positions of power and privilege to shape the perceptions of Latinas and the receptivity of dominant-culture providers toward them.

Language and culture are important factors in understanding health disparities to the extent that Latinas with low education and income levels are less likely to have access to health care services and the kind of assistance that facilitates full communication with their provider. These and other factors contribute to their being viewed as a subordinate group by public health systems (Zambrana, 2001). Data on English-language proficiency and citizenship status reveal that 75 percent of Latinos and Latinas speak English well to very well and that only 39 percent of Latinos are immigrants, with about half of those residing in the country for more than ten years (Lillie-Blanton and Hudman, 2001; Perez, 2000). Intersectional analyses argue that understanding the origins of these differences, as well as the multiple and simultaneous factors that contribute to them by Latino subgroup, is a vital step toward reducing disparities.

COMPLICATING IDENTITY

Intersectional analyses make us aware that both individual and group identity are complex—influenced and shaped not simply by a person's race, class, ethnicity, gender, physical ability, or nationality but by the confluence of all of those characteristics. Nevertheless, in a hierarchically organized society, some statuses become more important than others at any given historical moment and in specific geographical locations (King, 1995). Within groups, there is far greater diversity than appears when, for analytical purposes, people are classified with a single term. The term *Latina*—as a gendered, ethnic, and racial construct—is interconnected with multiple discourses on social stratification and political national identity. Its meaning varies depending on the social context in which it is employed and the political meanings associated with its usage. The term *Latino/Latina* emerged as a direct counterpoint to *Hispanic*. It challenged the privileging of Spanish or Hispano lineage over the other indigenous and African lineages of the Spanish-speaking individuals in the United States. The renaming was imperative as it centered the multiple roots of Latino and Latina cultural identity, and the dialogue surrounding this issue raised awareness of the multiple lineages and histories of Spanish-speaking people in the United States, particularly the historically underrepresented groups and more recent Caribbean immigrants. As Echazabal-Martinez (1998, p. 21) noted, "Mestizaje, the process of interracial and/or intercultural mixing, is a foundational theme in the Americas, particularly those areas colonized by the Spanish and Portuguese. Mestizaje underscored the affirmation of cultural identity as constituted by national character."

In the United States, Latinos have historically been classified as whites, although they have resisted racial categorization. The discourse on mixed race is constitutive of ethnic identity, although in Spanish-speaking countries, white-race Latinos have access to more economic and social capital than individuals of mixed or black race. Thus, whiteness continues in Latin America, as in the United States, to remain at the top of the economic and political hierarchy. Since the 1980s, Latinos have been provided the opportunity to identify both ethnic and racial category in census reporting, but the resistance continues. In the 2000 Census, 48 percent of Latinos described themselves as white, 2 percent as blacks, 6 percent as mixed, and 42 percent as "other." The resistance to racial categorization obscures the fact that Latinos have been historically perceived as people of color and thus have been economically and socially marginalized. The debate continues around the pressure to classify individuals based on race that is unique to the national character of the United States.

The reconstruction of racial and ethnic Latino and Latina identity as a discourse on national identity is subverted in the hegemonic currents of the black/white binary in the United States and the "Eurocentric glorification of a cultural sameness, of similarity in identity" (Echazabal-Martinez, 1998, p. 23). Furthermore, as

Duany (1998) argues, Caribbean immigrants and migrants confront a two-tiered division of racialized identity in the United States between whites and nonwhites derived from the rule of hypodescent—the assignment of the offspring of mixed races to the subordinate group. He states, "Caribbean societies tend to be stratified in terms of both class status and color gradations. Phenotype and social status rather than biological descent define a person's racial identity, especially in the Spanish-speaking countries" (p. 148). Therefore the reconstruction of one's racial and social status and cultural identity by the host society can generate significant social and psychological tensions within and across these groups.

As a result, Latino/Latina as a social construct needs to be problematized because its underlying political discourse is not understood by those self-identified Hispanics (who prefer to acknowledge only their Spanish roots) and is even less understood by health researchers who prefer neat categories for analyses of what is now perceived as the Latino or brown race. Thus, homogenizing all Latinos and Latinas into one category forecloses the discourse on national identity and overlooks the effects of the intersection of race, ethnic subgroup, and socioeconomic status on Latina health.[4]

Identity for Latinas is complicated by differences in national origin, citizenship, and class (within both the sending and host countries), as well as race and ethnicity. An intersectional approach necessitates acknowledging these differences and seeks to reveal and understand these differences. For example, the health of Latinos has been reported generally as an aggregate without much attention to ethnic subgroup or gender, and race has been completely omitted. The generalized view that all Latinos as an ethnic/cultural group are healthy—that is, the Hispanic epidemiological paradox—has kept Latinos as a group outside the debates on health disparities (De la Rosa, 2002; Franzini, Ribble, and Keddie, 2001; Fuentes-Afflick, Hessol, and Perez-Stable, 1999; Hunt and others, 2002; Palloni and Arias, 2003).

From an intersectional perspective, culture is considered only one of the multiple dimensions that shape health outcomes, and its influence is considered in the context of historical, economic, political, structural, and representational factors. When data have shown favorable or adverse health status for Latinas, cultural attributes are identified as causal factors. In the study of health outcomes, the Latino group becomes homogenized into a political category that is associated with a specific racial phenotype, economic status, and cultural attributes. Consequently, when public health researchers adopt Latinos as a political category for study, ignoring the group's heterogeneity, they inadvertently reinforce a cultural deficit model or the paradoxical finding of the poor as healthy. Using the term *Latina* as a political category impedes the accurate measurement of structural and political factors such as institutional racism, and the data serve only a limited purpose in advancing knowledge on health disparities within and across Latina subgroups.

DATA SOURCES AND LIMITATIONS

Available health data provide a glimpse of the status of Latino women's health in the United States, although trend data are not available in most cases. Data collection in all states and the District of Columbia did not occur until 1997 for Latinos. Difficulties in interpretation of the data remain, due to limited analyses by subgroup, gender, and socioeconomic status (see Zambrana and Carter-Pokras, 2001; Rodriguez, 2000). There are significant differences among Latinos associated with modes of historical incorporation, race, socioeconomic status, and place of residence. For example, available data for Puerto Rican women show that they have the least favorable health indicators, such as self-assessed health status and infant mortality rates, compared to other Latina subgroups and non-Hispanic white women (Hajat, Lucas, and Kington, 2000; Carter-Pokras and Zambrana, 2001). Multiracial Latina subgroups such as Puerto Ricans that experience poorer health outcomes illustrate the intersectional effects of racial and ethnic status on health disparities in the United States (Landale, Oropesa, Llanes, and Gorman, 1999). For example, while the infant mortality rate for all Latinos is 5.7 per 1,000 live births, the rates range from a low of 4.7 per 1,000 among Cuban Americans to a high of 8.3 per 1,000 among Puerto Ricans (National Center for Health Statistics, 2002).

Notably, recent national surveys collect data only on Mexican Americans and were administered only in English until the year 2000. Hence, the opportunity to understand the health status of approximately 40 percent of Latinas has been missed. Data may not be representative of the experiences of specific Latina groups, including immigrants and non-English-speaking citizens, low-income groups who reside in rural areas, migrant farm workers (of whom Latinos comprise nearly 80 percent), *colonia* residents living in the unincorporated areas along the 2,000-mile U.S.-Mexican border (which often lack sewers and running water) (Azevedo and Ochoa Bogue, 2002), and inner-city residents of distressed neighborhoods. Furthermore, data on Puerto Rican women who reside on the island of Puerto Rico are not readily available for national comparisons. Although most data in this chapter are presented as an aggregate, it is important to understand that in population-based and national studies, disaggregation reveals different health disparities for each group.

SOCIAL, EDUCATIONAL, AND ECONOMIC CORRELATES OF LATINA HEALTH

More than 90 percent of the Latino population lives in urban areas, and nearly 46 percent of those urban residents live in the central cities of metropolitan areas. Nearly 75 percent of all Latinos live in either the South (33 percent) or the West (44 percent), with one in three Latinos living in California. In 1990, California had 50 percent of the Mexican-descent population and more than one-third of the Central and South American population (Reyes, 2001). These geographical data reflect the historical, political, and economic position of Latinas in the United States. Table 7.1 presents selected sociodemographic and access variables by gender, race, and ethnicity. Latinas are a relatively young population, with close to 50 percent in the age range of fifteen to forty-four. Twenty percent of Mexican females, 17.6 percent of Puerto Rican females, and 9.3 percent of Cuban females are under age fifteen, while 5 percent of Mexican females, 7.2 percent of Puerto Rican females, and 23.6 percent of Cuban females are older than age sixty-five. Mexican American and Puerto Rican women are the least likely to have completed high school and college and the most likely to be unemployed, compared to Cubans and other racial and ethnic groups (U.S. Census Bureau, 2001).

Low educational attainment is associated with limited financial resources, barriers to improved employment opportunities, and

TABLE 7.1. SOCIODEMOGRAPHIC DATA ON WOMEN IN THE UNITED STATES

	Total Latinos	Mexican Americans	Puerto Ricans	Cuban Americans	African Americans	Non-Hispanic Whites
Total women (in thousands)	16,369	10,582	1,496	669	18,927	98,584
Percentage of total population	11.7	7.5	1.1	0.47	13.5	70.3
Age distribution of group						
Under 5 years old	11	12.7	8.5	6	8	5.9
5–14 years old	18.9	20.1	17.6	9.3	17.2	12.7
15–44 years old	48.7	49.3	48.7	37.9	47.2	41.6
45–64 years old	15	12.9	18	23.2	18.9	24.1
65 years old and over	6.3	5	7.2	23.6	8.8	7.8
Educational attainment, persons 25 years old and over						
Percentage high school graduates or higher	57.5	51.8	65.5	70.9	78.3	88.4
Percentage bachelor's or higher	10.6	7.1	12.3	21.8	16.7	25.5
Labor force status, civilians 16 years and over						
Percentage in labor force	38.7	36.1	42.9	41.1	41.7	48.7
Unemployment rate						
Male	7.7	6.1	8	6.7	3.8	3.6
Female	6.2	8.5	8.3	4.6	3.3	3.3
Access factors (both sexes)						
Percentage uninsured	32	39	19	21	18.4	12.9
Percentage without usual source of care	21	25	14	14	14	11

Source: Mills (2000); U.S. Census Bureau (Mar. 2000).

low rates of intergenerational upward mobility. In 1999, a quarter of Latinas had incomes below the poverty line, including 29 percent of Puerto Rican females and 26 percent of Mexican American females. In 2000, 17 percent of Latinas earned at least $35,000, compared to 33 percent of white women. Only 26 percent of non-Latino female-headed families had incomes below the federal poverty level, compared to 47 percent of Puerto Rican, 38 percent of Mexican, and 34 percent of Cuban female-headed households (Therrien and Ramirez, 2001).

Socioeconomic status is strongly linked with access to health insurance and health care services (American College of Physicians, 2000; Brown and others, 1996). Compared to white females (12.9 percent) and black females (18.4 percent), Latinas (32 percent) are the least likely to have health insurance (Collins, Hall, and Neuhaus, 1999). With data disaggregated by subgroup, 39 percent of Mexican Americans are uninsured, compared to 19 percent of Puerto Ricans and 21 percent of Cubans (National Center for Health Statistics, 2001). Lack of health insurance is in part accounted for by structural factors, such as the greater likelihood of Latinas having less education than non-Latinas, being employed in industries that do not provide health benefits, and having a partner who works in a similar employment sector (Commonwealth Fund, 2000; Schur and Feldman, 2001).

As groups with a high risk of experiencing access problems and barriers to care, both Latinas and uninsured women were the least likely to have had a doctor visit in the past year (31 percent and 24 percent, respectively) (Brown, Ojeda, Wyn, and Levan, 2000). Disaggregated by subgroup, Puerto Ricans and Cuban Americans have health care use rates comparable to whites, while Mexican American women have rates lower than whites (Office of Research on Women's Health, 2002). Interestingly, Puerto Rican women have access to health care equal to whites and more access than Mexican-origin groups, yet they have more adverse health outcomes. Social conditions such as high rates of unemployment and higher likelihood of concentration in inner-city neighborhoods, combined with being a racialized group, lead to poorer health status. These social conditions contribute to increased health risk and are compounded by limited access to quality health care. For example, institutional racism in the form of discriminatory practices by health providers, such as not making screening referrals or ensuring follow-up for a detected condition, may disproportionately and negatively affect the health status of Puerto Ricans. Their identity as a mixed-race, ethnic, and low-income group intersects with racialized structural and political factors to suggest why Puerto Ricans may experience less favorable health status when compared to whites and other Latinas. Among Mexican American and Puerto Rican women, who are disproportionately represented among the poor and near poor, the combined stresses of poverty and its attendant social conditions—lack of health insurance and poor quality of care for themselves and their children—represent significant precursors to poor health outcomes (Commonwealth Fund, 2000; Dalakar and Proctor, 2000; Office of Research on Women's Health, 2002).

HEALTH STATUS AND BEHAVIOR PROFILE

Health is broadly defined as a sense of well-being and freedom from disease and discomfort. Research on Latina health and disease has been sparse except for a disproportionate number of studies on pregnancy and pregnancy outcome. Of note is Giachello's observation (2001) that much reproductive health research has omitted representational and structural factors such as the effects of racial, ethnic, and gender biases of providers on outcomes. It has instead reinforced representational biases by focusing on high fertility, young age, and cultural explanations positing the beneficial effect of foreign-born status on Latina pregnancy outcomes, with the resultant epidemiological paradox. In effect, research on the factors that influence Latina women's health status at different developmental ages is almost nonexistent. Giachello (p. 12) notes the gaps in research on Latina health: "There is a need to study biological, behavioral, environmental and social processes, including community norms, that determine the physical, emotional and cognitive growth of Latinas from the moment of inception and through transitions of infancy, childhood and adolescence, which set the foundation for conditions, diseases, and behaviors that impact human reproduction and ultimately lead to disparities."

The following section draws on more recent information on health status, health behaviors, and chronic conditions among Latinas by age. Integrated in this section is work on adolescent Latino females that provides both retrospective and prospective insight into how health behaviors at a younger age may contribute to health behaviors and the presence of chronic conditions at later developmental stages. These data represent some preliminary baseline estimates, as they are derived from multiple data sources. The differences by race and ethnicity do not all appear to be significant. Yet for Latinas, issues regarding literacy in understanding survey questions, trust of interviewers, and limited knowledge of a medical condition may also bias study results due to underreporting of conditions. Thus, methodological issues related to the quality of the data and their representativeness warrant caution and limit our ability to interpret with confidence. These limitations strongly reflect the lack of progress concerning information on Latina health and the need for more rigorous data collection methods.

Figure 7.1 displays differences in health status by gender, race, and ethnicity. Latinas are the most likely to report fair or poor health (29 percent), including 27 percent of Puerto Ricans and 13 percent of Cubans, while African American women are the most likely to report a health condition that limited their activity (16 percent) (Henry J. Kaiser Family Foundation, 2001; National Center for Health Statistics, 2002). It is noteworthy that Latinas are less likely to report a chronic condition requiring ongoing medical care (19 percent) and taking prescription drugs regularly (33 percent). These data suggest that Latinas, who are the least likely to be insured and to have seen a doctor in the past year, may not be aware of existing medical conditions that contribute to their reported fair or poor health status. In addition, it appears that Latinas may be either self-medicating in order to manage their health conditions or experiencing psychosocial distress that affects their perceived health status.

The Latina respondents in this study were predominantly low-income Mexican-origin women who were simply categorized as Latina. Although on the surface supporting the epidemiological paradox that Latinas or Mexican-origin women are a healthy group in spite of their low socioeconomic status, these data may also suggest undetected chronic health conditions among Mexican American women. The "poor as healthy" paradox for Latinas is an artifact of aggregated data and further reflects a large body of literature that focuses on healthy, young, reproductive-age

FIGURE 7.1. DIFFERENCES IN HEALTH STATUS BY RACE/ETHNICITY:
WOMEN AGES EIGHTEEN TO SIXTY-FOUR

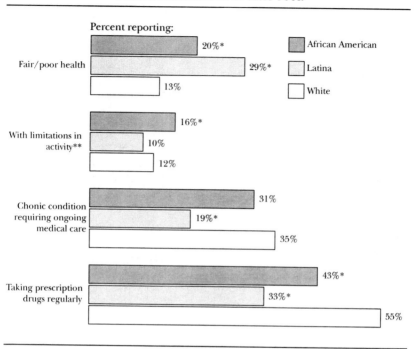

Note: *Significantly different from the reference group (white women) at $p < .05$.

**Limitations in activity were due to a disability, handicap, or chronic disease that kept respondents from participating fully in school, work, housework, or other activities.

Source: The Henry J. Kaiser Family Foundation (2001).

Mexican-origin women. Needed instead are rigorous studies of structural and political factors such as quality of care and its relationship to undiagnosed and misdiagnosed health conditions among Latinas of different ages and subgroups. The uncritical approach taken by many investigators promulgates the myth of health among Latinas, which is challenged by recent data on chronic conditions by subgroup.[5]

Table 7.2 presents data on selected health behaviors and chronic conditions for women by race and ethnicity. Urban and rural-dwelling Latinas, forty years old and older, report low rates of participation in moderate physical activity (Wilcox and others,

TABLE 7.2. Health Status and Health Behaviors Data on Women in the United States

	Total Latinos	Mexican Americans	Puerto Ricans	Cuban Americans	African Americans	Non-Hispanic Whites
Behaviors						
Moderate physical activity						
Adolescents	16.7%	—	—	—	17.8%	25.8%
Urban dwelling, ages 40 and older	11.6	—	—	—	7.5	11.9
Rural dwelling, ages 40 and older	20.7	—	—	—	4.7	7.8
Overweight	56.8	48	40	32	64.5	43
Current tobacco use	13.7	12.2	20.7	11.6	22.8	25.2
Frequent alcohol consumption (ages 18–44)	23.0	—	—	—	15.9	30.8
Mental health						
Moderate to severe depressive symptoms in the past week (ages 18 and older)	53	—	—	—	47	37

Screening Behaviors						
Mammogram within the past 2 years (40 years or older) and past 3 years (35 years and older)	67.0 46.0	54.0	43.0	41.0	72.9	71.4
Pap test in the past year and past 3 years	63.0 77.0	80.0	77.0	73.0	73.0	64.0
Blood pressure test in the past year	54.0	—	—	—	64.0	58.0
Physical in the past year	74.0	—	—	—	82.0	80.0
Chronic Condition						
Arthritis	33	—	—	—	40	32
Asthma	9	—	15.95	—	10	11
High serum cholesterol levels	—	17.7	23.0	17.0	19.9	20.7
Hypertension (20 and older)	—	22.3	17.6	13.6	36.4	19.7
Cardiovascular disease	26.9	—	—	—	29.4	31.0

(Continued)

TABLE 7.2. HEALTH STATUS AND HEALTH BEHAVIORS DATA ON WOMEN IN THE UNITED STATES

Whites	Total Latinos	Mexican Americans	Puerto Ricans	Cuban Americans	African Americans	Non-Hispanic Americans
Cancer, all sites, 1998, new cases per 100,000 population	284.8				390.8	438.1
Diabetes	17	—	—	—	16	9
Osteoporosis	12	—	—	—	10	21
AIDS case rate	19.7	—	—	—	57.7	21.7

Sources: Blackman, Eddas, and Miller (1999); Brown and others (1996); Centers for Disease Control and Prevention (2000); Collins, Hall, and Neuhaus (1999); Collins and others (1999); Crespo, Loria, and Burt (1996); Division of STD Prevention (2000); Hajat, Lucas, and Kington (2000); Henry J. Kaiser Family Foundation (2001); National Center for Health Statistics (2001, 2002); National Coalition of Hispanic Health and Human Services Organization (1996); Office of Research on Women's Health (2002); Wilcox and others (2000); Zambrana, Breen, Fox, and Gutierrez-Mohamed (1999).

2000). Other data show that almost 60 percent of Latinas and black women were sedentary, compared to 40 percent of white women (National Center for Health Statistics, 2002). Examining body weight, 48 percent of Mexican American females were overweight, compared to 40 percent of Puerto Rican women and 32 percent of Cuban women (Brown, Ojeda, Wyn, and Levan, 1996). Based on 1997 data, these rates are lower than those of black women (65 percent) and similar to those of white women (43 percent) (Office of Research on Women's Health, 2002; National Center for Health Statistics, 1997). Latino immigrants who have lived in the United States for more than fifteen years are more likely to be obese (35 percent) than Latino immigrants who have lived in the United States for less than fifteen years (25 percent) (Brown, Ojeda, Wyn, and Levan, 1996). Physical inactivity and being overweight are directly linked to medical conditions such as diabetes and cardiovascular disease. Little research has been conducted with Latinas regarding these risk factors and linked medical conditions.

We observe similar patterns of health behaviors by age among Latinas. Young Latinas are also more likely to be overweight and less likely to engage in physical activity than white girls (Kann and others, 2000; National Alliance for Hispanic Health, 2000). Not unexpectedly, among all racial and ethnic groups, an inverse relation between income and obesity is observed; that is, as personal incomes rise above the poverty level, obesity levels decrease (Office of Research on Women's Health, 2002). Health-promoting behaviors are closely linked to economic assets, safe environmental spaces, and early-age onset of chronic conditions.

Other health behaviors associated with health outcome include tobacco and alcohol use. Latinas are less likely to smoke than other racial/ethnic women. However, among Latina subgroups, Cuban women are less likely to be current smokers (11.6 percent) than either Puerto Rican women (20.7 percent) or Mexican American women (12.2 percent), but if they smoke, they are more likely to be heavy smokers (10 percent) than Puerto Rican women (7 percent) or Mexican American women (4 percent) (Hajat, Lucas, and Kington, 2000; Office of Research on Women's Health, 2002; Office of the Surgeon General, 2001). In contrast, Latinas aged eighteen to forty-four are more likely to consume alcohol than black women but less likely than white women (National Center for Health Statistics, 2001). Latina adolescents are more likely than black adolescents in the same age group to report having tried cigarette smoking and having drunk alcohol or driven with someone who had been drinking (Kann and others, 2000). Trend data suggest that patterns of risk behavior are increasing for Latina adolescents, and these health behaviors may influence their adult health status and onset of chronic conditions (National Center for Chronic Disease Prevention and Health Promotion, 2000). These risk behaviors may be associated with unfavorable health and mental health outcomes for Latinas (National Alliance for Hispanic Health, 2000).

Indicators of mental health for Latinas by developmental life stage and place of birth represent serious concerns as they are closely associated with health status and outcome. Among women ages eighteen and older, Latinas are more likely to report having experienced moderate to severe depressive symptoms in the past week (53 percent) than both African American women and white women (47 percent and 37 percent, respectively) (Collins, Hall, and Neuhaus, 1999). Latinas are more likely (24 percent) than whites (22 percent) and blacks (16 percent) to report depression in their lifetime (Rouse, 1995). However, low-income Latinas (17 percent) are less likely than low-income black women (36 percent) and low-income white women (58 percent) to report a mental health care visit (Alvidrez, 1999). Being born in the United States is associated with elevated risk for mental health problems. This perhaps occurs because the distress caused by low socioeconomic status, racism, and a subordinate position in the United States is greater without the experience of the low standard of living in another country to which to compare it (Golding and Burnam, 1990). It may also be the case that second-generation Caribbean and Latino immigrants, depending on their level of education and class status, are more likely to withstand the process of racialization in the United States and how it affects them or have a stronger sense of self-confidence that buffers the psychological impact of racism. In contrast, devaluing of a second-generation individual's culture and severe experiences with racism and discrimination can seriously affect that person's self-esteem. Variations in social and economic resources, strength of ethnic ties to parental generation, and experiences of discrimination are associated with racial/ethnic identity and mental well-being (see Chapter Six, this volume). Mexican American adolescents and adults living in the United States have higher rates of depressive symptoms, illicit drug use, and suicidal ideation than Mexican immigrants (Burnam and others, 1987). Latino girls have higher rates of attempted suicide than any other racial or ethnic group (National Alliance for Hispanic Health, 2000). High levels of economic, environmental, and interpersonal stress are most likely linked to the high level of psychosocial distress reported by Latina women and adolescents (U.S. Department of Health and Human Services, 1999; Schulz, Parker, Israel, and Fisher, 2001). These factors might be associated with less likelihood to engage in health-promoting and self-care behaviors among Latinas (Sanders-Phillips, 1996). Perceived social acceptance and receptivity of host society should be explored as possible predictors of service use, particularly preventive health services (Portes, 2000). Arcia, Skinner, Bailey, and Correa (2001) found that perceived social acceptance is a measure of perception, not of cultural behavior, and is therefore independent of language use, proficiency, and the cultural orientation of current or desired environments. Lack of social receptivity in the host society is a form of institutional discrimination and may influence individuals' choice of their degree of active participation in health behaviors, such as use of preventive screening.

Engaging in preventive health care behaviors is associated with being married, having a high school education, and having higher rates of screening behaviors (Collins and others, 1999; Zambrana, Breen, Fox, and Gutierrez-Mohamed, 1999). Consistent with prior studies, data in the lower panel of Table 7.2 show that Latinas are less likely to have had any screening tests, including blood pressure check and annual physical, compared to other racial/ethnic groups. Based on 1997 age-adjusted data, 67 percent of Latinas reported having a mammogram in the past two years, compared to 71.4 percent of white women and 72.9 percent of African American women (Blackman, Eddas, and Miller, 1999). For Pap smears, 63 percent of Latinas reported having one in the past year, compared to 64 percent of whites and 73 percent of blacks (Collins and others, 1999; Office of Research on Women's Health, 2002).

Yet these national screening rates may not represent actual screening practices of poor and limited English-language-proficiency Latinas. Lower screening rates among low-income Latinas in inner-city and rural areas are consistent with observations and experiences of providers and community-based organizations in those areas. Low rates of preventive screening behaviors are associated with low socioeconomic status, discriminatory provider attitudes, low literacy skills, and the often-attendant psychosocial distress (Brown and others, 1996; Zambrana, Breen, Fox, and Gutierrez-Mohamed, 1999). The intersection of these dimensions with structural factors such as limited access to health care and poor-quality health services limits opportunities for screening, early detection, and management of chronic medical conditions. We hypothesize that undiscovered health disparities among Latinas are strongly associated with quality of care as mediated by the doctor-patient relationship. Health disparities have been found to be associated with factors such as patients' perceived discrimination and mistrust of the health care system; representational factors (SES and racism) that contribute to poor or ineffective communication between patient and physician and health care clinicians' lack of cultural competence and sensitivity; and structural and political factors, such as access to care and poor-quality care (Smedley, Stith, and Nelson, 2003).

CHRONIC ILLNESS CONDITIONS BY GENDER, RACE, AND ETHNICITY

Table 7.2 displays selected chronic conditions by gender, race, and ethnicity. Latinas report slightly higher rates of arthritis, asthma, diabetes, and osteoporosis than do white women (Henry J. Kaiser Family Foundation, 2001). Although limited information is available on antecedents of chronic conditions and consequences in terms of quality of life among Latinas with chronic health conditions, it is known that Latinas are less likely to use health care services and to know when they have a chronic condition. The National Health and Nutrition Examination Survey found that 38 percent of Mexican Americans with diabetes were not previously aware that they had diabetes, compared to 33 percent of whites. Mexican American women (22.3 percent) are the Latino subgroup most likely to have high blood pressure, with higher rates than white women (19.7 percent) but lower rates than black women (36.4 percent) (National Center for Health Statistics, 2001). Latinas

(54 percent) were less likely than African American women (64 percent) or white women (58 percent) to have had their blood pressure checked in the previous year (Brown and others, 1996). Twenty-two percent of Mexican American women had hypertension, compared to 18 percent of Puerto Rican women and 14 percent of Cuban women (Crespo, Loria, and Burt, 1996). Although more than 95 percent of hypertensive Latinas knew of their condition, only 86 percent of Mexican American and Puerto Rican and 79 percent of Cuban women reported receiving necessary treatment. Of those who received treatment, only 44 percent of Mexican American, 42 percent of Puerto Rican, and 30 percent of Cuban women had their hypertension under control (Pappas, Gergen, and Carroll, 1990).

Although Latinas are reported to have low rates of cancer overall, the incidence of cervical cancer is almost one and a half times greater than the rate for white women (Wingo and others, 1998). Fewer Latinas are diagnosed with breast cancer than white women, but Latinas are more likely to be diagnosed at a more advanced stage and are therefore more likely to die from breast cancer. More Central and South Americans, Mexican Americans, and Puerto Ricans had tumors larger than 1 centimeter than did white women, which Heeden and White (2001) explained by the lower rates of mammography screening in the Latino population.

Latinas represent 12 percent of the U.S. female population but account for 20 percent of all reported AIDS cases (Centers for Disease Control and Prevention, 1998, 1999). Latinas predominantly contract HIV through heterosexual contact (47 percent), followed by intravenous drug use (40 percent), while intravenous drug use was the predominant mode of transmission for whites (42 percent) and blacks (41 percent) (Centers for Disease Control and Prevention, 2000). Among Latinas, Puerto Rican women report the most cases of HIV infection and AIDS (Zambrana, Cornelius, Boykin, and Salas Lopez, 2004). Explanations for the higher rate of AIDS among Puerto Rican women are that they tend to partner or marry largely within the subgroup, which contributes to the heterosexual spread of HIV/AIDS, and when they use intravenous drugs, they tend to do so within the context of needle-sharing networks that are racially and ethnically homogenous (Office of Research on Women's Health, 2002).

Disproportionate morbidity among Latinas from diabetes, HIV/AIDS, and cervical and breast cancer and high morbidity among Puerto Rican women due to high rates of serum cholesterol and asthma illustrate the intersection of race/ethnicity, poverty, gender, and institutional context (Delgado and Trevino, 1985; Ledogar and others, 2000). While access to quality health care, including detection and treatment, is crucial and undoubtedly plays a role in excess mortality, the excess morbidity is a function of the physical and psychological stressors related to economic and neighborhood conditions. In effect, the inequity in social conditions contributes to disparate risk of becoming ill, which is then compounded by disparate access to health care—including both screening and diagnosis, and treatment—once a person becomes ill.

Quality of Care: Medical Mistrust, Medical Errors, and Unequal Treatment

The quality of the institution-provider and patient relationship, particularly the content and tone of the communication, is strongly associated with continuity of care, management of care, and quality of life for the patient (Ashton and others, 2003). Women rely on their health care providers to answer their questions during a consultation that can have important effects on their adherence to treatment regimens and alleviate their apprehensions regarding emerging health conditions or secondary conditions or comorbidities. A study found that 34 percent of Latinas surveyed reported concerns about quality of care received, while only 20 percent of white women and 24 percent of African American women reported such concerns (Henry J. Kaiser Family Foundation, 2001). Although few women (10 percent) reported that their doctors did not take the time to answer their questions fully, Latinas (14 percent) were more likely than African American (8 percent) or white women (9 percent) not to have all their questions fully answered. These concerns may be related to language and literacy barriers and cultural expectations that the expert is not to be questioned. In addition to reporting that their questions were not fully answered, 17 percent of women reported that in the past two years, they had not understood or remembered information they received from their provider during a visit. Latinas (20 percent) were significantly more likely than African American women (14 percent) to have left a doctor's office without understanding or remembering their doctor's instructions (Henry J. Kaiser Family Foundation, 2001).

Although data are not available on the level of trust that Latina patients have in their providers and the institutions in which they receive health care services, trust is based on perceived competence, compassion, privacy and confidentiality, reliability and dependability, and communication (Pearson and Raeke, 2000). Reported barriers to health care by Latinos in general would suggest that trust is a central concern among Latinas. These data imply that Latinas are concerned about quality of care, questions left unanswered, and instructions not understood. Thus, low-income Latinas, who are less likely to challenge their providers or to have the language and literacy skills or health knowledge to explain their medical history and symptoms succinctly, may experience increased anxiety, less ability to comply with regimen, greater likelihood of incurring medical errors, and, in turn, less favorable health outcomes. To further our understanding of health disparities by gender and Latino ethnicity, factors such as institutional forms of racism, medical errors, and medical mistrust require inclusion and ethnic-specific measurement in future studies, supplementing the few studies identified by the Institute of Medicine report *Unequal Treatment* (Smedley, Stith, and Nelson, 2003).

IMPLICATIONS FOR INTERVENTIONS AND RESEARCH: AN ONGOING DIALOGUE

Disparities in Latino women's health are invariably connected to and affected by SES, race, ethnicity, and access to quality community-based institutional resources that are gender and family supportive. Two levels of interventions are required and have been consistently reported as ways to decrease disparities. First is improving social conditions by providing a living wage, universal health insurance, and quality health and human service resources in neighborhoods, which would decrease economic and social inequality. A second level of interventions involves structural and institutional changes, such as securing collaborative partnerships of public health institutions with the communities that they serve, increasing sociocultural competence of providers who are predominantly non-Latino and deliver health care to Latinos and Latinas, increasing financial opportunities for the education and training of underrepresented Latino subgroups, and implementing and enforcing antidiscriminatory health practices (Grantmakers in Health, 2000; U.S. Department of Health and Human Services and Grantmakers in Health, 1998). Both levels of intervention are imperative and only together can reduce disparities in health outcome for low-income, racial/ethnic women.

Attention to equity in the provision of health care services involves the design and delivery of services that are community based and at a literacy and language level consistent with the voiced and documented needs of low-income Latino women. Construing universalism as equity rather than advancing knowledge and policy on health disparities simply reinforces our current patterns of unequal distribution of resources and racial and ethnic disparities. At the institutional level, equity involves efforts to improve the core knowledge and skills of institutional providers with respect to socioeconomic, racial and ethnic, and cultural competence, with a particular emphasis on the importance of treating patients with equality and respect.

For the past three decades, the emphasis on the importance of training members of historically underrepresented Latino and African groups has been unrealized (Sullivan Commission, 2004). As noted in the Sullivan report, "The fact that the nation's health professions have not kept up with the changing demographics may be an even greater cause of disparities in health access and outcomes than the persistent lack of health insurance for tens of millions of Americans" (2004, p. 1). Increasing financial resources for the education and training of underrepresented racial/ethnic (African American, Mexican American, Puerto Rican, and Native American) health care professionals, physicians, nurses, and other allied health professionals who are more likely to serve their own community is key to improving quality of services and eliminating health disparities (U.S. Department of Health and Human Services, 1998, 2000; Zambrana, 1996; Boykin and others, 2003).

Existing health disparities are associated with discriminatory practices within the health care system. Consequently, antidiscrimination procedures must be clarified, monitored, and enforced at the state and local governmental levels to prevent the illegal diversion of eligible low-income Latino women from health insurance programs and services. Health care providers receiving state and federal funds must be monitored for racial profiling and other forms of discrimination so as to discourage and punish its occurrence. The responsibilities of service providers to patients with language barriers must also be clarified, monitored, and enforced in order to ensure access of limited-English-proficient individuals to health care services and programs. Extant knowledge confirms the detrimental effects of structural and institutional factors associated with health disparities among low-income Latino women. Yet effective remedies to eliminate these racial and ethnic disparities depend on a willingness to measure these nonmedical factors (social conditions and health care quality) in designing the next generation of research efforts.

RESEARCH DIRECTIONS

The next generation of research on Latino women's health requires contextualization within the economic and political realities of historically underserved and underrepresented Latino women's experiences in the United States. Such research is needed to obtain an accurate picture of the intersectionality of race, ethnicity, gender, culture, and socioeconomic status, taking into account both detrimental social conditions and discriminatory health care institutional practices (Smedley, Smith, and Nelson, 2003). A conceptual framework for understanding health disparities must part from prior assumptions so as to ensure that previously known associations and relationships are not reproduced as new knowledge—for example, the link between poverty and less favorable health outcomes or the Latino epidemiological paradox. Tautological arguments that overlook the racialized, gendered institutional inequities within public health systems contribute to stagnant theoretical approaches that fail to increase our knowledge of these groups. New conceptualizations must acknowledge the structural and political reality of poorly resourced institutions, particularly schools and health care facilities, in the urban, rural, and migrant communities where many Latinas live.

If data are to prove useful in improving quality of life and quality of care for Latino women, investigators must measure the quantity and quality of the services delivered by the public health infrastructure that serves the family and community (Smedley and Syme, 2000). Sufficient evidence suggests that low-income Mexican American and Puerto Rican women (with whom most studies have been conducted) have long reported extensive barriers to health care that have not changed substantially over three decades. Neglecting to acknowledge the links among race/ethnicity, family economic security, and health status and outcome propels a knowledge production process of disservice to our public health community and the subjects of study: low-income Latino women.

To accurately measure factors that contribute to health disparities among Latinas, the emerging intersectional approach must assess individual and institutional factors and the known consequences of poverty. This includes measures of level of education and income; continuous health insurance coverage with access to a comprehensive set of family-supportive public benefits, such as mental health, day care, and job development opportunities; as well as high-quality, community-based primary and preventive health services that are gender and family responsive. The research imperative is to look beyond the aggregate category of Latina and take into account the effects of individual demographic factors such as historical incorporation of Latina subgroups by region; SES; social conditions, such as community and neighborhood resources; institutional health care factors, such as medical errors, medical trust, and quality of care as measured by provider-patient communication; and the appropriateness of health care services provided.

Improving the quality of care available to Latinas requires transformation of governmental policies on research. The study of low-income Latinas requires a priority focus on key areas of disproportionate morbidity and mortality burden, including ambulatory-sensitive conditions, such as asthma and diabetes and other chronic conditions. Factors that are associated with the onset of these conditions and their effect on quality of life must be further explored to address the unique issues affecting Latinas by birthplace, race, socioeconomic status, and geographical location, including rural and border areas. In addition, intergenerational research is important, as the historic neglect of Latinas in research has left a void in our knowledge of family health patterns and conditions and community context that may help to explain some of the disparity in this group.

CONCLUSIONS

Some recent work represents a laudable improvement regarding information on Latinas (Aguirre-Molina and Molina, 2003; Aguirre-Molina, Molina, and Zambrana, 2001). These data are predominantly descriptive and may serve as a baseline for future comparative investigation. In contrast, past empirical inquiry may represent a less valuable source of health information as it has been conducted without taking into account important variables (noted throughout this chapter) in Latinas' lives that are associated with health outcomes. Concerns remain that available data may not be accurate indicators of morbidity, risk factors, and mortality among Latinas by subgroup, income, race, and ethnicity. Furthermore, data may not represent the health of Latinas due to misreporting or not reporting racial and ethnic identifiers and underreporting due to undiagnosed and misdiagnosed medical conditions of Latinas.

Yet many investigators persist in uncritically assuming that available data provide accurate information on Latinas. As scholars continue to debate the pathways of poverty, the value of racial and ethnic identifiers, and the indicators of unequal treatment, the economic divide between racial and ethnic underrepresented groups and majority groups widens, and the existing inequitable distribution of resources remains unchanged. Furthermore, the potentially fertile dialogue among social scientists and public health, clinical, and biomedical scholars remains stagnant. A shift of vision to a more interdisciplinary and intersectional lens that accounts for traditional inequities in our public systems can advance our knowledge on Latino women's health. Institutionalized knowledge production that has focused on either individual or group attributes has not permitted the public health community to build on the accumulated knowledge of the intersection of race, ethnicity, gender, SES, and institutional practices.

As Latinas, who represent a relatively young population, move through the developmental life cycle, it is unsettling to confront the stark fact that so little knowledge has been accumulated over the years on their health-promoting and health-debilitating resources and conditions. As Camarillo and Bonilla (2001, p. 131) observed, "Hispanics need to become an integral part of the movement to uncover the complex forces intensifying inequality, poverty, political passivity, exploitation, and social isolation, not only within their own ranks but in the United States as a whole." Unquestionably, the active involvement of Latino and Latina investigators who are committed and principled on issues of social inequality is essential to the production of knowledge on Latinas that can generate new and useful insights on health. The past decade has yielded a foundation for new work on Latina health (Aguirre-Molina and Molina, 2003). Its ability to compel new frameworks in future inquiry relies not only on increased representation of Latinos in health and medical fields but also on the national commitment to uncover with integrity "the complex forces intensifying [social] inequality" in the United States.

Notes

1. According to the 2000 Census, 70.3 percent of American women are non-Latino white, 13.5 percent are non-Latino African American/black, 11.7 percent are Latinas, and 5 percent are other (about 3 percent Asian/Pacific Islander, 1 percent American Indian/Alaskan Native, and 1 percent other) (U.S. Census Bureau, 2001). By the year 2050, Latinos are expected to constitute 25 percent of the U.S. population (Centers for Disease Control and Prevention, 1999).
2. Hereafter, non-Latino white will be referred to as white and non-Latino black will be referred to as African American or black.
3. For a more extended discussion of this issue in reference to Proposition 187 in California, see Dill, Baca Zinn, and Patton (1999) and Hondagneu-Sotelo (1996).
4. For an excellent historical account of the role of race and class and exclusionary racial practices in the United States and Latin American countries, see Rodriguez (2000).
5. See Carter-Pokras and Zambrana (2001) for a discussion of the epidemiological paradox and the reexamination of data for Mexican Americans from the San Antonio Heart Study.

References

Adler, N. E., and others. "Socioeconomic Inequalities in Health." *Journal of the American Medical Association*, 1993, *24*, 3140–3145.

Aguirre-Molina, M., and Molina, C. (eds.). *Latina Health in the United States.* San Francisco: Jossey-Bass, 2003.

Aguirre-Molina, M., and Pond, A.N.S. *Latino Access to Primary and Preventive Health Services: Barriers, Needs and Policy Implications.* New York: Columbia University Press, 2003.

Aguirre-Molina, M., Molina, C., and Zambrana, R. E. (eds). *Health Issues in the Latino Community.* San Francisco: Jossey-Bass, 2001.

Alvidrez, J. "Ethnic Variation in Mental Health Attitudes and Service Use Among Low-Income African American, Latina, and European Young Women." *Community Mental Health Journal,* 1999, *35*(6), 515–530.

American College of Physicians. *No Health Insurance? It's Enough to Make You Sick.* Philadelphia: American College of Physicians, 2000.

Arcia, E., Skinner, M., Bailey, D., and Correa, V. "Models of Acculturation and Health Behaviors Among Latino Immigrants to the U.S." *Social Science and Medicine,* 2001, *53*(1), 41–54.

Ashton, C. M., and others. "Racial and Ethnic Disparities in the Use of Health Services: Bias, Preferences, or Poor Communication?" *Journal of General Internal Medicine,* 2003, *18,* 146–152.

Azevedo, K., and Ochoa Bogue, H. "Health and Occupational Risks of Latinos Living in Rural America." In M. Aguirre-Molina, C. Molina, and R. E. Zambrana (eds.), *Health Issues in the Latino Community.* San Francisco: Jossey-Bass, 2002.

Blackman, D. K., Eddas, M. B., and Miller, D. S. "Trends in Self-Reported Use of Mammograms (1989–1997) and Papanicolaou Tests (1991–1997)— Behavioral Risk Factor Surveillance System." *Morbidity and Mortality Weekly Report,* Oct. 8, 1999, p. 11.

Bourdieu, P. "The Forms of Capital." In J. G. Richardson (ed.), *Handbook of Theory and Research for the Sociology of Education.* Westport, Conn.: Greenwood Press, 1985.

Boykin, S. D., and others. "Mentoring Underrepresented Minority Female Medical School Faculty: Momentum to Increase Retention and Promotion." *Journal of the Association for Academic Minority Physicians,* 2003, *14*(1), 15–18.

Brown, E. R., Ojeda, V. D., Wyn, R., and Levan, R. *Racial and Ethnic Disparities in Access to Health Insurance and Health Care.* Los Angeles: UCLA Center for Health Policy Research and Kaiser Family Foundation, Apr. 2000.

Brown, E. R., and others. *Women's Health Related Behaviors and Use of Clinical Preventive Services: A Report of the Commonwealth Fund.* Los Angeles: UCLA Center for Health Policy Research, 1996.

Burnam, M. A., and others. "Acculturation and Lifetime Prevalence of Psychiatric Disorders Among Mexican Americans in Los Angeles." *Journal of Health and Social Behavior,* 1987, *28,* 89–102.

Camarillo, A. M., and Bonilla, F. "Hispanics in a Multicultural Society: A New American Dilemma?" In N. J. Smelser, W. J. Wilson, and F. Mitchell (eds.), *America Becoming: Racial Trends and Their Consequences.* Washington, D.C.: National Academy Press, 2001.

Carter-Pokras, O., and Baquet, C. "What Is 'Health Disparity'?" *Public Health Reports,* 2002, *117,* 426–434.

Carter-Pokras, O., and Zambrana, R. E. "Latino Health Status." In M. Aguirre-Molina, C. Molina, and R. E. Zambrana (eds.), *Health Issues in the Latino Community.* San Francisco: Jossey-Bass, 2001.

Centers for Disease Control and Prevention. *HIV/AIDS Among Hispanics in the United States.* Atlanta: U.S. Department of Health and Human Services, 1998.

Centers for Disease Control and Prevention. *HIV/AIDS Surveillance Report: US HIV and AIDS Cases Reported Through June 1999.* Atlanta: U.S. Department of Health and Human Services, 1999.

Centers for Disease Control and Prevention. *HIV/AIDS Surveillance Report.* Atlanta: U.S. Department of Health and Human Services, 2000.

Chin, M. H., and Humikowski, C. A. "When Is Risk Stratification by Race or Ethnicity Justified in Medical Care?" *Academic Medicine,* 2002, *77*(3), 202–208.

Collins, K., Hall, A., and Neuhaus, C. *U.S. Minority Health: A Chartbook.* New York: Commonwealth Fund, 1999.

Collins, K., and others. *Health Concerns Across a Woman's Lifespan: The Commonwealth Fund 1998 Survey of Women's Health.* New York: Commonwealth Fund, 1999.

Commonwealth Fund. *Working Without Benefits: The Health Insurance Crisis Confronting Hispanic Americans.* New York: Commonwealth Fund, Mar. 2000.

Crenshaw, K. "Beyond Racism and Misogyny: Black Feminism and 2 Live Crew." In M. Matsuda, C. Lawrence, and K. Crenshaw (eds.), *Words That Wound.* Boulder, Colo.: Westview Press, 1993.

Crespo, C. J., Loria, C. M., and Burt, V. L. "Hypertension and Other Cardiovascular Disease Risk Factors Among Mexican Americans, Cuban Americans, and Puerto Ricans from the Hispanic Health and Nutrition Examination Survey." *Public Health Reports,* 1996, *111*(suppl. 2), 7–10.

Dalakar, J., and Proctor, B. D. *Poverty in the United States: 1999.* Washington, D.C.: U.S. Government Printing Office, 2000.

De la Rosa. "Perinatal Outcomes Among Mexican-Americans: A Review of an Epidemiological Paradox." *Ethnicity and Disease,* 2002, *12,* 480–487.

Delgado, J. L., and Trevino, F. M. "The State of Hispanic Health in the United States." In *The State of Hispanic America.* Oakland, Calif.: National Hispanic Center for Advanced Studies and Policy Analysis, 1985.

Dill, B. "Work at the Intersections of Race, Gender, Ethnicity and Other Dimensions of Identity in Higher Education." Unpublished report to the Ford Foundation, 2002.

Dill, B., Baca Zinn, M., and Patton, S. "Race, Family Values, and Welfare Reform." In L. Kushnick and J. Jennings (eds.), *A New Introduction to Poverty: The Role of Race, Power, and Politics.* New York: New York University Press, 1999.

Division of STD Prevention. *Sexually Transmitted Disease Surveillance, 1999.* Atlanta: Centers for Disease Control and Prevention, 2000. http://www.cdc.gov/nchstp/dstd/Stats_Trends/1999SurvRpt.

Duany, J. "Reconstructing Racial Identity: Ethnicity, Color, and Class Among Dominicans in the United States and Puerto Rico." *Latin American Perspectives,* 1998, *25*(3), 147–172.

Echazabal-Martinez, L. "*Mestizaje* and the Discourse of National/Cultural Identity in Latin America, 1845–1959." *Latin American Perspectives,* 1998, *25*(3), 21–42.

Ellen, I. G., and Turner, M. A. "Does Neighborhood Matter? Assessing Recent Evidence." *Housing Policy Debate,* 1997, *8*(4), 833–866.

Franzini, L., Ribble, J. C., and Keddie, A. M. "Understanding the Hispanic Paradox." *Ethnicity and Disease,* 2001, *11,* 496–518.

Fuentes-Afflick, E., Hessol, N. A., and Perez-Stable, E. J. "Testing the Epidemiologic Paradox of Low Birth Weight in Latinos." *Archives of Pediatric Adolescent Medicine,* 1999, *153,* 147–153.

Giachello, A. "The Reproductive Years—The Health of Latinas." In M. Aguirre-Molina, C. Molina, and R. E. Zambrana (eds.), *Health Issues in the Latino Community.* San Francisco: Jossey-Bass, 2001.

Golding, J. M., and Burnam, M. A. "Immigration, Stress, and Depressive Symptoms in a Mexican American Community." *Journal of Nervous Mental Disorders,* 1990, *178*(3), 161–171.

Grantmakers in Health. "Strategies for Reducing Racial and Ethnic Disparities in Health." Washington, D.C.: Grantmakers in Health, 2000.

Hajat, A., Lucas, J. B., and Kington, R. *Health Outcomes Among Hispanic Subgroups: United States, 1992–1995.* Hyattsville, Md.: National Center for Health Statistics, Feb. 2000.

Heeden, A. N., and White, E. "Breast Cancer Size and State in Hispanic American Women, by Birthplace: 1992–1995." *American Journal of Public Health,* 2001, *91*(1), 122–125.

Henry J. Kaiser Family Foundation. *Kaiser Women's Health Survey.* Washington, D.C.: Henry J. Kaiser Family Foundation, 2001.

Hernandez, D. J., and Charney, E. (eds.). *From Generation to Generation: The Health and Well-Being of Children in Immigrant Families.* Washington, D.C.: National Academy Press, 1998.

Hondagneu-Sotel, P. "Unpacking 187: Targeting Mexicans." In R. I. Rochin (ed.), *Immigration and Ethnic Communities: A Focus on Latinos.* East Lansing, Mich.: Julian Samora Research Institute, 1996.

hooks, b. *Black Looks: Race and Representation.* Boston: South End Press, 1992.

Hunt, K. J., and others. "All-Cause Mortality Among Diabetic Participants in the San Antonio Heart Study. Evidence Against the Hispanic Paradox." *Diabetes Care,* 2002, *25,* 1557–1563.

Kann, L., and others. "Youth Risk Behavior Surveillance—United States, 1999." *Morbidity and Mortality Weekly Report,* June 9, 2000, p. 49.

King, D. K. "Multiple Jeopardy, Multiple Consciousness: The Context of a Black Feminist Ideology." In B. Guy-Sheftall (ed.), *Words of Fire: An Anthology of African-American Feminist Thought.* New York: New Press, 1995.

Landale, N. S., Oropesa, R. S., Llanes, D., and Gorman, B. K. "Does Americanization Have Adverse Effects on Health? Stress, Health Habits, and Infant Health Outcomes Among Puerto Ricans." *Social Forces,* 1999, *78*(2), 613–642.

Ledogar, R. J., and others. "Asthma and Latino Cultures: Different Prevalence Reported Among Groups Sharing the Same Environment." *American Journal of Public Health,* 2000, *90*(6), 929–935.

Lillie-Blanton, M., and Hudman, J. "Untangling the Web: Race/Ethnicity, Immigration, and the Nation's Health." *American Journal of Public Health,* 2001, *91*(11), 1736–1739.

Mills, R. J. *Health Insurance Coverage 1999.* Washington, D.C.: U.S. Government Printing Office, 2000.

National Alliance for Hispanic Health. "The State of Hispanic Girls." Mar. 2000. http://www.hispanichealth.org.

National Center for Chronic Disease Prevention and Health Promotion. "Behavioral Risk Factor Surveillance System." 2000. http://apps.nccd.cdc.gov/brfss/race.asp?cat=WH&yr=2000&qkey=311&state=US.

National Center for Health Statistics. *National Health Interview Survey.* 1997. http://www.cdc.gov/nchs/nhis.htm.

National Center for Health Statistics. *Health, United States, 2001 with Urban and Rural Health Chartbook.* Hyattsville, Md.: U.S. Public Health Service, 2001. http://www.cdc.gov/nchs.

National Center for Health Statistics. *Health, United States, with Chartbook on Trends in the Health of Americans.* Hyattsville, Md.: U.S. Public Health Service, 2002. http://www.cdc.gov/nchs/nhis.htm.

Office of Research on Women's Health. *Women of Color Health Data Book.* Bethesda, Md.: National Institutes of Health, 2002.

Office of the Surgeon General. *Women and Smoking: A Report of the Surgeon General.* Rockville, Md.: U.S. Department of Health and Human Services, Public Health Service, 2001.

Palloni, A., and Arias, E. "A Re-Examination of the Hispanic Mortality Paradox." Working paper, Center for Demography and Ecology–University of Wisconsin, Jan. 2003.

Pappas, G., Gergen, P. J., and Carroll, M. "Hypertension Prevalence and the Status of Awareness, Treatment, and Control in the Hispanic Health and Nutrition Examination Survey (HHANES), 1982–1984." *American Journal of Public Health,* 1990, *80*(12), 1431–1436.

Pearson, S. D., and Raeke, L. "Patients' Trust in Physicians: Many Theories, Few Measures and Little Data." *Journal of General and Internal Medicine,* 2000, *15,* 509–513.

Perez, S. (ed.). *Moving Up the Economic Ladder: Latino Workers and the Nation's Future Prosperity: State of Hispanic America 1999.* Washington, D.C.: National Council of La Raza, 2000.

Portes, A. "The Two Meanings of Social Capital." *Sociological Forum,* 2000, *15*(1), 1–11.

Reyes, B. L. (ed.). *A Portrait of Race and Ethnicity in California: An Assessment of Social and Economic Well-Being.* San Francisco: Public Policy Institute, 2001.

Rodriguez, C. *Changing Race—Latinos, the Census and the History of Ethnicity in the United States.* New York: New York University Press, 2000.

Rouse, B. A. (ed.). *Substance Abuse and Mental Health Statistics Sourcebook.* Washington, D.C.: U.S. Government Printing Office, 1995.

Sanders-Phillips, K. "Correlates of Health Promotion Behaviors in Low-Income Black Women and Latinas." *American Journal of Preventive Medicine,* 1996, *12*(6), 450–458.

Schulz, A., Parker, E., Israel, B., and Fisher, T. "Social Context, Stressors, and Disparities in Women's Health." *Journal of the American Medical Women's Association,* 2001, *56*(4), 143–149.

Schur, C. L., and Feldman, J. *Running in Place: How Job Characteristics, Immigrant Status, and Family Structure Keep Hispanics Uninsured.* New York: Commonwealth Fund, 2001.

Smedley, B. D., Stith, A. Y., and Nelson, A. R. (eds.). *Unequal Treatment: Confronting Racial and Ethnic Disparities in Health Care.* Washington, D.C.: National Academy Press, 2003.

Smedley, B. D., and Syme, S. L. *Promoting Health: Intervention Strategies from Social and Behavioral Research.* Washington, D.C.: National Academy Press, 2000.

Stewart, A. L., and Napoles-Springer, A. M. "Advancing Health Disparities Research: Can We Afford to Ignore Measurement Issues?" *Medical Care*, 2003, *41*(11), 1207–1220.

Stryer, D., Clancy, C., and Simpson, L. "Minority Health Disparities:
AHRQ Efforts to Address Inequities in Care." *Health Promotion Practice*, 2002, *3*(2), 125–129.

Sullivan Commission on Diversity in the Health Care Workforce. *Missing
Persons: Minorities in the Health Professions.* A Report of the Sullivan
Commission. 2004. http://www.sullivancommission.org.

Therrien, M., and Ramirez, R. R. *The Hispanic Population in the United States:
March 2000.* Washington, D.C.: U.S. Bureau of the Census, 2001.

U.S. Census Bureau. *Current Population Survey, March 2000.* Washington,
D.C.: Ethnic and Hispanic Statistics Branch, Population Division.
Mar. 6, 2001. http://www.census.gov/population/www/socdemo/
hispanic/ho00–01.html.

U.S. Department of Health and Human Services. *Mental Health: A Report of
the Surgeon General—Executive Summary.* Rockville, Md.: U.S. Department
of Health and Human Services, Substance Abuse and Mental Health
Services Administration, Center for Mental Health Services, National
Institutes of Health, National Institute of Mental Health, 1999.

U.S. Department of Health and Human Services. *Healthy People 2010:
Understanding and Improving Health.* (2nd ed.) Washington, D.C.:
U.S. Government Printing Office, Nov. 2000.

U.S. Department of Health and Human Services and Grantmakers in
Health. *Elimination of Racial and Ethic Disparities in Health.* Washington, D.C.: U.S. Government Printing Office, 1998.

Weber, L. *Understanding Race, Class, Gender, and Sexuality: A Conceptual
Framework.* New York: McGraw-Hill, 2001.

Wilcox, S., and others. "Determinants of Leisure Time Physical Activity
in Rural Compared with Urban Older and Ethnically Diverse
Women in the United States." *Journal of Epidemiology and Community
Health*, 2000, *54*, 667–672.

Wingo, P. A., and others. "Cancer Incidence and Mortality, 1973–1995."
Cancer, 1998, *82*, 1197–1207.

Zambrana, R. E. "The Underrepresentation of Hispanic Women in
Health Professions." *Journal of the American Medical Women's Association*, 1996, *51*(4), 147–152.

Zambrana, R. E. "Improving Access and Quality for Ethnic Minority
Women." *Women's Health Issues*, 2001, *11*(4), 354–359.

Zambrana, R. E., Breen, N., Fox, S. A., and Gutierrez-Mohamed, M. L.
"Use of Cancer Screening Practices by Hispanic Women: Analyses
by Subgroup." *Preventive Medicine*, 1999, *29*, 466–477.

Zambrana, R. E., and Carter-Pokras, O. "Health Data Issues for Hispanics: Implications for Public Health Research." *Journal of Health Care for the Poor and Underserved,* 2001, *12*(1), 20–34.

Zambrana, R. E., Cornelius, L., Boykin, S., and Salas Lopez, D. "Latina and HIV/AIDS Risk Factors: Implications for Harm Reduction Strategies." *American Journal of Public Health,* 2004, *94*(7), 1152–1158.

Zambrana, R. E., Mogel, W., and Scrimshaw, S.C.M. "Gender and Level of Training Differences in Obstetricians' Attitudes Toward Patients in Childbirth." *Women and Health,* 1987, *12*(1), 5–24.

CHAPTER EIGHT

IMMIGRANT WORKERS

Do They Fear Workplace Injuries More Than They Fear Their Employers?

Marianne P. Brown

> *We are not safe . . . from the work you can get hurt,*
> *you understand me? Up until now I've been spared.*
> *But who says I'm "home free"? . . . Of course [I*
> *worry about getting hurt]! If I get hurt, what will*
> *become of me? So, I would have to go to Mexico*
> *because there I know they would take care of me. . . .*
> *You're always worried about that. . . . You just go,*
> *because you don't have a choice. We have to*
> *continue. . . . [All my coworkers] all of them, it's*
> *the same worry. It's impossible not to think like that.*
> *Even if we don't want to. That is, you can't avoid*
> *it, you have it on your mind already.*
> FRANCISCO, FORTY-FIVE YEARS OLD, FROM MEXICO, WHO
> HAS WORKED AS A DAY LABORER IN THE UNITED STATES
> FOR TEN YEARS (BROWN, DOMENZAIN, AND VILLORIA-
> SIEGERT, 2002)

The sweat and blood of immigrant, as well as slave, labor has played a critical role in U.S. economic development from the time Africans were brought here in the seventeenth, eighteenth, and nineteenth centuries. Northern Europeans of Irish and German descent arrived in the mid-1800s, followed by southern and eastern Europeans a few decades later. It was Chinese immigrants laying track from the West—and Irish immigrants laying track from the East—who braved extremely hazardous conditions to build the two rail lines that converged in Utah in 1869 to form the Transcontinental Railroad. Over time some of these immigrant groups have gained some protection; others remain in marginal positions due to race/ethnicity and legal status.

Historically, immigrant workers have often held dangerous jobs. It was immigrants who were the victims of the most infamous workplace disaster in New York City prior to September 2001, the Triangle Shirtwaist Factory fire, which killed 146 garment workers on the afternoon of March 25, 1911. About 60 percent of the Triangle workers, along with management, were East European Jews. Most of the rest came from Italy. At least 123 were women, and of these, at least 64 were teenagers (Von Drehle, 2003). The fire lasted only fifteen minutes, but workers were trapped because exits were locked, there was no sprinkler system, there were not enough stairways, there had never been fire drills, and the eighteen-inch-wide fire escape collapsed with dozens of people on it. Public revulsion at the conditions that led to the fire resulted in pathbreaking labor law legislation, which established the Factory Investigation Commission. In its first two months, the commission's ten inspectors visited two thousand factories in twenty industries to uncover unacceptable health and safety conditions.

Eighty years later, the Imperial Food Products fire in Hamlet, North Carolina, left fifty-six seriously injured and twenty-five dead—eighteen were women, and twelve were African American. There were no fire extinguishers, safety exits, or sprinkler system. In eleven years of business, the plant had never had an official inspection by its state Occupational Safety and Health Administration (OSHA). As a result of this tragedy, the North Carolina OSHA office was threatened with takeover by federal OSHA, and a host of new worker safety laws was passed.

The structure of employment in the United States has always placed those with little power—whether because of immigrant status, gender, race, or lack of other employment options—in employment where they have few options but to accept dangerous work with little or no protections. The search for cheap labor within capitalist systems places immigrant workers at particular risk. While which worker groups are most vulnerable may change over time because of their perceived "otherness" or "difference" (Harvey, 1996, p. 342), the forces that structure unequal protections remain essentially unchanged. Currently, male Hispanics hold this position, as evidenced by high rates of immigrant worker mortality.

Immigrant workers enter a workforce that is already stratified by race, sex, age, ethnicity, and educational level, with most taking the least desirable jobs. And Native Americans and African Americans who have low incomes and educational levels also tend to work in jobs that are less desirable and have fewer protections; they are part of this continuum of vulnerability. Immigrants face special issues. Although there has not been a high-profile tragedy for immigrant workers since the Triangle fire, low-profile tragedies occur every day. More than two Hispanic workers, many of them recent immigrants, die of work-related injuries each day.

Immigration at an All-Time High

Currently, more immigrants come to the United States than to any other country (Bean and Lowell, 2003). In 2000, an estimated 1.2 million foreign-born were added to the U.S. population; 850,000 entered legally and some 350,000 illegally (United Nations Population Division, 2003). During the 1990s, 11 percent came from the Caribbean, 30 percent from Asia, and 36 percent from Latin America, with Mexico by far the largest source.

Immigrants are now 11 percent of all U.S. residents—but 14 percent of all workers and 20 percent of low-wage workers (those who earn less than 200 percent of the minimum wage). In certain metropolitan areas such as Los Angeles, New York, Chicago, and Miami, the concentration is much higher. A recent study conducted by the Center for Labor Market Studies at Northeastern University concluded that recent immigrants were critical to our nation's growth in the past decade, accounting for half of all new wage earners (Sum, Fogg, and Harrington, 2002).

In spite of immigrants' contribution to the U.S. economy— the services and products they provide—many native-born Americans display ambivalence about their presence. Immigrants serve as scapegoats for many Americans' anger about the erosion of wages, rising job instability, and declining social benefits (Abel, 2004).

Employers in certain sectors make special efforts to recruit immigrant workers, accepting their word that they are legal—that is, have legal working papers. In fact, illegal immigrants are more appealing to some employers because they will work in conditions unacceptable to native-born workers. For example, janitorial companies that clean Wal-Mart stores have recruited illegal immigrants, paying many off the books. One night, one of Wal-Mart's workers "sliced his hand open on a floor-scraping blade and was rushed to a hospital. He had problems paying the bill because his job did not provide health insurance and his employer shunned the workers' compensation system" (Greenhouse, 2003). In another case, the world's largest processor of chicken, beef, and pork, Tyson Foods, was charged in U.S. district court with having recruited hundreds of illegal immigrants from Mexico and Guatemala to work in plants in at least twelve states. Notably, according to company reports, employee turnover at all Tyson's poultry plants runs at about 100 percent per year. Much of the work is difficult and dangerous, and some say this largely accounts for the high turnover rate. The court found the company not guilty, although one of its employees served two years in prison for assisting the transport of illegal immigrants. And a personnel manager who was indicted for immigrant law violations agreed to cooperate with prosecutors but subsequently committed suicide (Rosenbloom, 2003).

Because illegal immigrants often work in what they consider unacceptable conditions, many native-born resent their presence and relocate. For example, in California urban areas that have experienced increased immigration, native-born workers have fled to smaller towns or other states (Briggs, 2004).

When examining the history of racial oppression in America, Blauner (1972) noted that America has used workers of color for the cheapest labor, concentrating people of color in the most unskilled jobs. People of color provided much of the hard labor that built up the base necessary for industrialization (Blauner,

1972). Workers of color, particularly immigrants without legal working status, are preferred because they have the least power and the fewest protections. Furthermore, their lower status in the workforce where there are native-born workers results in a hierarchy that minimizes action based on common interests. This creates a dynamic that Bonacich (1994) calls a "split labor market." White employers interviewed by Wilson (1996) in the early 1990s, as well as Waldinger and Lichter's later surveys (2003), found employers preferred hiring Hispanics over African Americans because of employer perceptions of their work ethic, migration networks that bring in other similar workers as needed, social skills, consumer orientation, and tendency when dissatisfied with their jobs to leave rather than speak up or be disruptive at work. This last point reflects the power differential employers prefer, particularly since 1973, where changes in the labor market have resulted in "flexible accumulation," which requires a large contingent workforce with little job security (Harvey, 1996).

HISPANIC IMMIGRANTS IN VULNERABLE POSITIONS

This chapter focuses on Hispanic immigrants because they are the largest immigrant group in the United States—a population that continues to grow—and because recent governmental reports show that there are higher rates of fatal work injuries for Hispanic workers than for any other racial/ethnic group. Also, foreign-born Hispanics bear a disproportionate share of the fatal work injury burden (National Research Council, 2003). Notably, while fatal work injury rates for other workers in the United States are declining, fatality rates for Hispanic male workers are increasing. In addition, nonfatal injury and illness rates are higher among Hispanic workers than any other group (National Research Council, 2003).

This chapter examines the factors that contribute to these higher work-related fatality, injury, and illness rates for Hispanics—with a particular emphasis on Hispanic immigrants and their disempowered position in the labor force—and proposes some policy changes to address this problem.

RISING FATALITY, INJURY, AND ILLNESS RATES

The U.S. Census Bureau predicts that by the year 2050, Hispanics will represent one out of every four persons in the United States, up from about one in eight in 2000 (National Research Council, 2003). This increase is due to immigration into the United States and high birth rates for this population. Dispersion trends tell us that the public health challenges, such as workplace health and safety risks, cannot focus only on states with traditionally large Hispanic populations: California, Texas, New York, Florida, and Illinois. Hispanic communities now are growing rapidly in the Carolinas, Arkansas, Georgia, Tennessee, Nevada, Alabama, Kentucky, Minnesota, Nebraska, and other states.

The kinds of fatalities, injuries, and illnesses Hispanics experience vary from state to state, depending on the kinds and density of industries. Overall, between 1998 and 2000, service industries and the retail trades employed the most Hispanic men and women, followed by construction for Hispanic men (National Research Council, 2003). Over 29 percent of working Hispanic women were private household workers, 14.8 percent worked in nondurable goods manufacturing (for example, food processing), 11.2 percent in agriculture, forestry, and fishing, and another 11.2 percent in the wholesale trades.

FATALITIES

From 1995 to 2000, as many as 4,167 Hispanics died as the result of a fatal job injury. The industries with the most deaths, in descending order, were construction, agriculture, forestry and fishing, transportation and public utilities, retail trade, and services. Males accounted for 94 percent of the total. An example in the agriculture industry occurred in rural California in 2001. An undocumented worker from Mexico was required to climb down into a sump hole full of farm detritus (which can give off a lethal gas), fell into the liquid, and drowned. A rescuer, also an illegal immigrant, also fell in and drowned. The employer had received training about the hazards of this kind of work and the required safety procedures. Yet no safety procedures were in place: no training, no air testing, no respirators, no air harnesses, not even a ladder (Barstow, 2003b). Furthermore, the workers tasked with this dangerous work had not received the "confined space" training legally required by OSHA.

Hispanic females, the remaining 6 percent who were fatally injured, were employed in technical, sales, administrative support, or service occupations at the time of their deaths. The total number of fatal work injuries in these two last occupations accounted for nearly 60 percent of the recorded fatalities. For Hispanic females, the primary fatal event was workplace homicide (42 percent), followed by highway incidents (25 percent). Although the Bureau of Labor Statistics does not specify the causes of these homicides, they most likely occurred in the course of robberies in the sales and service occupations, the most common cause of violent deaths in the workplace. The second most likely cause of such homicides is domestic violence, with women's partners coming to the workplace to attack them. Although it is not known to what extent this is true for immigrant women, there is evidence to suggest this may be a significant factor. To support this, Crenshaw (1995) notes that although 1990 amendments to the Immigration and Nationalities Act were designed to protect women from abusive men whom they come to the United States to marry, many are still vulnerable to such violence. In order to leave the abusive relationship, they have to gather evidence from police, medical personnel, psychologists, and others. This requirement, along with cultural barriers to reporting abuse, results in women continuing to live with their abusers, nonreporting of abusive acts, and the consequent escalation of abuse in some cases. Consequently, such immigrant women are at increased risk for physical abuse, including homicide, at home as well as at work.

It is important to note that fatality statistics are relatively accurate, as it is not easy to hide a death in a workplace; most get reported to OSHA and the Bureau of Labor Statistics. However, the same is not true for work-related injuries and illnesses; many are never reported for a variety of reasons that will be discussed below.

INJURIES AND ILLNESSES

The Bureau of Labor Statistics estimates that each year between 1998 and 2000, there were approximately 182,000 injuries to Hispanic males and 66,000 injuries to Hispanic females. Seven occupations that ranked in the top ten for nonfatal injuries and illnesses for Hispanic males were the same occupations with the most fatalities: construction and nonconstruction laborers, truck drivers, farm workers, freight stock and material handlers, janitors and cleaners, groundskeepers and gardeners, miscellaneous machine operators, carpenters and apprentices, and cooks. For Hispanic females, the occupations with the most nonfatal injuries and illnesses were nursing aides, orderlies, and attendants; maids; janitors and cleaners; laborers except construction; assemblers; miscellaneous food preparation occupations; miscellaneous machine operators; cashiers; cooks; and sales workers.

As with fatalities, Hispanic men have a higher risk of nonfatal workplace injury or illness than any other gender/race-ethnicity group in the United States. Hispanic women have a higher risk of a nonfatal injury than white women, but their risk is slightly lower than for black women. The reasons are unclear but are probably related to the kinds of high-risk jobs they held, reflecting their undesirable position on a continuum of vulnerability.

It is generally accepted that official injury and illness statistics are undercounts for a variety of reasons. With respect to Hispanics, it is recognized that there is underreporting in the census and the Current Population Survey (National Research Council, 2003). This is particularly true for mobile or migrant populations, populations without telephones or stable residences, and illegal immigrants, who may not respond to surveys for fear of being turned in to immigration officials. One strong indication of underreporting for Hispanics is the disparity between their increasingly higher-than-average fatality rates and their lower-than-average reported lost work time injury rates.

Also, many Hispanic immigrants are self-employed and thus exempt from most occupational safety and health regulations, including fatality, injury, and illness reporting requirements (employers must report these annually). Furthermore, new entrants into the U.S. labor market increasingly are employed through temporary employment agencies or small contractors for work in construction, manufacturing, clerical, janitorial, house cleaning, home care, and other services, and these temporary employment agencies or small employers do not always report injuries and illnesses. In addition, many are working in the informal labor sector, where they are paid in cash, under the table and off the books, by employers who are not complying with many laws that cover wage and hours, workers' compensation, health and safety, and other labor laws.

There are also disincentives for employers to report injuries and illnesses, even though they are required to under OSHA, because increases can have a negative impact on the employer. Increased injuries and illnesses can result in increased workers' compensation premiums, being targeted by OSHA for inspections, or receiving higher fines when they receive citations if their injury rates suggest a bad-faith effort to make their workplace safe. Furthermore, if they employ undocumented or illegal workers (those without legal working papers) who become injured, they may not want to report those injuries because it could reveal that they employ such workers. One such case is that of a New Jersey foundry owned by McWane, the nation's largest manufacturer of cast-iron pipe. With a blue-collar workforce composed largely of immigrants, the company has been charged with repeatedly exposing workers to unsafe conditions and regularly deceiving environmental and workplace safety regulators. "The managers took other steps to evade regulators. . . . They falsified injury logs, submitted false pollution monitoring reports and burned incriminatory evidence in . . . a furnace that turns scrap metal into molten iron." The Environmental Protection Agency charged that the company gave the workers a harsh choice: "Perform an unreasonable work task or lose your job; work injured or lose your job; lie to OSHA or lose your job; lie to environmental regulators or lose your job; forgo filing workers' compensation claims or lose your job" (Barstow, 2003a).

Hispanic workers themselves have disincentives to report injuries and illnesses to their employers. Not the least of these is that if they are undocumented, they feel vulnerable to possible harassment, dismissal, or deportation. Some 500,000 Mexicans come to the United States each year, and an estimated 60 percent are undocumented (Faux, 2003). It has been estimated that two out of every five low-wage workers (those who earn less than 200 percent of the minimum wage) are undocumented (Capps and others, 2003).

In addition, workers who toil in low-skilled, low-income jobs often feel that if they raise these issues, they can easily be replaced by others. Immigrants, in particular, feel vulnerable because of their race, class, and immigration status, as well as their wider family net, with people in their towns of origin depending on their income. Indeed, many immigrant workers regularly send portions of their wages to their families in their birth countries to help cover living expenses. Across Latin America, the dependence on these remittances is staggering. The total "tops all international development assistance and is increasing by an average of 11 percent a year" (Thompson, 2002).

Also, these workers are marginalized because most do not have health insurance as part of their job, and many do not know they have a right to workers' compensation insurance if they suffer a job-related injury or illness. Consequently, if they report an injury and have to miss work, there will be no income replacement during their absence.

AN OPPORTUNITY TO DISCUSS WORKPLACE EXPERIENCES

Because little has been done to obtain a true picture of U.S. immigrant workers' lived reality, in 2001 we conducted an ethnographic "Voices" study of seventy-five such workers in Los Angeles County (Brown, Domenzain, and Villoria-Siegert, 2002). The goal was to hear their perceptions of health and safety conditions and the situations they face regularly on the job. Workers were recruited through worker centers and labor unions over a ten-month period for in-depth interviews—ranging from thirty minutes to two hours—in their native languages, mostly Spanish. Their names are confidential, and pseudonyms have been used when quoting from these interviews. Workers were chosen from six industries with low-paid, low-skilled jobs for which they were often compensated under the table and off the books: day labor (construction and gardening work), domestic (house cleaners), garment manufacturing, home care (personal assistance for the ill, elderly, and disabled), hotel (room cleaners), and restaurant (waitresses and kitchen help) work. The method chosen—in-depth interviews away from the workplace—was consistent with that promoted by feminist-informed health research (Whittle and Inhorn, 2001). The intent was to listen actively to workers who are structurally marginalized because of their race, class, gender, and immigration status, and document their diverse experiences, understand their everyday working lives, and connect their workplace safety and health experiences to larger political and economic forces. It is important to recall that since the mid-1800s, California's white male immigrants have obtained middle-class jobs, while Mexican, Japanese, Chinese, and Indian male populations have been ensconced at the bottom of the class structure as unskilled manual workers (Almaguer, 1994).

Risky Jobs

It is generally acknowledged by occupational health experts that one of the reasons Hispanic immigrants are at a greater risk for job-related fatality, injury, and illness is that they tend to work in more hazardous jobs than the average U.S. worker. Fatalities, injuries, and illnesses for Hispanic males occur in construction, agriculture/forestry/fishing, transportation and public utilities, retail trade, and services. These are known to be high-risk occupations—particularly the first three. In addition, Hispanic males do the riskier tasks in these industries because they perceive that they do not have other options. In construction, Hispanic immigrants are usually given the heavier work and jobs that require working on high places, such as roofing. In agriculture, forestry, and fishing, they are given the more dangerous jobs, as with the men who went into the toxic sump on the farm described earlier. In the areas of transportation and public utilities, they are at risk of highway accidents and other hazards.

Fatalities for females occur in sales and service occupations, where they do work that involves the exchange of money and security is lax, or where they are involved with transportation related to their work. Hispanic immigrant females also work in sales, where there is an increased risk of robbery, combined with physical violence, and service, where there are ergonomic- and toxic-chemical-related disorders in the health care, home care, housekeeping, hotel, and janitorial sectors. They also experience ergonomic-related problems in the manufacturing sector, such as in food processing, garment manufacturing, and various kinds of other assembly work.

LITTLE HEALTH AND SAFETY TRAINING
OR PROTECTIVE EQUIPMENT

Hispanic immigrant workers receive little or no training on how to do their jobs safely. And if training is provided, it is most often not in their first language. Also, they are frequently not given personal protective equipment to wear—such as respirators, gloves, or eye protection—which their employer is legally obligated to provide. The farm worker example mentioned earlier is such a case.

The Voices research revealed that employers in the six industries studied provided little or no health and safety training, and workers themselves had to purchase the protective equipment that California law says employers must supply. Instead, these workers relied on each other for guidance on how to do their jobs safely, as Serafin, a thirty-six-year-old day laborer from Mexico, noted:

> We talk about the normal things that one talks about with friends, right? With coworkers we say, "You know what? Be careful when you do that job because you could fall down or something. When you are doing something that can cause you an accident be very cautious." . . . They hire you in other places and, "You know what? You are going to do this." But they never explain to you, "Look, do it like this, or like that." Or for example, "There is some danger here with this machine." No, they never tell us that. Our coworkers explain to us, but the employer never explains anything [Brown, Domenzain, and Villoria-Siegert, 2002, p. 28].

Domestic workers taught themselves about the hazards of the job through their own experiences; reading the labels on the liquids they used; "intuition"; advice from other workers from their country of origin; family members; brochures, TV, Internet, and magazines; and sometimes they let each other know about the health symptoms they experienced after they used certain cleaning liquids. Soledad, a domestic worker from Mexico who had done house cleaning for one year, said, "When I want more information regarding health and safety issues, I get it in many different places . . . in bookstores. You can find brochures, or books too, which can be helpful, books that teach us how to. . . . There is always information on the computer, there could be information there. . . . On the Internet. . . . Well, my son is the one who helps me to do that" (Brown, Domenzain, and Villoria-Siegert, 2002, p. 28).

The garment workers could not cite one example of employer-provided training on health and safety, although one did mention there were safety posters on the walls. They relied on the media—TV and radio—coworkers, themselves, or a worker advocacy center that provided assistance to garment workers. Socorro, a forty-five-year-old female garment worker from Guatemala who had worked one year in this industry, said, "Well, based on my studies I protect myself, because nobody else does. For example, regarding the [sewing] machine's dust that I was telling you about, well I have bought my mask to protect myself from it. . . . And to protect myself from an accident with the machine. Well, all my years of experience have helped me a lot. You can get many important things from the news too. . . . The rest I got from working experience, studying, and reading" (Brown, Domenzain, and Villoria-Siegert, 2002, p. 23).

For home care workers, those who belonged to a union received health and safety information from it. They and the nonunionized home care workers also got such information from coworkers and their own personal experience. Marianela, a thirty-eight-year-old Latino with ten years of experience working as a home care worker, said, "I would say home care workers get information from their peers. If I need to know any more, I know that I can ask the union . . . or go to the library. . . . I've learned a lot more because of the class [conducted by the union] I'm taking. And also I took another class on how to protect yourself from HIV and other blood transferring diseases, and hepatitis and things like that" (Brown, Domenzain, and Villoria-Siegert, 2002, p. 30).

For hotel workers, employer training, such as kitchen sanitation rules, was usually calculated to protect the consumer. Workers sometimes turned to coworkers for safety information. In the cases where there was a union, it provided information about worker rights but not health and safety rights. Alfonso, a fifty-five-year-old hotel worker from Mexico who had done this work for sixteen years, said, "We want more information about how to protect and take care of ourselves at the workplace . . . that's one of my questions. Because we do not know . . . we do not know . . . how can we say, 'This is happening, what can we do?'" (Brown, Domenzain, and Villoria-Siegert, 2002, p. 31).

For restaurant workers, the main source of information on health and safety was coworkers and friends. Employers did not generally provide health and safety training and were not identified as a source to go to with a health or safety problem. Jen, a thirty-two-year-old restaurant worker from Guatemala who had worked in restaurants for eleven years, had this to say: "The few things that I have learned, I learned them from the TV . . . how to protect yourself from liquids and things . . . because there was a time that the meat, I do not know what disease they transmitted . . . but I got scared, because I saw it on the news. So from there on I handled the meat with care" (Brown, Domenzain, and Villoria-Siegert, 2002, p. 22).

ENGLISH PROFICIENCY AND LEVEL OF EDUCATION AS BARRIERS TO SAFETY

Immigrant workers feel particularly vulnerable in their jobs because many do not know any English, or their level of proficiency is very low. If employers provide training or materials on health and safety, they are usually in English. Ofelia, a sixty-five-year-old Hispanic domestic worker for twenty-one years, had this to say:

> Since one doesn't know English or anything, it's what the [employers] say. That's the way it is for a lot of people, and a lot don't know their rights. They used to make them [cleaning liquids] slightly milder. Nowadays they are too strong. And there are a lot of people who do not know English. And if you don't read what it says on the label, it's worse. You have to know what liquid to use for one thing or another. Because if you mix two liquids that are opposites, you can get—the container has the information—you can choke. Like an attack, because since both liquids are not supposed to be together. . . . You have to read the label, and if a domestic worker doesn't know how to speak English, she can't read it. So she can mix two liquids and get harmed [Brown, Domenzain, and Villoria-Siegert, 2002, p. 26].

Thirty-one-year-old Consuelo from Guatemala worked in the garment industry for eight years and said this about the importance of knowing English: "Yes, I'm interested in learning English. But me, I have been here for so long, and I haven't done the effort to study. That's also why I am going through this situation at work, because if I knew English, I think I would have a better job" (Brown, Domenzain, and Villoria-Siegert, 2002, p. 26).

Carlota, a forty-two-year-old from Mexico with thirteen years working as a room cleaner in hotels, talked about one way the employer took advantage of workers who did not speak English:

> As I told you, my arms hurt because of the work. They hurt a lot, and only recently . . . we left [were laid off], they gave us a paper . . . to sign that we had left the hotel . . . that we didn't have an accident. The manager gave it to us to sign, but since we often . . . don't know how to read English, I think that they only say what's in their interest and leave it to us to interpret. Many signed it, many, the majority . . . people that really did have injuries! For example, there was a woman who had an accident when one of the carts . . . turned over on her. Those carts are very heavy! And in steering the cart like this, she twisted her back. And the doctor told her she was injured for life . . . and, for example, she signed the paper that day . . . that they brought to the meeting. Because she was on light duty, and another one was on light duty. And . . . they signed the paper! They washed their hands of it . . . they don't speak English, and they're not sure how it works. There was a woman who spoke English. And when we asked the woman what the paper said after we had already signed it, she told us that it was a paper that said that . . . the hotel was giving it to assure that no one had come out injured. That's what the woman told us [Brown, Domenzain, and Villoria-Siegert, 2002, p. 27].

According to Census 2000, almost half (46 percent) of all foreign-born workers are limited English proficient (LEP). Nearly three-quarters (73 percent) of LEP workers speak Spanish; much smaller percentages speak other languages. Strikingly, 29 percent of workers who have been in the United States for twenty years or more are still considered LEP.

It is clear that limited English proficiency is closely linked to limited education. According to the Urban Institute's findings from the 2002 Current Population Survey, 18 percent of the immigrant labor force have less than a ninth-grade education. Another 12 percent have completed the ninth grade. The educational level for Mexican males is particularly low. Those who have immigrated to the United States since 1985 average fewer than six years of schooling (Bean and Lowell, 2003). Notably, there are significant gender differences among immigrant men and women who take low-wage jobs. More than three-quarters (76 percent) of female low-wage immigrant workers hold a high school diploma, compared with 66 percent of male low-wage immigrant workers. Women are also more likely to be proficient in English than foreign-born male workers (59 percent versus 50 percent). These factors help explain the different kinds of jobs immigrant men and women hold and their associated risks.

Another important phenomenon is the bimodal educational distribution of immigrants in recent years. "Immigrants coming to the country have had either a high level of education (that is, a college degree) or a low level (that is, without a high school diploma)" (Bean, Chapa, Berg, and Sowards, 1994). This educational distribution mirrors the change in the labor market: a substantial growth in the number of high- and low-end jobs, with lesser increases in the middle range (Milkman and Dwyer, 2002).

Their limited English proficiency and little formal education limit the kinds of jobs immigrant workers can hold and also put them at risk for employer abuse regarding health and safety, as well as other labor law protections. Such workers are also at a disadvantage if they wish to report health and safety or other infractions in the workplace to governmental agencies. For example, a worker who dials 911 in south Florida is answered by an English-only-speaking dispatcher, and the Department of Labor's Wage and Hour Division in Fort Myers, Florida, has a prerecorded message that relays in English "bureaucratese" the few types of complaints the office does handle (Bowe, 2003).

IGNORANCE OF RIGHTS AND RESOURCES TO ASSIST WITH HEALTH AND SAFETY PROBLEMS

Immigrant workers do not have easy access to regulatory agencies. Of the seventy-five workers interviewed in the Voices study, only seven had heard of Cal-OSHA, and none had contacted the agency for assistance. Cal-OSHA is the state-run agency in California that issues workplace health and safety standards, enforces those standards when they inspect workplaces, and provides information to workers and employers about workplace health and safety issues and their respective rights and responsibilities. Cal-OSHA and federal OSHA laws specify that it is the employer's responsibility to provide a safe and healthful workplace. In addition, almost none of the workers were familiar with their rights to workers' compensation, which is handled by the Division of Workers' Compensation in California.

Although they were unfamiliar with Cal-OSHA and its protections, many garment and restaurant workers were familiar with the state labor commissioner's responsibility to enforce wage and hour laws because immigrant worker advocacy centers had told them about this agency. Some did not contact governmental agencies because of their immigration status (they were undocumented) and also because of experiences in their home countries that made them think governmental agencies were unfriendly to workers. Also, those without legal work authorization incorrectly thought that workplace health and safety laws in California did not apply to them. Most did not know where to go for treatment if they got hurt or sick on the job. Thirty-two-year-old restaurant worker Jen, who had worked for eleven years in this industry, had this to say: "I have heard there are laws in California. . . . But if there were really laws, they would be checking, wouldn't they? They would go to see the workers to check if they are treated well. . . . But there isn't. I worked seven years in a restaurant, and I never saw . . . I think that since they don't check on the employer, he feels in a higher status. He takes advantage of the situation. . . . The law is not being enforced" (Brown, Domenzain, and Villoria-Siegert, 2002, p. 22)

Another restaurant worker, Jairo, twenty-two years old, who had worked in this industry for two and a half years, talked about workers' ignorance about their right to report injuries to their employer: "Well, I think that the one who knows the California law is more likely to report it to the employer. But some people don't know anything. And, well, if you don't know, if you just arrived and you have an accident, and the employer knows you just arrived, he is going to scare you, and you refrain from supporting it" (Brown, Domenzain, and Villoria-Siegert, 2002, p. 20).

Thirty-eight-year-old Marianela, who worked in home care for ten years, did not know that workers' compensation provides wage replacement: "The reason why I think they [workers] do not report it is because they're not aware of what they're entitled to . . . their rights. They don't report it also because there's a language barrier.

And because they won't get paid. Basically, it's because they won't get paid. . . . Or you know, they [employer] might think they're lying. They [workers] probably feel like they have to be dying in bed in order to report it" (Brown, Domenzain, and Villoria-Siegert, 2002, p. 18).

Thirty-one-year-old Consuelo, who had worked as a garment worker for eight years, had no knowledge of Cal-OSHA:

> Well, in this country, I don't know much about local laws. But I think that . . . there would have to be a good organization, and with the president, the city council, and all those people who have to create an organization . . . and someone has to tell them, "Worry about those people." Every once in a while, like the Health Department has to come and check if they have water, the conditions of the bathroom. . . . But it would have to be the people who are powerful, I think. It depends on them, the mayor, and the city council. The employers are responsible too, because when you have a business, you know that you have to be responsible to your employees. And if they can't, then they shouldn't have a business, I think. But despite that, they do what they do with one [the worker] because of their ambition for money [Brown, Domenzain, and Villoria-Siegert, 2002, p. 21].

RELUCTANCE TO SPEAK UP

Immigrant workers are reluctant to speak up about dangerous health and safety conditions or to report injuries and illnesses because their marginal status makes them feel vulnerable at work. Also, they do not think speaking up will result in any change in conditions. In addition, workers come to the workplace with cultural mores or attitudes that sometimes prevent them from taking action. Many low-skilled workers feel vulnerable because of their legal status, their educational level, and their lack of English proficiency. Fifty-year-old Ciro, who had worked as a day laborer for two years and was currently on the staff of a worker advocacy center, had this to say:

> That's something that we [immigrant worker advocacy center] also have to teach the day laborers—to get education—we have to teach them not to be afraid. Just because they have no papers

[legal worker status] doesn't mean they don't have the right to. . . . Like my brother, he told the employer, "Are you going to fire me? First you pay me . . . you pay me first, then you throw 'la migra' [the former immigration agency, the Immigration and Naturalization Service] on me. . . . I don't care." I say, "There are laws. If you don't have a mode of surviving, there are offices where they can help you. If you don't have the means and you get hurt and you can't work, and you can't pay the rent, there are offices where they can help you, even though you don't have papers." Many workers get scared. They go, "No, what if we go there and then they call 'la migra?'" [Brown, Domenzain, and Villoria-Siegert, 2002, p. 25].

Ofelia, a sixty-five-year-old domestic worker of twenty-one years, talked about the fear of speaking up:

They [other domestic workers] fall down the stairs; a friend fell down. Another friend says that she slipped when she was waxing the floor. But, as I told you, they don't say anything because it's a danger for us, because since they don't have insurance and maybe they don't have legal documents. I think that an illegal person has to shut her mouth. But a person who does have legal documents, well, it's very important that she reports it if something happens to her. Whether they help them or not, but she has the right to speak up [Brown, Domenzain, and Villoria-Siegert, 2002, p. 25].

Thirty-nine-year-old Milagros had worked as a garment worker for nine and a half years. She had this to say about employers' preference to hire workers without legal documents in order to avoid workers who might express dissatisfaction:

The owners of the factory, they just like to have undocumented people . . . because they pay them whatever they want. . . . For example, if you've been working in a factory for three months and you say something to the boss like, "Go away!" or something, then you [are] asking to get fired or something. So it's not in the best interest to have people with papers working because they can demand their rights. . . . So that's what happened in the factory. . . . [The owner] thought that I could talk to some people from the government, from the state, or, for example, the Labor Commission . . . and tell them what was happening in that factory [Brown, Domenzain, and Villoria-Siegert, 2002, p. 26].

Li, a twenty-seven-year-old who had worked in restaurants for one year, noted that both lack of legal documents and inability to speak English hampered speaking out: "One of the most nagging problems is that many workers . . . don't have a Green Card. . . . Because my status is not legal, I can't request any benefit as well as an inspection. . . . But another problem is that it's very difficult for many . . . to visit this kind of public entity [Cal-OSHA] because of language barrier" (Brown, Domenzain, and Villoria-Siegert, 2002, p. 27).

Originally from Guatemala, thirty-four-year-old Selena, a hotel worker for thirteen years, observed that employers fire workers if they report injuries:

> They had fired a coworker who had reported it [an injury], I do not know how many days later. They fired her because they didn't believe her. They do not believe the worker because they say that, "If you got hurt, and it hurt at the moment, why didn't you come to the office or to security to report it?" No, they [employer] do not report it, and then . . . they say, "No, she got hurt at home, and now she wants to file a complaint or a suit." Maybe they [workers] do not report it because they have seen how the doctor is [Brown, Domenzain, and Villoria-Siegert, 2002, p. 31].

This last reference to the company doctor shows a lack of faith in the doctor who is hired by the company. There is a belief that the doctor will not say the injury is work related, and for that reason they feel it is useless to tell the employer they were hurt.

Sometimes cultural mores keep workers from speaking up. For example, researchers in California who were conducting a study of ergonomic-related disorders in a horticulture plant with Spanish-speaking immigrants found they were very reluctant to use the term *dolor* (pain) when describing their health condition but would easily refer to a *molestia* (discomfort), downgrading the level of severity. It should be noted that the Voices study found no difference between men and women in acknowledging risks and injuries. There was no support for the assumption that machismo interfered with obtaining a true sense of whether Spanish-speaking male workers acknowledge risk or suffer injuries or illnesses.

EMPLOYERS APPARENTLY UNINTERESTED

Another reason immigrant workers are reluctant to speak up about health and safety problems is that they think that their employers are not interested in these issues and wish them to just go away. Also, some employers have instituted "safety incentive programs" that reward workers or groups of workers if they do not experience or report work-related injuries or illnesses. Fifty-one-year-old Javier from Mexico, with three years as a day laborer, expressed this feeling: "[We do not report because] to be honest, I think the employer is not going to do anything. Because we are 'informal' [that is, part of the informal labor sector], we come and go, so we do not get to have a doctor or anything" (Brown, Domenzain, and Villoria-Siegert, 2002, p. 17).

Monica, a fifty-four-year-old domestic worker for four years from Nicaragua, said this about her client-employer: "And one thinks, if I tell the client [ill, disabled, or elderly person], she is going to tell me not to come back. So to avoid losing the job, I shut up. I do not say anything. . . . Then, one just shuts up, one doesn't say anything because one thinks, well, I do not have any chance to win, I am not going to waste my time. And I just try to heal it and keep on working" (Brown, Domenzain, and Villoria-Siegert, 2002, p. 17).

Forty-three-year-old garment worker Mateo from Mexico, who had worked in this industry for twenty-five years, expressed how reluctant employers are to assist them when they are hurt:

> They do not have insurance. They do not have any. So you need to look out for yourself. . . . They do not pay attention to you, because they do not have enough insurance to cover us. . . . If a person's fingers gets pierced, you're taken to the doctor. . . . When you injure a finger, yes, they take you. . . . Whether they pay depends on how you claim it. Because really, if you do not claim it [under workers' compensation law], you won't get paid anything—not even your days that you stopped working—because, well it's impossible for you to work with an injured finger. But if you demand it, maybe they'll pay. I, at least, was one of the people who *did* demand it. But you always run into problems, always, always [Brown, Domenzain, and Villoria-Siegert, 2002, p. 18].

Some who will not tell their employers tell their coworkers. Such was the case with thirty-two-year-old Fabio from Mexico, who had a bad fall at work. He had worked for a little over a year in a restaurant kitchen:

> I just told the cook. I mean, he picked me up. Because at the beginning I couldn't get up, and I asked him to help me to get up. . . . He lifted me, and he asked me what had happened. "No, I slipped." I went to the back. My leg hurt all afternoon. It was numb from the blow. I didn't say anything to her [the employer]. I mean, since I am supposed to not be . . . I didn't say anything [to the employer]. She just knew that I had fallen down, but she didn't know I got hurt. They do not care! That's the only accident I have had. I fell down in the kitchen [Brown, Domenzain, and Villoria-Siegert, 2002, p. 19].

Employer-sponsored "safety incentive programs" are increasingly being used in many workplaces. They create competition among workers or work groups to reduce their reported injury and illness rates. In the hotel industry, for example, they are quite popular. This is what fifty-three-year-old Benita, a hotel worker from El Salvador with three years working in this field, had to say about such programs:

> Yes, we have a system where if during the whole month. . . . This is kind of new. We didn't have this before, but lately they were giving a $30 bonus that . . . if a worker didn't complain about any pain, or didn't miss a workday, or if there were no accidents, they would give us that bonus. Sometimes they [the workers] get hurt, and they do not say anything for the sake of getting the $30. But I think that's not loving herself. . . . How can I get hurt, or fall down, and not report it? Just to receive that? No, that's not right. Yes, it *did* happen. Or, if someone missed one workday, they would say, "No, now they won't give you anything because you missed that day." For example, in my group there were about eight to ten people. And we would always try to not miss one day, but the manager always misses a day. And he is in this person's group; they wouldn't get anything [no bonus]. If one person missed one day, the other workers wouldn't get anything [Brown, Domenzain, and Villoria-Siegert, 2002, p. 31].

In summary, immigrant workers, and particularly low-wage, low-skilled immigrant workers, clearly recognize their marginality—their lack of power—in the workplace. Employers also recognize this marginality, see it as to their advantage, and consequently often prefer hiring immigrant workers for low-wage, low-skilled jobs, which are also often high risk. More often than not, these employers do not provide employees with health insurance, which is not legally required, or workers' compensation insurance, which is legally required. Or if they do, they often do not let the workers know they have the right to use it if they are hurt or made ill by the job. These immigrant workers have virtually no access to OSHA. These conditions apply to documented as well as undocumented workers.

The gendered nature of their work results in higher risks for males. Also, the different education and language proficiency levels between females and males result in differing risks. Immigrant females on average have attained higher education and language proficiency levels compared with immigrant males, which contributes to immigrant males' working in jobs with higher risks.

For these reasons and others, male immigrant workers in particular fear their employers more than they fear work-related injuries. They are taking a gamble that they will not be injured—even though they tend to work in some of the most dangerous jobs. And if they are injured, they will not report it in order to avoid their employer's wrath—which may be expressed in illegal harassment, firing, or being turned in to immigration authorities.

WHAT IS TO BE DONE?

Strategies ranging from a better-informed public to better information and education for immigrant workers to labor law reform can help address the issues outlined in this chapter.

NEED FOR A NATIONAL DEBATE

In order for there to be policy changes that provide significant health and safety protections for immigrant workers, the American public needs to be made aware of their current working conditions. Perhaps more important, in order to build support for new protective policies, the American public needs to be educated about how the lack of protections for these workers directly affects them as well.

By analogy, in fall 2003, California voters were asked to vote on a proposition that would prevent the state from asking a person's race or national origin when collecting data about public education, health issues, contracting, and employment. Designed to promote a race-blind society, this proposition would have eliminated the collection of race/ethnicity information by all state agencies in California. The immediate public response was, "That sounds fine, since such information should be a privacy issue." But when a public health awareness campaign's key message was that passage of this proposition could affect all Californians if patterns of disease by race/ethnicity could not be tracked and followed up with prevention programs, then the public's attitude changed. The measure was soundly defeated (Blanco, 2003).

If employers of immigrant workers do not carry workers' compensation insurance or do not let their employees know when they do have it, then many injured immigrant workers will use public sector–financed health services when they are hurt on the job. In this case, the taxpayer pays even though the employer is legally responsible. And for the minority of immigrant workers who do have employer-provided health insurance and use this benefit for work-related injuries, this practice also contributes to the rise of health care premiums for everyone. These issues are relevant for all Americans.

Native-born workers who work for employers who primarily employ immigrants and avoid implementing required safety protections are equally at risk—the phenomenon of a sinking tide lowering all ships. For instance, if no respirators are provided to immigrant workers in a lead battery plant, then it is unlikely they will be provided to any native-born workers since the inequity would be obvious to everyone on the shop floor. Conversely, if employers are forced to implement safety protections in places where immigrants work, native-born workers will also benefit.

Raising public awareness of immigrants' job health and safety requires initiatives that focus on ways these workers can speak out without putting their employment at risk. Avenues for this include providing regulatory agency hot lines where immigrant workers can call to report—in their native language—unsafe conditions;

public hearings held by elected officials; and more in-depth, open-ended interview studies, such as the Voices research, where immigrant workers describe the health and safety conditions under which they toil.

Immigrant Workers' Need for Information

In addition to increasing public awareness of their plight, immigrant workers need to be informed about their health and safety rights. Some would argue that this is the task of governmental regulatory agencies. Because of the rising toll of fatalities and injuries for Hispanic workers, federal OSHA director John Henshaw has declared that OSHA will communicate needed information in Spanish through employers, the media, and trade associations, as well as working with people at the state level (Vavra, 2003). However, Henshaw has not proposed targeted inspections in workplaces where immigrants are employed. Instead, his focus has been on providing more OSHA materials in Spanish and making these available through the Internet, despite evidence that most Spanish-speaking immigrants do not have easy access to the Internet. At the state level, virtually every state is experiencing a budget crisis, and there is a great deal of variation among the executive branches of each state regarding whether this issue is a priority. Therefore, it is more realistic to focus on the local community level for informing workers of their rights. Furthermore, immigrant workers are wary of governmental agencies for a number of reasons. They often do not perceive them as having helped workers in their country of origin, they are afraid such agencies may be linked to immigration authorities, and staff members in these agencies are perceived as "different" from them.

Avenues that are perceived as friendlier by immigrant workers are unions, worker advocacy centers, immigrant service centers, community clinics, town-of-origin clubs, churches, and other such affiliations. The number of unionized workers in the United States has dropped significantly since 1980, when President Reagan broke the air traffic controllers' union. The private sector is only about 11 percent organized now. Some unions are targeting immigrant workers in their organizing drives. Unions also need to build bridges between workers of color who are immigrants and those who are native born. The UNITE HERE union, whose members are mostly Hispanic immigrants, is doing this. A summer 2004 contract proposal submitted to Los Angeles hotel owners asked them to hire ombudsmen and establish a diversity task force to reach out to African American communities and eliminate hiring barriers (Bacon, 2004). At the same time, San Francisco UNITE HERE's contract proposal called for increasing the diversity of the hotel workforce by hiring African American workers. This was prompted by the fact that since the 1960s, African American employment in San Francisco hotels has dropped to less than 6 percent.

Worker advocacy centers that serve immigrant workers are increasingly reaching out to these workers. These organizations need more funding and technical assistance in order to provide such information and serve as bridges to governmental agencies (by anonymously reporting health and safety violations and injury and illness cases). The Voices from the Margins report and the Working Immigrant Safety and Health Coalition report (Teran, Baker, and Sum, 2002) both recommend these avenues to reach immigrant workers about health and safety protections.

Another avenue for reaching Hispanic immigrant workers with information about their workplace rights is the public schools. The proportions of working youth and recent immigrants are increasing in the United States. Teen workers have a two times greater risk of work-related injuries than working adults in general. Thus, both groups are at high risk. Furthermore, many immigrant workers have children who attend public schools. If information about workplace injury and illness prevention and health and safety rights were part of the regular high school curriculum, as it is in many Canadian provinces, these students could impart what they have learned to their parents in their native language.

In a limited way, this has been attempted, with positive results, at the Labor Occupational Safety and Health (LOSH) Program at UCLA. LOSH's work was predicated on the work of Kim and McKenry (1998), researchers who have studied social networks and observed that among African Americans, Asian Americans, Hispanics, and Caucasians, the first three were significantly more likely to call on children for help and advice. They observed that such networks can help provide pathways for intervention and suggested children should be the focus of intervention and attempts to build linkages to other groups. Also, with respect to the Mexican immigrant community, Valenzuela's work (1999) underscores the importance of immigrant family networks and the role children play in their families' attempts to cope with the hardships of immigration, poverty, and minority status. His in-depth interviews revealed that children often act as bridges to the larger society by obtaining information and advocating on their families' behalf as tutors, advocates, and sometimes surrogate parents.

ENGLISH PROFICIENCY

One major factor preventing immigrants from being informed about workplace health and safety issues and from speaking up is that too many cannot speak English. In fact, one study in California found that over 40 percent of new immigrants are struggling with the English language and do not speak English well or at all (Hill and Hayes, 2003). Such workers are at a great disadvantage in a workplace where most communication is in English. Providing easily accessible English as a Second Language (ESL) or related programs (literacy, citizenship, or vocational training) for this population could improve their integration into the general workforce.

ESL classes are offered in communities where immigrants predominate—through adult schools, private language schools, in churches, in unions, and in other community-based venues. But the demand for such classes far outweighs their availability. Consequently, there still is a need to develop new, innovative methods for providing English classes for recent, and sometimes not so recent, arrivals.

TARGETING WORKPLACE INSPECTIONS AND PROTECTING WHISTLE-BLOWERS

It is important that federal OSHA and states with their own OSHA plans target industries where immigrant workers predominate to conduct what are called unannounced "programmed" or "scheduled" inspections. Most OSHA worksite inspections are complaint driven. That is, a worker files a complaint with the OSHA office saying the employer is not providing a safe workplace and asks for an inspection. Because immigrant workers are reluctant to file such complaints for the same reasons they are reluctant to speak up about hazards or injuries and illnesses on the job, it is unlikely they will do so. Therefore, federal and state OSHA programs need to develop a strategic plan for making unannounced visits to industrial sectors where immigrants work. Such sweeps have been conducted by Cal-OSHA (in collaboration with the state labor commissioner and the Division of Workers' Compensation) in the agricultural, construction, and garment manufacturing sectors in California. Many violations of safety standards have been uncovered, and numerous fines have been levied. But these sweeps have been few, and they are not often reported in the media to serve as a warning to other employers.

Of course, it is illegal for employers to retaliate against workers who exercise their rights to report workplace injuries, illnesses, and unsafe conditions to management and to file complaints with OSHA. But most states that have their own OSHA plans and those that are covered by federal OSHA have a poor record when it comes to protecting whistle-blowers who exercise these rights. Although workers who are discriminated against for exercising these rights can file complaints with a governmental agency, there is no aggressive program to investigate these complaints. But immigrant workers feel particularly vulnerable to retaliation for addressing health and safety concerns. There need to be specific whistle-blower protection laws in place to protect these workers regardless of their immigration status.

LONG-TERM REFORM

Many big-picture labor policy issues need reform today. We need labor laws that make it easier to organize into unions, city and state living-wage laws and ordinances, mandatory employer-based health insurance, and workers' compensation reform that increases wage replacement ceilings, caps medical payments, and reduces or eliminates the need for a lawyer. All these reforms are increasingly difficult to institute as corporations relocate away from communities that make such demands to set up shop in communities that are not making such demands.

The policy that would have the most profound impact on immigrant workers is immigration law reform that grants permanent legal status to immigrants who have lived in the United States a certain length of time so that they would no longer toil under the threat of retaliation if they speak up about unacceptable conditions at work. In the 108th Congress, Representative Sheila Jackson from Texas introduced such a bill, which also proposed funding job training programs for unemployed native-born workers (Bacon, 2004).

CONCLUSION

It is clear that immigrant workers have continued to make a major contribution to the economic development of the United States since the founding of this country. At the same time, many are putting their lives and safety at risk. This class of workers is by virtue of their position in U.S. society most at risk for injuries, illnesses, and fatalities in the workplace. In most cases, immigrant workers fear their employers more than they fear workplace injuries, even though they are dying or becoming injured at rates significantly higher than native-born workers. Currently, these workers are largely without voice. They need opportunities to speak out without retribution. This chapter suggests some legal protections that are needed as well as channels through which immigrant workers could speak out—if given the opportunity. Most important, others not at risk, such as the general public, regulatory agencies that cover workplace health and safety, and elected representatives, now need to speak out on behalf of these workers as it is a human rights issue.

There will continue to be a need for immigrant workers in the fields of service, retail, construction, agriculture, and some types of manufacturing in the United States. Most of these jobs are not likely to go overseas or over the border. Health and safety protections for these workers will continue to be an issue as long as employers take advantage of their marginal status. Now is the time to address this pressing need before more workers are killed or maimed.

References

Abel, E. "'Only the Best Class of Immigration': Public Health Policy Toward Mexicans and Filipinos in Los Angeles, 1910–1940." *American Journal of Public Health*, 2004, *94*(6), 932–939.

Almaguer, T. *Racial Fault Lines: The Historical Origins of White Supremacy in California.* Berkeley: University of California Press, 1994.

Bacon, D. "Black/Migrant Rivalry for Jobs Can Be Eased." *Los Angeles Times,* Aug. 22, 2004, p. M2.

Barstow, D. "Officials at Foundry Face Health and Safety Charges." *New York Times,* Dec. 16, 2003a, p. 22.

Barstow, D. "California Leads Prosecution of Employers in Job Deaths." *New York Times,* Dec. 23, 2003b, p.1.

Bean, F. D., Chapa, J., Berg, R. R., and Sowards, K. A. "Educational and Sociodemographic Incorporation Among Hispanic Immigrants to the United States." In B. Edmonston and J. S. Passel (eds.), *Immigration and Ethnicity.* Washington, D.C.: Urban Institute Press, 1994.

Bean, F. D., and Lowell, L. B. "Immigrant Employment and Mobility Opportunities in California." *State of California Labor,* 2003, *3,* 87–117.

Blanco, M. "Why Proposition 54 Was Defeated." Presentation at the Annual Meeting of the American Public Health Association, San Francisco, Nov. 16, 2003.

Blauner, R. *Racial Oppression in America.* New York: HarperCollins, 1972.

Bonacich, E. "A Theory of Ethnic Antagonism: The Split Labor Market." In R. Takaki (ed.), *From Different Shores—Perspectives on Race and Ethnicity in America.* (2nd ed.) New York: Oxford University Press, 1994.

Bowe, J. "A Shameful Harvest." *American Prospect,* 2003, *14*(7), 38–39.

Briggs, V. M., Jr. "The Economic Well-Being of Black Americans: The Overarching Influence of U.S. Immigration Policies." In S. Shulman (ed.), *The Impact of Immigration on African Americans.* New Brunswick, N.J.: Transaction, 2004.

Brown, M. P., Domenzain, A., and Villoria-Siegert, N. *Voices from the Margins: Immigrant Workers' Perceptions of Health and Safety in the Workplace.* Los Angeles: University of California at Los Angeles, Labor Occupational Safety and Health Program, 2002.

Capps, R., and others. "A Profile of the Low-Wage Immigrant Workforce." Oct. 27, 2003. http://www.urban.org/url.cfm?ID=310880.

Crenshaw, K. W. "Mapping the Margins: Intersectionality, Identity, Politics, and Violence Against Women of Color." In K. W. Crenshaw, N. Gotanda, G. Peller, and K. Thomas (eds.), *Critical Race Theory: The Key Writings That Formed the Movement.* New York: New Press, 1995.

Faux, J. "How NAFTA Failed Mexico." *American Prospect,* 2003, *14*(7), 35–37.

Greenhouse, S. "Illegally in the U.S., and Never a Day Off at Wal-Mart." *New York Times,* Nov. 5, 2003, p. 5.

Harvey, D. *Justice, Nature and the Geography of Difference.* Cambridge, Mass.: Blackwell, 1996.

Hill, L. E., and Hayes, J. M. *California's Newest Immigrants.* San Francisco: Public Policy Institute of California, 2003.

Kim, H. K., and McKenry, P. C. "Social Networks and Support: A Comparison of African Americans, Asian Americans, Caucasians and Hispanics." *Journal of Comparative Family Studies,* 1998, *29*(2), 313–334.

Milkman, R., and Dwyer, R. E., "Growing Apart: The 'New Economy' and Job Polarization in California, 1992–2000." *State of California Labor,* 2002, *2,* 3–31.

National Research Council. *Safety Is Seguridad.* Washington, D.C.: National Academy Press, 2003.

Rosenbloom, J. "Victims in the Heartland." *American Prospect,* 2003, *14*(7), 29–31.

Sum, A., Fogg, N., and Harrington, P. *Immigrant Workers and the Great American Job Machine: The Contributions of New Foreign Immigration to National and Regional Labor Force Growth in the 1990s.* Boston: Northeastern University, Center for Labor Market Studies, 2002.

Teran, S., Baker, R., and Sum, J. *Improving Health and Safety Conditions for California's Immigrant Workers.* Berkeley: University of California's Labor Occupational Health Program, 2002.

Thompson, G. "Big Mexican Bread Winner: The Migrant Worker." *New York Times,* Mar. 25, 2002.

United Nations Population Division. *International Migration Report: 2002.* New York: United Nations Population Division, 2003.

Valenzuela, A., Jr. "Gender Roles and Settlement Activities Among Children and Their Immigrant Parents." *American Behavioral Scientist,* 1999, *42,* 720–742.

Vavra, B. "Do You Understand? Overcoming Language, Cultural Barriers in the Workplace." National Safety Council: *Safety + Health,* May 2003.

Von Drehle, D. *Triangle: The Fire That Changed America.* New York: Atlantic Monthly Press, 2003.

Waldinger, R., and Lichter, M. I. *How the Other Half Works: Immigration and the Social Organization of Labor.* Berkeley: University of California Press, 2003.

Whittle, K. L., and Inhorn, M. C. "Rethinking Difference: A Feminist Reframing of Gender/Race/Class for the Improvement of Women's Health Research." *International Journal of Health Services,* 2001, *31*(1), 147–165.

Wilson, W. J. *When Work Disappears: The World of the Urban Poor.* New York: Knopf, 1996.

PART FOUR

STRUCTURING HEALTH CARE

Access Quality and Inequality

CHAPTER NINE

HEALTH DISPARITIES
What Do We Know? What Do We Need to Know? What Should We Do?

H. Jack Geiger

One of the most persistent facts of life—and death—in the United States is that African Americans, Native Americans, Hispanics, and members of many Asian subgroups live sicker, die younger, and more often experience inferior health care, in comparison with the white majority. These are the phenomena frequently described as "health disparities," a term that has multiple meanings and is used too often without precise definition. Its major categories are disparities in health status and disparities in health care, but it is sometimes employed to refer to disparities in access to care, and frequently it is used nonspecifically to describe any or all three of these categories. It is worth observing, furthermore, that *disparities* carries at best a faint connotation of moral concern—stronger than the studiously neutral *differences* but weaker than *inequality* or *inequity*. These stronger terms place such phenomena more clearly in the broader American social context of differentiation—by race, ethnicity, social class, and gender—in power, privilege, and resources, and in the different life experiences and life opportunities that result.

In this chapter, I briefly review the evidence of disparities in health status—the burdens of excess morbidity, mortality, and health-related quality of life that characterize poor and minority population groups in the United States. Next, I review disparities in health care—the differences in the quality, intensity, and comprehensiveness of the medical care afforded to patients of these same poor and minority populations. I point out that these two kinds of disparities are only indirectly related, since the medical care of any population makes only a modest contribution to its mortality experience or life expectancy. Both, however, are deeply rooted in, and reflect, a larger context: the pervasive and continuing power of race, social class, and gender as divisive and differentiating forces in defining the social determinants of health and the social, biological, and physical environments in which different American groups live. I examine the existing evidence of causation for each type of disparity and identify important gaps in our knowledge and critical needs for further research. Finally, I propose policy changes, health system actions, and research programs that should be undertaken now to begin the process of eliminating inequity in both health status and health care.

DISPARITIES IN HEALTH STATUS

At no time in the history of the United States has the health status of African Americans, Native Americans, Hispanics, and members of many Asian subgroups equaled or even approximated that of white Americans (Geiger, 2001; Byrd and Clayton, 2000; National Center for Health Statistics, 2003). While the health of all American racial, ethnic, and social class groups has improved dramatically over that long time span, and particularly during the past six decades, people of color and the less affluent continue to experience excess morbidity and mortality (Arias and Smith, 2003; Hajat, 2000). These facts of illness, disability, and premature death continue to be particularly severe for African Americans, whose mean life expectancy is almost six years shorter than that of non-Hispanic whites, and on some indicators, such as infant mortality rates, the black-white gap has recently been increasing (National Center for Health Statistics, 2003; U.S. Department of Health and Human Services, 2000; National Center for Education in Maternal and Child Health, 2000).

These gaps have been stubbornly resistant to change and have profound individual and social costs. If African Americans instead had experienced the same age-adjusted mortality rates as whites during the decade 1991–2000 alone, according to one recent estimate, as many as 866,000 black deaths would have been averted (Woolf, 2004). This is the cumulative toll of excess African American deaths (as compared with whites) from cardiovascular disease, cerebrovascular disease, cancer, diabetes, HIV, pneumonia and influenza, and complications of pregnancy (National Center for Health Statistics, 2001). Comparable cumulative estimates for preventable premature death could be made for Hispanic Americans, who have higher death rates than non-Hispanic whites for diabetes, liver disease, and HIV, and for many categories of excess mortality for Asian/Pacific Islanders and Native Americans/Alaska Natives.

These data and countless other findings of health status disparities by race, ethnicity, social class, gender, migration, acculturation status, and other variables are described and analyzed in detail in thousands of peer-reviewed journal articles, numerous government reports, and other chapters in this book. What is of further significance is the evolution of explanations for these differences over time.

What Causes Disparities in Health Status?

Throughout the nineteenth century and well into the twentieth, the conventional public wisdom, buttressed by elaborate, pseudo-scientific articles in the medical literature, was that there were biologically and genetically distinct human races—and that African Americans (along with southern and eastern Europeans, Chinese, and any darker-skinned immigrants of other nationalities) were biologically and intellectually inferior, more susceptible to disease (Cartwright, 1851), and, implicitly, a threat to the health of the body politic. The American eugenics movement of the 1920s, incorporating these beliefs, presaged the later full-blown claims of Nazi theories of racial superiority. Alleged biological inferiority and attendant racist stereotyping in turn were used to justify "the settled fact" of rigid segregation and second-class status in citizenship, education, employment, housing, and health (Finnegan, 2003).

Minority scholars throughout this period offered vigorous arguments rejecting biological determinism, but for the most part, this work was ignored by mainstream science and most of the public. In 1944, however, Gunnar Myrdal and his colleagues published

An American Dilemma, a comprehensive examination of the conflict between the nation's formal commitments to equality and the reality of its racial practices. It offered a powerful argument for the social and structural causes—in particular, racism and discrimination—of the massive disparities it documented in education, employment, economic achievement, and other major sectors. It included a presentation of the then-current data on African American health status and explained that "area for area, class for class, Negroes cannot get the same advantage in the way of prevention and cure of disease that whites can. . . . Discrimination increases Negro sickness and death both directly and indirectly, and manifests itself both consciously and unconsciously" (pp. 171–172). "Discrimination" referred to both de jure and de facto practices in the larger society and to the structure of a segregated health care system. In the light of what we now know, these were astonishingly prescient statements.

Other, more variegated explanations of disparities in health status have dominated health policy and social science research in more recent decades. Health status disparities have been associated with socioeconomic status (SES) as measured by income, education, and employment; childhood poverty and social position; geographical variation; lack of access to health care; exposure to environmental and occupational hazards; racial/ethnic residential segregation and its effects on income, wealth, social isolation, and access to resources and opportunities; institutional and individual discrimination; lifestyle choices and behavioral risks; inferior housing and poor nutrition; differing beliefs about health and illness; and the consequences of income inequality (Williams, 2004; Berkman and Kawachi, 2000; Hofrichter, 2003; Krieger, 2004; Kawachi, Kennedy, and Wilkinson, 1999). Collectively, these give substance and detail to what has become classic public health doctrine: that the major determinants of population health status, and the primary explanations of disparities among population groups, lie in the social, physical, biological, economic, and political environments, which are determined by the larger society's norms, values, social stratification systems, and political economy (King, 1996; Menefee, 1996). These are, in effect, contemporary articulations of principles first expressed by Rudolf Virchow, the father of social medicine, and John Simon, the first health officer of London, more than 150 years ago.

Finally, in the early years of the twenty-first century, explanatory theories came full circle. Elements of the old biological determinism reappeared, this time in the form of (fiercely disputed) claims that new genetic data support the existence of biologically distinct human "races" (or "groups of continental origin") that offer at least partial explanations for population group differences in susceptibility to (or manifestations of) specific diseases, including common ailments of complex genetic origin. (For critiques of this perspective, see Schwartz, 2001; Goodman, 2000; Graves, 2001; Cooper, 2003.) Challenges to the prevailing scientific view that "race" is a social rather than a biologically meaningful construct have their parallel in conservative critics of the social determinants of health, who tend to select minority lifestyle choices and behavioral risks, alleged health illiteracy, inappropriate use of health care, or "lack of personal responsibility" as the noteworthy causes of differing population group morbidity and mortality (Satel, 2000). These contentions ignore elegant studies of attributable risk that estimate that lifestyle choices can account for less than 30 percent (at most) of the excess mortality of the poor and minorities (Lantz and others, 1998) and overlook the fact that lifestyle choices themselves are shaped in part by social and environmental factors that significantly constrain choice. Furthermore, an earlier U.S. surgeon general's report estimates that medical care explains only 10 percent of variation in health status (U.S. Department of Health, Education and Welfare, 1979), and more recent studies indicate that ensuring medical care for all would reduce premature deaths by only 10 to 15 percent (McGinnis, Williams-Russo, and Knickman, 2002). These factors thus leave at least 60 percent of the disparities in health status unexplained. (Further evidence of the limited effect of health care on mortality is provided by the persistence of health status disparities by social class and race/ethnicity in nations, such as the United Kingdom, that provide universal access to care.)

RACISM, SOCIAL CLASS, AND THE SOCIAL CONTEXT OF DISPARITIES IN HEALTH STATUS

Multiple national studies of majority beliefs about minorities affirm that negative racial and ethnic characterizations, though often subtle in open expression, continue to be widely held and have been stubbornly resistant to significant change. The ideology of white superiority and minority inferiority is used to attribute the causes of disparities in minority health status to the alleged behavior of people of color and ethnic minorities, rather than to the realities of the nation's social class and racial stratifications and the hazardous social, economic, and physical environments they have created. In 1990, for example, 29 percent of white respondents characterized blacks and Hispanics as "unintelligent"; 44 percent said blacks were "lazy," and 33 percent said the same of Hispanics; 56 percent and 42 percent, respectively, said blacks and Hispanics "prefer welfare," and 50 percent and 38 percent, respectively, believed blacks and Hispanics were "violence prone" (National Opinion Research Center, 1990). Five years later, a similar study reported almost identical responses (Survey Research Center, 1995), and in 2001 some 60 percent of white respondents agreed that "most blacks don't have the motivation or willpower to pull themselves up out of poverty" (Washington Post/Kaiser Foundation/Harvard University, 2001). In that survey, 51 percent said that African Americans "have about the same opportunities in life as whites have," and 49 percent said the same of Hispanics. (In this view, the old civil rights song now comes in the past tense, as "We *Have* Overcome.") In a 2004 poll, more than two-thirds of Americans overall rejected the statement "We should make every possible effort to improve the position of blacks and other minorities, even if it means giving them preferential treatment," a view that has not varied since 1987, and nearly half of whites asserted that efforts to promote equal rights have "gone too far" (Pew Research Center for the People and the Press, 2004). In this view, the civil rights song should say "We Have *Overshot.*"

Numerous studies and a long stream of recent books offer evidence that the United States has been in a decades-long period of rebounding individual and institutional racism. They include *Racism Without Racists: Color-Blind Racism and the Persistence of Racial Inequality in the United States* (Bonilla-Silva, 2003); *Whiteout: The Continuing Significance of Racism* (Doane and Bonilla-Silva, 2003); *White Men on Race: Power, Privilege and the Shaping of Cultural Consciousness* (Feagin and O'Brien, 2003); *Race in the Schoolyard* (Lewis, 2003); and *Jim Crow's Children: The Broken Promise of the* Brown *Decision*

(Irons, 2002). Conservative critics, in contrast, specifically dismiss the contribution of institutional and individual racism to disparities in health—indeed, to deny the very existence of any current racism (D'Souza, 1996; Thernstrom and Thernstrom, 1999).

Race and ethnicity, of course, are not the only variables affecting the failure to achieve anything approaching health equity. Social class differences in health status within racial/ethnic groups are often larger than between such groups, and gender differences within and between racial/ethnic groups are also significant, as I note below.

In a society that likes to pretend that social class stratification does not really exist and that unlimited upward mobility is available to all, social class has been relatively underemphasized as a determinant of health status, despite substantial evidence that it is a significant contributor (Isaacs and Schroeder, 2004; Krieger and Fee, 1994). The traditional components of socioeconomic status—income, education, and occupation—all have been found to be independently associated with health status. In the United Kingdom, where social class stratification is a routine tool of epidemiological investigation, job classification predicted cardiovascular mortality more effectively than cholesterol level, hypertension, or smoking in London civil servants, all of whom had access to the National Health Service (Marmot, Rose, Shipley, and Hamilton, 1978). In the United States, individuals with less than a high school education have far higher rates of cardiovascular, gastrointestinal, pulmonary, and renal disease than those with a high school diploma (Pincus, Callahan, and Burkhauser, 1987). Socioeconomic status is a major contributor to the higher mortality of African Americans versus whites, and education is important in that gradient; indeed, the health status of educated minorities is far closer to that of educated white populations than to that of poor and less educated minorities (Guralnik and others, 1993). The social class gradient in mortality has increased in recent decades (Pappas, Queen, Hadden, and Fisher, 1993), as has income inequality.

Since race and ethnicity are deeply confounded with income, wealth, education, and occupation in American society, these combined factors are major determinants of disparities in health status. Health care is not immune to these larger social forces.

Disparities in Health Care: Unequal Treatment

The American health care system has its own long history of racial and class segregation and discrimination. Well into the seventh decade of the twentieth century, it was "embedded in intense racism and discrimination" (Thomson, 1997, p. 910). North and south, de jure and de facto, it was legal and often customary for hospitals flatly to refuse admission to black patients or house them separately in basement wards. Facilities and systems of care for the poor, the "charity hospitals" and public health clinics, were often physically inferior, underfunded, and overcrowded, and nursing homes were—and remain—highly segregated. Black and other minority physicians were routinely denied hospital staff appointments and membership in whites-only local, state, and national medical associations. One review of this history concluded that "discrimination was everywhere, including among the medical and health professionals who furnished care and ultimately determined the structure, design, and operation of the health system" (Rosenbaum, Markins, and Darnell, 2000).

The Civil Rights Act and the Medicare and Medicaid legislation of 1965 accomplished profound changes in these institutional patterns, although physicians' private offices were shielded from the full mandate for integration. At the same time in the 1960s, scattered studies began to appear in peer-reviewed medical literature noting differences in the quality and comprehensiveness of the individual diagnostic and therapeutic medical care provided for African Americans. Such findings were hardly new—similar observations predated the founding of the nation (Byrd and Clayton, 1992)—but they signaled a double violation: of basic American concepts of fairness and, more specifically, of the ethical and egalitarian commitments of medicine. During the next three decades, larger-scale quantitative evidence that racial/ethnic inequities occurred frequently in American medical care flowed into the literature when researchers gained access to large administrative and clinical databases from Medicare, the Health Care Financing Administration, the Department of Veterans Affairs, other federal and state agencies, and multicenter clinical studies. In 1990, the American Medical Association formally acknowledged the existence of such black-white disparities in health care and noted that "disparities in treatment decisions may reflect the existence of subconscious bias. . . . The health care system, like all other elements of society, has not fully eradicated this [racial] prejudice" (American Medical Association, Council on Ethics and Judicial Affairs, 1990, p. 2346.) Yet these findings did not command national public attention until the publication in 2001 of the Institute of Medicine's (IOM) landmark study *Unequal Treatment: Confronting Racial and Ethnic Disparities in Health Care* (Smedley, Stith, and Nelson, 2003).

Numerous exhaustive reviews now document the range and magnitude of inequities in diagnosis and treatment. The IOM volume included a ninety-page bibliography of more than one hundred key peer-reviewed studies. A forty-page commissioned paper examined the voluminous evidence in just six major disease and treatment categories (Geiger, 2001). A published review and analysis of racial disparities in the diagnosis and treatment of cardiovascular disease (Kressin and Petersen, 2001) reappeared on the Internet as "The Weight of the Evidence," a Web site sponsored by several foundations, the American College of Cardiology, and the American Heart Association (Kaiser Family Foundation, 2002a). A sampling of other studies reviewed the evidence of racial/ethnic variations in the treatment of cancer (Shavers and Brown, 2002), pediatric disease (Hahn, 1995; Stevens and Shi, 2003; Lieu and others, 2002), and stroke (Oddone, Horner, Monger, and Matchar, 1993; Mitchell and Bollard, 2000). Similar findings have been summarized for the treatment of HIV/AIDS, diabetes, and other diseases. An annotated bibliography prepared for the report of an expert panel commissioned by Physicians for Human Rights listed more than eight hundred studies covering seventeen disease and treatment categories (Sohler, Walmsley, Lubetkin, and Geiger, 2003).

In sum, the evidence of differential treatment for African Americans, Hispanics, Native Americans, and Asian/Pacific Islanders is credible and robust, in studies that are appropriately controlled for such major confounding variables as insurance status, income and education, age, gender, stage and severity of disease, and presence or absence of comorbid illness. Furthermore, these studies examine the care of patients who are already in the health care system, minimizing access to care as a factor. This pattern has been found not only for such high-technology interventions as angioplasty and coronary artery bypass grafting, advanced cancer chemotherapy, and renal transplantation but also for such routine processes as general medical and surgical procedures and the treatment of asthma, diabetes, congestive heart failure, and pneumonia. Disparities have been noted even in such basic elements of the clinical care of minority and poor patients as the adequacy of clinical history taking, physical examinations, and routine laboratory procedures (Kahn and others, 1994). A growing literature is documenting failure to provide adequate pain medication for minority patients—for example, for Hispanics with bone fractures (Todd, Samarov, and Hoffman, 1993) and African Americans with colorectal cancer (Cleeland and others, 1997).

These are not rare or aberrant events, and they often have serious consequences. There is good evidence that denial of appropriate treatment to African Americans with coronary artery disease has included patients who were most seriously ill and were most likely to have benefited, and that those differences in care contributed to significant differences in their five-year mortality (Peterson and others, 1997). Black and Hispanic patients who have suffered heart attacks are less likely than whites to receive the appropriate drugs—even aspirin. Minority children with asthma are less likely to be given the most effective modern medications. African American patients with end-stage renal disease, all of whom are insured under a federal program, are less likely than their white counterparts even to be offered a discussion of the possibility of a kidney transplant (Klassen and others, 2002).

What is going on here? While professional medical societies have responded with vigorous affirmations of the need for change and specific proposals to accomplish it (American College of Physicians, 2004), the responses of physicians have been slow to evolve. Despite the overwhelming weight of the evidence, a Kaiser Foundation National Survey of Physicians in 2002 found that 55 percent of doctors asserted that the health care system "rarely" treats people unfairly on the basis of race or ethnicity, 10 percent said "never," and less than 30 percent said "at least sometimes" (Kaiser Family Foundation, 2002b). In contrast, 77 percent of African American physicians and 52 percent of Hispanic physicians reported that unfair treatment occurs at least somewhat often. Asked about the causes of any differential treatment by race/ethnicity, 58 percent of surveyed physicians said it was largely due to "too few physicians being available in minority communities," a statement that is largely irrelevant to the fact of profession-wide quality variations in the care of minority patients. Physicians (and other health workers) are reluctant to believe that their own behaviors, those of their peers, and the policies of their institutions may often violate their conscious commitments to equity.

GENDER, RACE, AND CLASS: INTERSECTORAL CLUES

Analyses of variations in health status by the major categories of race and class are important and enormously informative, but they are relatively crude approaches to understanding their causes, the wider social contexts in which they are embedded, or their impact on (or origins in) the everyday life experiences of women and men in these groups. Many categories are absurdly broad. "Hispanics" lumps together women of Puerto Rican, Dominican, Cuban, Central American, and Mexican origin (along with Brazilians, Chileans, Argentinians, and some actual Spaniards)—groups that vary in both social circumstance and various aspects of health status. "Asians" may refer to Chinese, Japanese, Korean, Vietnamese, Cambodian, Laotian, or Hmong groups, as well as to women of Indian, Pakistani, Bangladeshi, or other origins. The life experiences and health status of African Americans vary along an urban-rural continuum and differ from those of immigrants born in Africa or the Caribbean. In sum, every individual has multiple social identities— by "race," social class, age, primary language, cultural belief system, geographical region and neighborhood residence, and other variables—that affect health status in ways that may be cumulative, differentiated, or contradictory.

"Gender" is now understood as a social construct, a composite of assigned social roles and behaviors and ascribed qualities, rather than as a reference to biological identity, though in most current medical literature, the term is used in the latter sense. In any case, medical, sociological, and epidemiological data illuminate the complex intersections of women's health with issues of race and class.

In every population group, women live longer than men but report more chronic illness during their lifetimes, but those figures vary by race and ethnicity. A recent Kaiser Foundation study (2004) found that nearly 20 percent of African American women and 29 percent of Latinas described their health status as only "fair" or "poor," compared with 13 percent of white women. Nearly 60 percent of African American women aged forty-five to sixty reported a diagnosis of hypertension, compared with 28 percent of white women in the same age group, and 40 percent of African American women of all ages said they had arthritis, as did 33 percent of Latinas and 32 percent of white women. Almost twice as many African Americans and Latinas as white women had diabetes (16 percent, 17 percent, and 9 percent, respectively), and women of color were far likelier to suffer limb amputations, blindness, and end-stage renal disease. In contrast, roughly 25 percent of all women have been diagnosed with depression, but there is little variation by race/ethnicity (Kaiser Family Foundation, 2004). While low-income women of all race/ethnicity groups were twice as likely as the more affluent to be in fair or poor health, they also reported experiencing more barriers to health care because of lower health insurance coverage, problems with transportation, and the demands of work and child care. While I have previously noted that medical care makes only a small contribution to group health status, it has powerful effects on disability, pain and suffering, and quality of life.

A wide variety of methodologically different studies illustrate the diversity of approaches necessary to further our understanding of causation and the lived experiences of patients from different racial/ethnic groups. Age-adjusted breast cancer mortality rates among white and African American women in the United States have been diverging during the past twenty years, a finding that many investigators have speculated is due to inadequate African American access to health care and high-quality treatment, presentation at later stages of disease, or as yet undefined behavioral choices. But a recent epidemiological study of white and African American breast cancer survival in the U.S. Department of Defense Healthcare System—in which equal access to care is assured and insurance status and income are not relevant issues—found the same worsening survival for African American women, even when age and stage of disease were accounted for (Jatoi, Becher, and Leake, 2003). Relatively little is known, however, about differences in the psychosocial impact of breast cancer, health-related quality of life, and social context of survivorship. An intensive focus group study of African American, Asian American, Latina, and Caucasian survivors found significant variation by race/ethnicity in beliefs about health and illness, dietary practices, and coping strategies among these groups and identified them as priority areas for further research (Ashing-Giwa and others, 2004). Such beliefs, practices, and strategies, however, are themselves shaped (and constrained) by the larger social context.

Krieger has explored the effects of racial discrimination as a risk factor for hypertension in black and white women and men (Krieger and Sidney, 1996) and the effects of both racial and gender discrimination on blood pressure in African American women (Krieger, 1990). These were among the first of an ongoing series of research studies showing that the experience of perceived discrimination on the basis of race or gender is associated with increased risk of hypertension, an effect especially marked among those who failed to speak out or take action against such unfair treatment and, presumably, internalized their anger. No such associations were noted for white women, suggesting a unique risk for women of color. A study of Canadian native women proposed a model for understanding their impaired health that has some relevance for all minority groups in the United States. Their health, the author argued, "should be seen in a fourth world context," in which "a minority population exists in a nation where institutionalized power and prestige are held by a colonizing, subordinating majority" (O'Neil, 1986).

Age, gender, race, and social circumstance intersect dramatically in the HIV/AIDS epidemic in the United States. AIDS has become the leading cause of death for African American women aged twenty-five to forty-four (Bernstein, 2003). In government studies of twenty-nine states, an African American woman was twenty-three times as likely to be infected with AIDS as a white woman, and black women accounted for roughly 72 percent of all new HIV cases in women from 1999 to 2002. Most of the studies exploring the causes of these findings have focused on individual-level risk factors, with relatively little consideration of social context. A recent study, in contrast, argues for the primacy of structural violence and community-level factors to explain racial and ethnic differences in infection rates. These include the disproportionate incarceration rates of African men, creating an African American sex ratio in which women outnumber men in many local communities; residential segregation and constraints on access to sexually transmitted disease services; and social norms stigmatizing homosexuality, among other factors (Lane and others, 2004).

Similar interactions of race, age, gender, and health status among African American men and women are examined in some detail in Chapter Five in this volume, with particular attention to variation by social class. A full understanding of these data will require further consideration of social and community context, the intersection of race and gender roles, strengths as well as vulnerabilities, coping strategies, and access to institutional supports.

What Do We Need to Know?

Our knowledge of the existence of these inequities in care outstrips our understanding of their causes, though research has provided strong clues. Most of the earlier studies documenting unequal treatment included rather cursory and speculative discussions of possible causes but offered no hard data on what really influenced these specific and inequitable clinical decisions. Research in recent years has made it clear that there is no single smoking gun; causation, in the academic phrase, is multifactorial, and many different forces are in play (Smedley, Stith, and Nelson, 2003; Physicians for Human Rights, 2003; van Ryn and Fu, 2003). There is general agreement that these can be grouped into five broad categories: patient factors, provider factors, institutional factors, community factors, and geographical factors (Fiscella, 2004).

Patient factors frequently cited to explain disparities in care include patient choice or preference, usually implying a patient's refusal to accept a clinician's recommendation (Katz, 2001; Ayanian, Cleary, Weissman, and Epstein, 1999); cultural beliefs about health and medical care thought to be held by members of different minority groups; minority mistrust of the medical care system, based at least in part on high reported rates of perceived past discrimination (Corbie-Smith, Thomas, and St. George, 2002); language barriers (Fiscella, Franks, Doescher, and Saver, 2002); difficulties in cross-racial/ethnic, cross-gender, and cross-class physician-patient communication (Horowitz, Davis, Palermo, and

Vladeck, 2000); inadequate health literacy (American Medical Association, 1999); and alleged biological differences in clinical presentation.

While the data fall far short of justifying a convenient victim-blaming explanation of disparities, there is evidence for each of these factors. Two of them—the idea that patient preference accounts for disparities in care and the idea that minority distrust of the health care system accounts for such disparities—thus deserve special comment. First, in careful studies, the effect of patient preferences has never been sufficient to account for more than a small fraction of the observed disparities in care (Ayanian, Cleary, Weissman, and Epstein, 1999; Hannan and others, 1999). While many studies found evidence that some minority patients chose not to accept a physician's recommendation for a course of treatment or an intervention procedure, these decisions made only a minor contribution to the observed differences in the care that was provided, which in most cases was determined by the physician alone. Patient refusal, in turn, is in part the product of physician-patient communication, patient's level of health literacy and prior knowledge of a treatment or procedure, anticipation of out-of-pocket costs, and beliefs about the appropriateness and effectiveness of different courses of action in response to an illness. Second, recent research suggests that the depth and scope of minority mistrust, in all likelihood a reflection of past experiences of perceived racism in both the health care system and everyday life, have been underestimated. While mistrust is especially intense with regard to participation in clinical trials, it also is evident in everyday medical care. In one such study of a representative sample, 63 percent of African Americans and 38 percent of whites believed their physicians often prescribed medication as a means to experiment on people without their consent; 25 percent of African Americans and 8 percent of whites believed that their doctors had given them an experimental treatment without their consent. More than 45 percent of African Americans and approximately 35 percent of whites said they believed their doctors might expose them to unnecessary risks (Corbie-Smith, Thomas, and St. George, 2002). Such disproportionate levels of minority mistrust obviously may affect adherence to prescribed regimens and may interact with a patient's beliefs about the illness. If one's physician is not regarded as trustworthy and ethical, alternative theories of causation and treatment may seem safer and more credible. But trustworthiness is itself affected by physician behavior, especially with regard to listening, explaining, sharing decision making with the patient, and treating the patient with respect (Blanchard and Lurie, 2004).

Provider factors include lack of cultural competence—that is, a physician's familiarity with systems of belief about health and illness among both majority and minority patients of different racial or ethnic groups, socioeconomic position, primary language, gender roles, sexual orientation, and age. It also includes some understanding of the physical and social environments in which different patients live, the wide varieties of family structure, and the constraints of time and money that affect the working poor, as well as an understanding that physicians and other providers bring to the consulting room their own cultural backgrounds and beliefs (Carillo, Green, and Betancourt, 1999). Provider factors also involve physicians' participatory decision-making practice styles (Kaplan and others, 1996); clinical uncertainty about the findings in the medical history or symptom presentation of minority patients, especially for conditions in which there are no clear treatment guidelines (van Ryn, 2002; Balsa and McGuire, 2001; Bloche, 2001); overt racism (Finucane and Carrese, 1990); and both conscious and unconscious racial/ethnic bias and negative racial stereotyping influencing clinical decisions (van Ryn and Fu, 2003).

The issue of bias, racial/ethnic stereotyping, and other forms of stereotyping by gender, social class, sexual orientation, or any combination of these, is central to understanding inequities in care and intersectoral concerns. As I have noted, bias and stereotyping are vehemently denied by many physicians, who are committed to the belief that they, their peers, and their institutions treat everyone fairly. And they are methodologically difficult to establish, since direct solicitation of providers' racial/ethnic views is likely to elicit socially acceptable answers and since a rich literature in cognitive psychology affirms that such stereotyping can occur in the absence of conscious prejudice and, indeed, below the level of conscious awareness. These studies also show that stereotyping is facilitated by time pressure and cognitive overload—having to think about many things at once—an apt description of clinical work.

Two studies in recent years are particularly useful in illustrating the impact of "bias"—a term often used in the belief that flat-out charges of "racism" are counterproductive and only provoke indignant professional denials—on clinical decision making. A prospective study that enabled researchers to interview physicians about their reasons for the treatment decisions they had made documented the projection of classic negative racial stereotypes on African American patients with coronary artery disease. They were viewed as unlikely to participate in cardiac rehabilitation, insufficiently energetic, unlikely to understand clinical regimens, lacking in social supports, and not having stressful jobs—all on the basis of brief physician-patient interviews mostly concerned with clinical data. And these judgments were associated with physicians' decisions to deny a recommendation for bypass grafting even in some cases in which standard clinical criteria defined the need as urgent (van Ryn and Burke, 2000). The second study, also about coronary artery disease, reviewed the clinical decisions made by Veterans Affairs cardiologists, who were given all the relevant clinical information but—in more than nine hundred cases—were effectively blinded to each patient's race. There was no significant black-white difference in the decisions for angioplasty or bypass grafting. Removing that single variable from clinical awareness was associated with care that depended only on clinical characteristics, not race, in contrast to the findings in scores of studies in which patient race was known (Okelo and others, 2001).

Institutional factors include workforce diversity; availability of interpreters; geographical location of hospitals, physicians' offices, and other facilities; attitudes of nonphysician support staff; culturally appropriate signs, written materials, and health promotion programs; policies with regard to copayments, deductibles, and other out-of-pocket costs; and the presence or absence of intensive quality monitoring programs (Fiscella, 2004). The constraints on time for each patient visit, overall patient load, paperwork requirements, and other administrative burdens in managed care settings may also affect racially disparate outcomes in primary care, reducing the content and quality of physician-patient communication and increasing stereotyping (Barr, 1995).

Community factors include the proximity and availability of providers, the availability of regular sources of care (other than emergency rooms or walk-in clinics), the opportunities for continuity of care, the presence or absence of safety net providers, community levels of health knowledge and trust in the health care system, and community rates of insurance. A recent finding speaks to the power of residential segregation—and a previously unrecognized de facto segregation of medical care itself. In a national cross-sectional study of black and white Medicare patients, most primary care visits by black patients were with a small group of physicians (80 percent of their visits were accounted for by 22 percent of physicians), who provided only a small percentage of their care to white patients (Bach and others, 2004). In effect, to a large extent, these insured black and white patients were treated by different physicians. Furthermore, the physicians treating black patients were much more likely than those visited by white patients to report great difficulty in obtaining access for their patients to high-quality subspecialists, high-quality diagnostic imaging, and admission to the hospital, thus limiting the overall ability to provide high-quality care. These findings, it should be noted, deal primarily with ambulatory care and have no direct relation to the previously described overwhelming evidence of racial/ethnic disparities in inpatient care. Rather, they speak to the limitations of the primary care facilities and physicians' offices (whether the physicians were black or, as is the case, mostly white) available to most patients in residentially segregated inner-city and rural communities. They reflect the fact that a health care system organized on principles of a market economy inevitably produces an inequitable distribution of health care resources (Fernandez and Goldstein, 2004).

A recent cluster of geographical studies revealed yet another dimension of variation in the quality of care. In the United States, one study found, the overall quality of care (for all patients) varies significantly from one geographical area or metropolitan center to another, but variations in racial/ethnic disparities in the quality of care varied independent of the overall quality level. For black patients living in some predominantly black geographical communities, the quality of their care might be low even if black/white disparities were minimal. Pooled national data mask these regional differences. Here too it seems clear that residential racial segregation plays a role in the care that black patients receive (Baicker, Chancra, Skinner, and Wennberg, 2004).

What is insufficiently recognized is that all of these factors interact and may influence one another. Patient behavior, often rooted in community customs, cultural beliefs, and past experience, influences physician responses. Physician practice styles, often similarly influenced by community customs, cultural beliefs, and the cultures of undergraduate and graduate medical training, affect patient preferences. Lack of physician-patient concordance by race, gender, or social class affects communication, clinical decision making, and patient satisfaction. Stereotyping can operate in both directions: physicians' rote ascription of characteristics to minority patients and patients' beliefs that they are being treated with disrespect on the basis of race rather than as part of the frictions and insensitivities that afflict everyone in the health care system. The whole clinical encounter occurs in the context of a society that has multiple systems of social stratification, not least of which is the power imbalance between physicians and patients.

What we do not know is which one (or combination) of these causal factors is associated with each major type of racial/ethnic disparity in clinical decision making and health care. Are they the same for children and adults? For members of different minority groups? For different categories of disease? Why are disparities seen in some areas and not others? Which causal factors are most frequently operative in gender disparities, race/ethnicity disparities, social class disparities, and their combinations or intersections? Without such knowledge, how can we design effective interventions? These questions dictate both research and policy agendas.

WHAT SHOULD WE DO?

There are two broad approaches to intervention to reduce disparities in health care. The first is neutral on race/ethnicity, class, and gender: it focuses on the rigorous monitoring of quality of care and implementation of standardized expert guidelines and evidence-based clinical practices for all patients in all types of health care institutions. It draws on mounting evidence of appalling deficiencies in the quality of medical care, including a finding that barely half of the preventive and curative treatments provided to adults in the United States met recommended standards (Kerr and others, 2004; McGlynn and others, 2003; Institute of Medicine, 2001).

The second approach, focused on the specific disparities documented by *Unequal Treatment* and so many other sources, proposes both research and policy actions to deal with the issues of race/ethnicity, gender, and class. They are not mutually exclusive, and both types of efforts are already under way.

A minimal but essential requirement is that all clinical records in every health facility be coded by the patient's self-reported race/ethnicity and, possibly, by primary language and indicators of social class. Without such information, it will not be possible to monitor disparities effectively; identify problem providers, institutions, or areas of care; search more precisely for causes; and design interventions. Resistance to such identification is manifested in "color-blindness" ballot initiatives to eliminate all governmental collection of these data, it raises minority suspicions of racial profiling, and it will inevitably contain some imprecision, but it is necessary—in medical care as in multiple other areas of American life—to count race until race no longer counts. Multiple organizational efforts are already under way by hospital associations, managed care organizations, health insurance companies, and others, but such efforts are still in their infancy. Federal and state government leadership—and mandates—will be essential, especially for Medicare and Medicaid records, but that will require political will (and, in all probability, a different national administration). When the Agency for Healthcare Research and Quality (2004) produced a congressionally mandated first national report card on the scope and magnitude of racial/ethnic disparities in health care, for example, the Office of the Secretary of Health and Human Services attempted to censor it, downplay the findings, and remove all suggestions of discrimination (Geiger, 2004). It is important that racial/ethnic data on disparities should not be merely collected but routinely and consistently analyzed, as a responsibility of providers and of quality assurance oversight agencies.

Other efforts include widespread programs to teach cultural competency to physicians and other health providers practicing in a nation that is increasingly diverse and will soon reach "minority majority" status. We do not yet know which types of such education are most effective and at which stages of training, and there is no evidence yet of the effect of such provider education on the clinical care they provide, but such research also is in early stages of development and implementation. We know far too little of the values and attitudes students bring to their health professional training, how they may change in the course of that training, the relevant characteristics of the institutions in which they train, and the extent to which they vary by the social and personal characteristics of providers themselves.

Because race-based disparities in American medical care are, almost by definition, civil rights and human rights issues, Physicians for Human Rights, as part of numerous recommendations for congressional, judicial, and administrative action, urged full-scale monitoring by the Offices of Civil Rights in the federal Department of Health and Human Services and the Department of Justice.

What is perhaps of most interest to those concerned with intersectoral issues, finally, is an ongoing research agenda. The very nexus of disparities in medical care is the clinical encounter. That is where most inequities in diagnosis and treatment are generated. We need intense observational studies of race- and gender-discordant and -concordant physician-patient clinical encounters, in combined or parallel efforts by medical anthropologists and sociologists, cognitive psychologists, clinical educators, and quality assurance evaluators. Similarly, we need a new round of studies of the culture of medicine, focused on the behaviors and expressed attitudes toward race, ethnicity, and gender in ward rounds, medical and surgical residents' meetings, and both the overt and latent content of the instruction of medical and nursing students and other providers in training. Specifically, we need studies of what has been termed the natural history of social categorization in health professional education and practice. An enormous volume of such studies already exists, but too little of it is focused specifically on these issues.

It is only through this combination of quantitative and qualitative studies that we are likely to advance our understanding of intersectoral effects on health care and ultimately design effective interventions. Such efforts will have only a modest effect on the disparities in health status of disadvantaged and socially marginalized population groups, but they can have a powerful effect on the health-related quality of life—the lived experiences—of individuals. And at the very best, they can serve as a model for what it will take to reduce disparity in other sectors of American society, one step in the unsteady march toward equity.

References

Agency for Healthcare Research and Quality. *National Healthcare Disparities Report: Summary.* Rockville, Md.: Agency for Healthcare Research and Quality, 2004. http://www.ahrq.gov/qual/nhdr03.nhdrsum.htm.

American College of Physicians. "Racial and Ethnic Disparities in Health Care: A Position Paper of the American College of Physicians." *Annals of Internal Medicine,* 2004, *141,* 226–232.

American Medical Association, Council on Ethical and Judicial Affairs. "Black-White Disparities in Health Care." *Journal of the American Medical Association,* 1990, *263,* 2344–2346.

American Medical Association, Council on Scientific Affairs, Ad Hoc Committee on Health Literacy for the Council on Scientific Affairs. "Health Literacy: Report of the Council on Scientific Affairs." *JAMA,* 1999, *281,* 552–557.

Arias, E., and Smith, B. L. "Deaths: Preliminary Data from 2001." *National Vital Statistics Report,* 2003, *51,* 1–44.

Ashing-Giwa, K. T., and others. "Understanding the Breast Cancer Experience of Women: A Qualitative Study of African American, Latina and Caucasian Cancer Survivors." *Psychooncology,* 2004, *13,* 408–428.

Ayanian, J. Z., Cleary, P. D., Weissman, S., and Epstein, A. M. "The Effect of Patients' Preferences on Racial Differences in Access to Renal Transplantation." *New England Journal of Medicine,* 1999, *341,* 1661–1669.

Bach, P. B., and others. "Primary Care Physicians Who Treat Blacks and Whites." *New England Journal of Medicine,* 2004, *351,* 575–584.

Baicker, J., Chancra, A., Skinner, J., and Wennberg, J. E. "Who You Are and Where You Live: How Race and Geography Affect the Treatment of Medicare Beneficiaries." *Health Affairs Web Exclusive.* 2004. http://www.healthaffairs.org.

Balsa, A. I., and McGuire, T. G. "Statistical Discrimination in Health Care." *Journal of Health Economics,* 2001, *20,* 881–907.

Barr, D. A. "The Effects of Organizational Structure on Primary Care Outcomes Under Managed Care." *Annals of Internal Medicine,* 1995, *122,* 353–359.

Berkman, L. A., and Kawachi, I. *Social Epidemiology.* New York: Oxford University Press, 2000.

Bernstein, L. A. "Achieving Equity in Women's and Perinatal Health." Dec. 12, 2003. http://www.Medscape.com/womenshealthhome.

Blanchard, J., and Lurie, N. "R-E-S-P-E-C-T: Patient Reports of Disrespect in the Health Care Setting and Its Impact on Care." *Journal of Family Practice,* 2004, *53,* 721–730.

Bloche, G. "Race and Discretion in Medical Care." *Yale Journal of Health Policy, Law and Ethics,* 2001, *1,* 95–131.

Bonilla-Silva, E. *Racism Without Racists: Color-Blind Racism and the Persistence of Racial Inequality in the United States.* Lanham, Md.: Rowman and Littlefield, 2003.

Byrd, W. M., and Clayton, L. A. "An American Health Dilemma: A History of Blacks in the Health System." *Journal of the National Medical Association,* 1992, *84,* 189–200.

Byrd, W. M., and Clayton, L. A. *An American Health Dilemma.* New York: Routledge, 2000.

Carrillo, J. E., Green, A. R., and Betancourt, J. R. "Cross-Cultural Primary Care: A Patient-Based Approach." *Annals of Internal Medicine,* 1999, *130,* 829–834.

Cartwright, S. A. "Report on the Diseases and Physical Peculiarities of the Negro Race." *New Orleans Medical and Surgical Journal,* 1851, *8,* 28–37.

Cleeland, C. S., and others. "Pain and Treatment of Pain in Minority Patients with Cancer." *Annals of Internal Medicine,* 1997, *127,* 813–816.

Cooper, R. S. "Race, Genes and Health—New Wine in Old Bottles?" *International Journal of Epidemiology,* 2003, *32,* 23–25.

Corbie-Smith, G., Thomas, S. B., and St. George, D. M. "Distrust, Race and Research." *Archives of Internal Medicine,* 2002, *162,* 2458–2463.

Doane, A. W., and Bonilla-Silva, E. (eds.). *Whiteout: The Continuing Significance of Racism.* New York: Routledge, 2003.

D'Souza, D. *The End of Racism: Principles for a Multiracial Society.* New York: Simon & Schuster, 1996.

Feagin, J., and O'Brien, E. *White Men on Race: Power, Privileges, and the Shaping of Cultural Consciousness.* Boston: Beacon Press, 2003.

Fernandez, A., and Goldstein, L. "Comment: Primary Care Physicians Who Treat Blacks and Whites." *New England Journal of Medicine,* 2004, *351,* 2126–2127.

Finnegan, W. "The Fire Last Time." *New York Times Book Review,* Mar. 23, 2003, p. 12.

Finucane, T. E., and Carrese, J. A. "Racial Bias in Presentation of Cases." *Journal of General Internal Medicine,* 1990, *5,* 120–121.

Fiscella, K. "Within Our Reach: Equality in Health Care Quality." Paper presented at the Roundtable on Racial and Ethnic Disparities in Health Care Treatment, Harvard Law School Civil Rights Project, Boston, May 18, 2004.

Fiscella, K., Franks, P., Doescher, M. P., and Saver, B. "Disparities in Health Care by Race, Ethnicity and Language Among the Insured: Findings from a National Sample." *Medical Care,* 2002, *40,* 52–59.

Geiger, H. J. "Racial and Ethnic Disparities in Diagnosis and Treatment: A Review of the Literature and a Consideration of Causes." In

B. D. Smedley, A. Y. Stith, and A. R. Nelson (eds.), *Unequal Treatment: Confronting Racial and Ethnic Disparities in Health Care.* Washington, D.C.: National Academy Press, 2003.

Geiger, H. J. "Why Is HHS Obscuring a Health Care Gap?" *Washington Post,* Jan. 27, 2004, p. A8.

Goodman, H. A. "Why Genes Don't Count (for Racial Differences in Health)." *American Journal of Public Health,* 2000, *90,* 1699–1702.

Graves, J. L., Jr. *The Emperor's New Clothes: Biological Theories of Race at the Millennium.* New Brunswick, N.J.: Rutgers University Press, 2001.

Guralnik, J. M., and others. "Educational Status and Active Life Expectancy Among Older Blacks and Whites." *New England Journal of Medicine,* 1993, *329,* 110–116.

Hahn, B. A. "Children's Health: Racial and Ethnic Differences in the Use of Prescription Medications." *Pediatrics,* 1995, *95,* 727–732.

Hajat, A. "Health Outcomes Among Hispanic Subgroups: Data from the National Health Interview Survey, 1992–1995." *Vital Health Statistics,* 2000, *310,* 111–114.

Hannan, E. L., and others. "Access to Coronary Artery Bypass Surgery by Race/Ethnicity and Gender Among Patients Who Are Appropriate for Surgery." *Medical Care,* 1999, *37,* 68–77.

Hofrichter, R. (ed.). *Health and Social Justice: Politics, Ideology, and Inequity in the Distribution of Disease.* San Francisco: Jossey-Bass, 2003.

Horowitz, C. R., Davis, M. M., Palermo, A. S., and Vladeck, B. C. "Approaches to Eliminating Sociocultural Disparities in Health." *Health Care Financing Review,* 2000, *21,* 57–73.

Institute of Medicine. *Crossing the Quality Chasm: A New Health System for the Twenty-First Century.* Washington, D.C.: National Academy Press, 2001.

Irons, P. *Jim Crow's Children: The Broken Promise of the* Brown *Decision.* New York: Viking Penguin, 2002.

Isaacs, S. L., and Schroeder, S. A. "Class—The Ignored Determinant of the Nation's Health." *New England Journal of Medicine,* 2004, *351,* 1137–1141.

Jatoi, I., Becher, H., and Leake, C. R. "Widening Disparity in Survival Between White and African-American Patients with Breast Carcinoma Treated in the U.S. Department of Defense Health Care System." *Cancer,* 2003, *98,* 894–899.

Kahn, K. L., and others. "Health Care for Black and Poor Hospitalized Medicare Patients." *Journal of the American Medical Association,* 1994, *271,* 1169–1174.

Kaiser Family Foundation. "The Weight of the Evidence." Feb. 2002a. http://www.kff.org/whythedifference.html.

Kaiser Family Foundation. *National Survey of Physicians: Part I: Doctors on Disparities in Medical Care.* Menlo Park, Calif.: Kaiser Family Foundation, 2002b.

Kaiser Family Foundation. "Kaiser Women's Health Survey." Mar. 2004. http://www.kff.org/womenshealth.

Kaplan, S. H., and others. "Characteristics of Physicians with Participatory Decision-Making Styles." *Annals of Internal Medicine,* 1996, *124,* 497–504.

Katz, J. N. "Patient Preference and Healthcare Disparities." *Journal of the American Medical Association,* 2001, *286,* 1506–1509.

Kawachi, I., Kennedy, B. P., and Wilkinson, R. C. (eds.). *Income Inequality and Health.* New York: New Press, 1999.

Kerr, E. A., and others. "Profiling the Quality of Care in Twelve Communities: Results from the CQI Study." *Health Affairs,* 2004, *23,* 247–256.

King, G. "Institutional Racism and the Medical/Health Complex: A Conceptual Analysis." *Ethnicity and Disease,* 1996, *6,* 30–46.

Klassen, A. C., and others. "Relationships Between Patients' Perception of Disadvantage and Discrimination and Listing for Kidney Transplant." *American Journal of Public Health,* 2002, *92,* 811–817.

Kressin, N. R., and Petersen, L. A. "Racial Differences in the Use of Invasive Cardiovascular Procedures: Review of the Literature and Prescription for Future Research." *Annals of Internal Medicine,* 2001, *135,* 352–366.

Krieger, N. "Racial and Gender Discrimination: Risk Factors for High Blood Pressure?" *Social Science and Medicine,* 1990, *30,* 1273–1281.

Krieger, N. "Self-Reported Experiences of Racial Discrimination and Black/White Differences in Preterm and Low Birth Weight Deliveries: The CARDIA Study." *Journal of Epidemiology and Community Health,* 2004, *58,* 938–943.

Krieger, N., and Fee, E. "Man-Made Medicine and Women's Health: The Biopolitics of Sex/Gender and Race/Ethnicity." *International Journal of Health Services,* 1994, *24,* 265–283.

Krieger, N., and Sidney, S. "Racial Discrimination and Blood Pressure: The CARDIA Study of Young Black and White Adults." *American Journal of Public Health,* 1996, *86,* 1370–1378.

Lane, S. D., and others. "Structural Violence and Racial Disparity in HIV Transmission." *Journal of Health Care for the Poor and Underserved,* 2004, *15,* 319–335.

Lantz, P. M., and others. "Socioeconomic Factors, Health Behaviors, and Mortality: Results from a Nationally Representative Prospective Study of Adults." *Journal of the American Medical Association,* 1998, *279,* 1703–1708.

Lewis, W. E. *Race in the Schoolyard.* New Brunswick, N.J.: Rutgers University Press, 2003.

Lieu, T. A., and others. "Racial/Ethnic Variation in Asthma Status and Management Practices Among Children in Managed Medicaid." *Pediatrics,* 2002, *109,* 857–865.

Marmot, M. G., Rose, G., Shipley, M., and Hamilton, P. J. "Employment Grade and Coronary Heart Disease in British Civil Servants." *Journal of Epidemiology and Community Health,* 1978, *32,* 244–249.

McGinnis, J. M., Williams-Russo, P., and Knickman, J. R. "The Case for More Active Policy Attention to Health Promotion." *Health Affairs,* 2002, *21,* 78–93.

McGlynn, E. A., and others. "The Quality of Health Care Delivered to Adults in the United States." *New England Journal of Medicine,* 2003, *348,* 2635–2645.

Menefee, L. T. "Are Black Americans Entitled to Equal Health Care? A New Research Paradigm." *Ethnicity and Disease,* 1996, *6,* 56–68.

Mitchell, J. B., and Bollard, D. J. "Racial Variation in Treatment for Transient Ischemic Attacks: Impact of Participation by Neurologists." *Health Services Research,* 2000, *34,* 1413–1428.

Myrdal, G. *An American Dilemma.* New York: HarperCollins, 1944.

National Center for Education in Maternal and Child Health. *Knowledge Path: Infant Mortality.* Mar. 2000. http://www.necmh.org/pubs.

National Center for Health Statistics. "Deaths from 113 Selected Causes, by Ten-Year Age Groups, Race, and Sex: United States, 2000." 2001. http://www.cdc.gov/nchs/data/dvs/tab1250a.pdf.

National Center for Health Statistics. *Health, United States, 2003.* Hyattsville, Md.: National Center for Health Statistics, 2003.

National Opinion Research Center. University of Chicago, *General Social Survey.* Chicago: University of Chicago, 1990.

Oddone, E. Z., Horner, R. D., Monger, M. E., and Matchar, D. B. "Racial Variations in the Rates of Carotid Angiography and Endarterectomy in Patients with Stroke and Transient Ischemic Attack." *Archives of Internal Medicine,* 1993, *153,* 2781–2786.

Okelo, S., and others. "Race and the Decision to Refer for Coronary Revascularization: The Effect of Physician Awareness of Patient Ethnicity." *Journal of the American College of Cardiology,* 2001, *38,* 698–704.

O'Neil, J. "The Politics of Health in the Fourth World: A Northern Canadian Example." *Human Organization,* 1986, *45,* 119–128.

Pappas, G., Queen, S., Hadden, W., and Fisher, G. "The Increasing Disparity in Mortality Between Socioeconomic Groups in the United States, 1960 and 1986." *England Journal of Medicine,* 1993, *329,* 163–169.

Peterson, E. D., and others. "Racial Variation in the Use of Coronary Revascularization Procedures: Are the Differences Real? Do They Matter?" *New England Journal of Medicine*, 1997, *336*, 480–486.

Pew Research Center for the People and the Press. *Survey of the Political Landscape 2004, Part 5: Social and Political Attitudes About Race.* July 7, 2004. http://www.prc.org.

Physicians for Human Rights. "The Right to Equal Treatment: An Action Plan to End Racial and Ethnic Disparities in Clinical Diagnosis and Treatment in the United States." 2003. http://www.phrusa.org/righttoequaltreatment.pdf.

Pincus, T., Callahan, L. F., and Burkhauser, R. V. "Most Chronic Diseases Are Reported More Frequently by Individuals with Fewer Than 12 Years of Formal Education in the Age 18–64 United States Population." *Journal of Chronic Diseases*, 1987, *40*, 865–874.

Rosenbaum S., Markins, A., and Darnell, J. "U.S. Civil Rights Policy and Access to Health Care by Minority Americans: Implications for a Changing Health Care System." *Medical Care Research and Review*, 2000, *57*(suppl. 1), 237–248.

Satel, S. *PC MD: How Political Correctness Is Corrupting Medicine.* New York: Basic Books, 2000.

Schwartz, R. S. "Racial Profiling in Medical Research." *New England Journal of Medicine*, 2001, *244*, 1392–1393.

Shavers, V. L., and Brown, M. L. "Racial and Ethnic Disparities in the Receipt of Cancer Treatment." *Journal of the National Cancer Institute*, 2002, *94*, 334–357.

Smedley, B. D., Stith, A. Y., and Nelson, A. R. (eds.). *Unequal Treatment: Confronting Racial and Ethnic Disparities in Health Care.* Washington, D.C.: National Academy Press, 2003.

Sohler, N., Walmsley, J., Lubetkin, E., and Geiger, H. J. "An Annotated Bibliography of Racial and Ethnic Disparities in Health Care." In Physicians for Human Rights, *The Right to Equal Treatment*. Sept. 2003. http://www.phrusa.org/righttoequaltreatment/bibliography.

Stevens, G. D., and Shi, L. "Racial and Ethnic Disparities in the Primary Care Experiences of Children: A Review of the Literature." *Medical Care Research Review*, 2003, *60*, 3–30.

Survey Research Center. University of Michigan. *Survey on Race and Ethnicity.* Ann Arbor: University of Michigan, 1995.

Thernstrom, S. A., and Thernstrom, A. M. *America in Black and White: One Nation Indivisible.* New York: Simon & Schuster, 1999.

Thomson, G. E. "Discrimination in Health Care." *Annals of Internal Medicine*, 1997, *126*, 910–912.

Todd, K. H., Samarov, N., and Hoffman, J. R. "Ethnicity as a Risk Factor for Inadequate Emergency Department Analgesia." *Journal of the American Medical Association,* 1993, *269,* 1537–1539.

U.S. Department of Health, Education and Welfare. *Healthy People: The Surgeon General's Report on Health Promotion and Disease Prevention.* Washington, D.C.: Government Printing Office, 1979.

U.S. Department of Health and Human Services. *Healthy People 2010.* Washington, D.C.: Government Printing Office, 2000.

van Ryn, M. "Research on the Provider Contribution to Race-Ethnicity Disparities in Medical Care." *Medical Care,* 2002, *40,* 140–151.

van Ryn, M., and Burke, J. "The Effect of Patient Race and Socioeconomic Status on Physicians' Perception of Patients." *Social Science and Medicine,* 2000, *50,* 813–828.

van Ryn, M., and Fu, S. S. "Paved with Good Intentions: Do Public Health and Human Service Providers Contribute to Racial/Ethnic Disparities?" *American Journal of Public Health,* 2003, *93,* 248–255.

Washington Post/Kaiser Family Foundation/Harvard University Survey Project. "Race and Ethnicity in 2001: Attitudes, Perspectives, and Experiences." Aug. 2001. http://www.kff.org/newsmedia/washpost.cfm.

Williams, D. R. "Racial Disparities in Health." Paper presented at the Conference on Racial/Ethnic and Socioeconomic Disparities in Health: Implications for Action, Washington, D.C., Apr. 29, 2004.

Woolf, S. "Society's Choice: The Tradeoff Between Efficacy and Equity and the Lives at Stake." *American Journal of Preventive Medicine,* 2004, 49–56.

CHAPTER TEN

FROM CONSPIRACY THEORIES TO CLINICAL TRIALS

Questioning the Role of Race and Culture versus Racism and Poverty in Medical Decision Making

Cheryl Mwaria

Nowhere can the intersections of race, class, and gender be more clearly pictured than when viewing, through an ethnographic lens, medical decision making concerning the participation of underserved populations in clinical trials. Race/ethnicity, income, gender, and gender orientation are categories that can be used to analyze health data and identify health disparities in that they reflect social inequalities that often lie at the root of such disparities. This is particularly true in the United States because of its history of discrimination based on race/ethnicity, gender, gender orientation, and class—a history that includes unethical and occasionally forced participation in medical experiments based on these categories. That history has resulted in patients' and physicians' holding differing sets of behavioral expectations, which in themselves can at best lead to less than satisfactory clinical encounters and at worst serve to reinforce stereotypes and exacerbate disparities in health status.

Feminist scholars have long recognized that analyses based on these categories are often merely additive—that is, more categories of discrimination may be included for analysis rather than any attempt made to analyze the compound effect of such discrimination—and thereby tend to be overly simplistic. I believe a more useful approach is found in the interactive model, which, as articulated by King (1995, p. 298), demonstrates that "the relative significance of race, sex, or class in determining the conditions of black women's lives is neither fixed nor absolute, but, rather, is dependent on the socio-historical context and the social phenomenon under consideration." The same is true of other categories of underserved populations suffering inequities of access to health care, as can be seen when examining the participation of women and minorities in clinical trials.

Clinical trials, which have brought scientific rigor to clinical decision making (Novick, 1990), are critically important in clinical oncology, where they foster state-of-the-art medical care. However, without adequate minority enrollment in clinical trials, researchers cannot learn about differences among groups and cannot ensure the generalizability of results. Nevertheless, racial and ethnic minorities are underrepresented in all areas of clinical research. As Swanson and Ward (1995, p. 1747) argue, "Obstacles to recruiting are rarely published; when the information is available there is usually a lag of 5–15 years before the recruitment phase of a trial and the appearance of a published report." This forty-year trend of underrepresentation of minority patients can be seen in clinical trials for cancer prevention, detection, and treatment despite the disproportionate cancer burden in minority populations. Recruitment efforts in the National Cancer Institute's (NCI) Clinical Trials Program had yielded low patient accrual since its beginning in 1955, yet it was not until 1990 that the NCI directed its attention to the problem of low participation of racial/ ethnic minority patients (Roberson, 1994). Similarly, it was not until 1994 that the National Institutes of Health (NIH; 1994) published guidelines on the inclusion of women and minorities as subjects in clinical research.

The guidelines issued by NIH resulted in a flurry of studies, most of which argued that there were real barriers to minority recruitment for clinical trials and that the research paradigm needed to be expanded. Hughes, Tsark, Kenui, and Alexander (2000) found in a review of published literature a paucity of cancer data and clinical cancer research among Native Hawaiian and

Pacific Island communities; Hodge, Weinmann, and Roubideaux (2000) found many challenges in recruiting American Indians and Alaska Natives into cancer clinical trials and argued that for researchers and health care providers, the challenges center primarily on patient-provider communication, as well as sociocultural barriers; Kagawa-Singer (2000) argued for the expansion of the cancer research paradigm to improve the validity and generalizability of studies with underserved U.S. populations. Indeed, a workshop sponsored by NCI had only one study demonstrating that a minority population's participation in cancer-related clinical trials was generally representative: Alexander, Chu, and Ho (2000) found that Asian American accrual in NCI-supported trials is representative of the cancer burden of Asian Americans in the United States, but that those sixty-five and older were still unrepresentative.

Few studies focus on barriers to the recruitment of minority participants in clinical trials, and those that have been undertaken tend to stress structural and behavioral characteristics of the minority groups themselves. Structural, cultural, and linguistic factors have been identified as possible impediments to minority participation in cancer screening and research (Giuliano and others, 2000). Distrust of the medical system, based on personal experience and a history of racial discrimination and abuse in medical experiments, has frequently been cited as a barrier to participation (Gamble, 1997; Shavers-Hornaday, Lynch, Burmeister, and Torner, 1997).

Roberson's study (1994) of both cancer survivors and asymptomatic African American, Hispanic American, and Native American subjects found that the subjects, while familiar with the term *experimental studies,* were less familiar with the term *clinical trials.* Moreover, they knew of no one who had participated in clinical trials, agreeing that a lack of information was the primary reason that people like them did not participate in these trials. According to Roberson, members of each ethnic group expressed concern about "mistrust of white people and the feeling of being treated like guinea pigs" (p. 2689). Notably, while most (twenty-two out of twenty-eight) respondents in Roberson's study had no opportunity to participate in clinical trials, they believed such trials could be beneficial. Roberson noted that "African Americans, Hispanics, and Native Americans believed that the benefits of participating in clinical trials were to 'help find a cure,' 'help others,' 'assist with medical coverage,' and 'educate families'" (p. 2689).

Given the emphasis on cultural barriers to clinical trial participation on the part of minorities in medical literature (Fouad and others, 2000; Hodge, Weinmann, and Roubideaux, 2000; Holcombe, Jacobson, Li, and Moinpour, 1998; Kagawa-Singer, 2000; Shavers-Hornaday, Lynch, Burmeister, and Torner, 1997), it is not surprising to find a widespread notion that members of minority communities not only mistrust the medical community but often believe medical conspiracy theories (Herek and Capitanio, 1994; Hopkins, 1997; Parsons, Simmons, Shinhoster, and Kilburn, 1999). Mistrust as exhibited through the belief in medical conspiracy theories is assumed to be responsible in part for the low minority patient accrual in clinical trials and even to lead to failure to seek medical attention. This chapter challenges that notion through an examination of the often synergistic effect of race, class, and gender on medical decision making pertaining to clinical trial participation, both historically and in contemporary data collected through participant observation in an urban research hospital and outpatient clinic.

RACE, CLASS, AND GENDER IN MEDICAL DECISION MAKING

My own ethnographic observations over a six-month period at a major urban cancer center in New York City illustrate the ways in which medical decision making evolves between patients and physicians in an ethnically and economically diverse population. The study involved over 650 hours of field observations. Fifty-seven patients were drawn from a convenience sample to be interviewed both formally and informally during this period, as were fourteen staff research physicians, five research nurses, and the data management staff. As an ethnographer, I was able to immerse myself in the day-to-day activities of the research facility and develop interactive relationships with both patients and their health care providers.

The cancer center under study is located in an area where 20 to 32 percent of the population lives in poverty, but it is adjacent to some of the wealthiest neighborhoods in the city (U.S. Bureau of the Census, 2000). The center draws patients from all of its surrounding neighborhoods and other boroughs. A high immigrant population characterizes the neighborhoods from which the patient population is drawn. The demographics of the patient population reflect this diversity, including men and women who identified as African Americans, Asians, Latinos (Hispanics), Pacific Islanders, and recent immigrants from the former Soviet Union, Poland, Ghana, Japan, China, and the Caribbean. More than one-third of all New Yorkers were born outside the United States (compared with 11 percent nationwide), and of those, half are from Latin America. At the same time, a greater proportion of Asians in New York City are foreign born than any other racial or ethnic group (U.S. Bureau of the Census, 2000). Overall, people who are black, Hispanic, and poor in New York City experience the highest disease burdens (Frieden and Karpati, 2004).

Race/ethnicity and income have long been used to identify and analyze health disparities, as have gender and gender orientation. It should be remembered that these categories are socially, not biologically, determined. Although racial groupings tend to be identified by vague phenotypic characteristics, such as skin color, eye shape, or hair texture, they cannot be scientifically measured, nor do such characteristics divide the human population into discrete units. The complexities of using the concept of race to categorize human populations are made clear by Last (2001, p. 150), who defines race as follows:

> In biology a breed or variety of animals, plants, micro-organisms; a major division of humankind having distinct physical characteristics. Biologic classification of human races is difficult because of significant genetic overlaps among population groups. Social scientists have challenged the biologic definition of race, arguing that the concept of race most often reflects social and ideological conventions. Economic, social, cultural and behavioral differences are more important than biological differences in determining health status. However, race is a useful concept from the public health perspective because some diseases are strongly correlated with biological aspects of race; this may relate to gene-environment interaction or to the presence of specific genes—which may be due to environmental exposures of prior generations. Useful insights into human biology and genetics derive from analysis by racial group of large data sets such as the census and national health surveys.

While diseases with a clear genetic component may be more frequent in specific populations, they account for only a small fraction of racial disparities in health. Furthermore, it was only as of 2000 that the U.S. Census allowed people to identify themselves by more than one racial category. In the United States, race and class have historically been intertwined in complex ways, and the role of each is significant with respect to understanding health disparities. This can be seen in the following example from a recent report on health disparities in New York City:

> Black and Hispanic New Yorkers are generally poorer than White New Yorkers. As a result, racial/ethnic comparisons are usually a comparison of a poorer to a wealthier group. For some health outcomes, when income is taken into account, apparent racial/ethnic differences fall away. This means that, in each income category, Whites face similar health conditions to their Black and Hispanic counterparts. For other indicators, however, the racial/ethnic gaps persist in ways not accounted for by income alone. This means that race and ethnicity influence health in ways not measured by income alone [Frieden and Karpati, 2004, p. 1].

Underrepresentation of women and minorities in clinical trials is another example of disparities in access to health care. However, some studies have shown that the compound category of minority women is less well represented than either category alone (Brown, Fouad, Basen-Engquist, and Tortolero-Luna, 2000; Lillie-Blanton, Martinez, Taylor, and Robinson, 1993; Schulman and others, 1999; Stone and others, 1996), thereby illustrating an intersectional exacerbation of inequities in access to health care.

My study focused on one area of concern regarding health disparities, particularly with respect to cancer burden and cancer survival rates: minority participation in cancer-related clinical trials. One of the most striking findings of my six-month ethnographic study of the cancer center's patients is that of the fifty-seven patients interviewed, forty of whom were offered clinical trials, none of the forty refused to participate in a trial. Of the twenty-six African American and Hispanic American patients interviewed, the most compelling reason for participating in a clinical trial was the sincere hope that the trial would benefit themselves and others. A typical response was one given by Mr. E.L., a sixty-year-old African

American man with prostate cancer: "The help I get, I'm happy to give back." Mrs. B.B., a fifty-six-year-old African American woman with breast cancer, said, "I've heard of the Tuskegee experiment, but it could not really influence my decision to participate in a clinical trial. No one takes your care as seriously as you yourself do. You have to take control and push people to do for you." A young Hispanic male reasoned, "Why not take a chance?" A seventy-seven-year-old African American man opined, "My overall impression is that clinical trials are essential." One seventy-year-old African American man, Mr. P., was a veteran of three clinical trials. He explained:

> I've had experimental medicine three times—for stroke, high
> blood pressure, and now for my cancer. The blood pressure medi-
> cine didn't work; it even made my pressure higher. I did away with
> that experiment, but I've had A1 care and the best doctors in the
> world. I've heard some fellas talk about having gone to the clinic
> and been experimented on. Some came out well, but one was a
> "negative talker." He had arthritis and didn't feel helped by his
> experimental medicine. My doctors explained everything, and
> now they work together. I've been treated like family by my four
> doctors. I've been wonderful blessed.

Mr. P.'s analysis of his own experiences belies the characterization of poor minority patients as unable to make reasoned, intelligent decisions about their own medical care in the context of risks. It also belies the characterization of poor minority patients as mistrustful of medical care.

Although many patients were "willing to take a chance," they did so only when the clinical trial being offered was patiently, rather than patronizingly, explained to them. This applied to the seventeen patients interviewed who were receiving standard care as well as those on a clinical trial. They all appreciated honesty on the part of their physicians, particularly with respect to warnings about what to expect during the course of their treatment. Patients repeatedly told me that their fears were diminished when the physician or the research nurse told them how the treatment would proceed, even when they were told to expect pain or discomfort. Mrs. L.G., a fifty-year-old African American woman, said that she was initially suspicious of her physician's offer of a clinical trial and reported having "great anxieties"; however, "When Dr. H.

saw my face, he explained everything. He took my fears away."
What patients did not want to hear from medical personnel or
friends were negative prognoses. Mrs. Z.M. asserted, "A lot of people warned me not to do this or that, and it made me nervous, so I
just don't listen to them. I move away, even in the waiting room."

The study suggested that continuity of care and personal affect
on the part of the medical staff were of primary importance and
that minority patients, particularly those who were poor, often
made medical decisions on the basis of identification with a staff
member. This does not mean, however, that such patients were
willing to accept everything their physicians said. None of the
patients reported that they felt coerced into a trial or indeed into
any treatment strategy. The case of Mrs. N.R., a fifty-six-year-old
divorced Hispanic woman who was referred to an oncologist,
Dr. K., for follow-up treatment after a mastectomy, illustrates this:

> Dr. K. said I wouldn't last two years, but he isn't God, and he doesn't
> know! I cursed him out and walked out. I told my surgeon and he
> apologized; so did Dr. K. after that. I decided to work with him
> because he's an excellent oncologist. We still fight. We even hung
> up on each other when he called me in Aruba. I left him briefly,
> but I came back because I had lost a lot in terms of family relations
> and finances due to my illness. I would have died if I hadn't fol-
> lowed Dr. K.'s recommendations—not that I follow them com-
> pletely. I cut down on my steroids, after researching them on the
> Net. I told Dr. K. and he asked me why, so I told him. He said he
> would watch me for two weeks, and if there was no change, he'd
> agree to the reduced dosage. There was no change, and he
> reduced my dosage. I was right.

Mrs. N.R.'s story demonstrates the value of patience, perseverance,
and shared medical decision making between physician and patient.
Ten years after her initial diagnosis, she is still a private patient of
Dr. K. She is an attractive, well-educated woman who is proud of
her "stubborn" nature. Another "stubborn" woman, less well educated, decidedly poorer, and a former substance abuser, but equally
sharp and outspoken, fared considerably worse. As a clinic patient,
Mrs. S., a fifty-six-year-old African American woman with lung cancer, complained of her poor treatment. Although her chart indicated that she was married and her husband accompanied her to
the center, she was never addressed as *Mrs.* S. but rather by her first

name. Her husband, her friend, and this researcher all attested to the validity of her complaint:

> They just act like they don't care about you. I can never catch Dr. M.; he just vanishes. Dr. M. [a fellow] doesn't listen. I complain about pain, and he ignores me. I'm wheezing and have thick mucus in my throat. Anyone worth their salt would ask me about it, but here I have to tell them! Dr. S. [an attending physician] is too excited about her new baby to be bothered. She's scattered anyway. God help the child; when I told her about my pain, she said she'd write a prescription, but she completely forgot about it. Then instead of talking to me—she asks to talk to my husband like I'm not in my right mind! Nothing has ever been explained to me.

Mrs. S. was an astute observer. Dr. M. confessed the following to me about her: "I'm trying to pawn her off to one of the [junior] fellows, but I don't think she'll last another three months. She should know she's dying." To several of her colleagues, "scattered" was a "kind" description of the other physician's behavior. They reported that she was known to lose her temper and yell at staff members she considered her "inferiors," though they agreed she was gifted in her field. Mrs. S. was never offered a clinical trial, believed to be effective for palliative care for lung cancer patients, although she fit the eligibility criteria for the protocol.

The minority patients in this study, whether African American, Asian American, Latino (Hispanic), or of recent immigrant status, did not complain of overt racism, but African Americans and Latinos remained alert to subtle signs of it. Moreover, minority patients were far more likely to be uninsured and to express anxiety over their ability to pay for their treatment than white patients who were citizens. Illegal immigrants also faced these fears. Their fear was not irrational; it was based on the witnessed experiences of friends and acquaintances whose treatment was delayed or who were turned away because of inadequate medical insurance.

Yet another barrier faced by minority patients in enrolling in clinical trials was the frequent delay in treatment due to the failure of a local nonteaching hospital to make a timely correct diagnosis of cancer. Several African American and Latino patients reported such experiences, and the research nurses verified them. The experience of Mrs. C.J., a forty-six-year-old African American woman, illustrates this:

I began to feel sick in the early fall, so I went to my primary care physician. He wasn't alarmed, but the pain kept growing worse until I had to stop working in October. I worked with children with behavioral problems in a hospital setting. My doctor sent me to a surgeon, but the biopsy was inconclusive. I was sent home twice before being sent to a radiologist, who made two attempts to diagnose my condition but failed. Finally I met Dr. C., a liver specialist who performed a biopsy himself. He was the one to diagnose my pancreatic cancer. By then I was very weak. I couldn't eat, and I had lost a lot of weight. The pain was unbearable. Dr. C. referred me to my present doctor at the cancer center. I had already undergone six biopsies over a period of two months. That was very discouraging. I wanted an answer, but I couldn't start treatment without a diagnosis. I was very frustrated and frightened. I blame my local hospital because they kept me there too long without a diagnosis.

Mrs. C.J. was too ill and weak to qualify for a clinical trial when she arrived at the cancer center, but her physician started an aggressive therapy, closely following a clinical trial protocol for her disease. His efforts paid off, and she survived to go into remission and visit her relatives in the Caribbean. Her experience of a delayed diagnosis is all too common among minority patients and recent immigrants, many of whom seek medical attention early in the course of their disease but are stymied by restrictions imposed by insurance companies, lack of insurance altogether, or the limitations of physicians and hospitals without broad-based expertise in cancer diagnosis and treatment. Mr. J.V., a forty-year-old Hispanic man, had a similar experience that almost cost him his life: "I went to my neighborhood hospital with a golf-ball-sized tumor in my neck. I was petrified. I was told not to worry, that it was an infection of some kind, and antibiotics were prescribed. At first they seemed to do the trick; the tumor went down, but it soon returned, bigger than ever. Months went by before my wife and I got fed up and sought a second opinion at the cancer center. It took only two days for the doctors here to diagnose my disease—Burkett's lymphoma. They explained it to me and began aggressive treatment immediately."

There are other serious time-consuming constraints which explain how structural constraints, rather than delay in seeking care, limit the enrollment of minority patients in cancer-related clinical trials when they are also economically disadvantaged and restricted by insurance coverage or lack thereof. These involve the preparatory work—blood tests, X-rays, scans, dental work, or numerous other procedures—on patients prior to establishing their eligibility for a given clinical trial. Medicaid will pay only a capped amount per day, regardless of the number of medical procedures performed. Therefore, hospitals tend to order exams on different days to maximize their payment. This forces the poor to make more visits, which many find difficult or impossible given their illness. It discourages people from keeping appointments and may result in their being characterized as "noncompliant."

The real insight of this study came from interviews with research physicians at the cancer center. Here it became evident that patients were prescreened during recruitment on the basis of "educability" and "likeliness of compliance." Although this did not eliminate patient access to clinical trials based on race, class, or gender, physicians' perceptions of appropriate roles specific to these categories could clearly influence their recruitment practices. Physicians, in other words, often make implicit assumptions about the behavior of patients based on appearance and, in this case, class.

The physicians at the research center were as diverse as the patient population with respect to their racial/ethnic identification and the social class in which they were raised. They thereby represent a slice of the slowly changing face of American medicine. Although I observed all of the physician staff members during the course of the study, not all were formally interviewed. Of the fourteen physicians who were interviewed, six were foreign born and raised. Women too were represented in this research physician population. While all of the staff physicians had a significant amount of training in the United States, several had initial medical training outside the United States as well.

The physicians interviewed were all committed to clinical research, but most expressed frustration with what they perceived as a growing trend in structural constraints on clinical trials. The most common complaint was the amount of time it took to enroll patients in clinical trials. Familiarizing oneself with clinical trial protocols, particularly with eligibility criteria for patients, is time-consuming. Designing one's own study is even more so. Moreover, this relatively small research center, though comprehensive, generally had forty to fifty clinical trials in progress at a time. Consent forms for an average protocol may run anywhere from fifty to more than a hundred pages, and this does not include the recently enacted Health Information Protection Act (HIPA) forms, which have extended the time it takes to explain consent forms considerably. In the words of one young physician, "HIPA is definitely a disincentive to engage in clinical trial research." Given the perception of an increasingly laborious consenting process and the time pressures associated with clinical practice (physicians at the center spent five to seven minutes with a patient per visit), it is perhaps not surprising that the majority prescreened patients for "educability." One physician expressed this sentiment as follows: "The person with a high education can understand the purpose of the research and will be more compliant if they agree—otherwise they won't consent. They also ask more questions, which they have a right to do. Doctors should be prepared to answer them."

These sentiments were echoed by another oncologist, who declared, "I won't approach those who aren't smart enough or who won't be compliant. I try to explain protocols in simple terms, but some don't get it." The time and costs of enrolling patients in clinical trials in his view justified his approach. It should be noted, however, that while these constraints are primarily expressed in terms of class, overall blacks and Hispanics in New York City tend to be poorer and less well educated than whites. Ethically, physicians are correct not to enroll anyone in a clinical trial who does not clearly understand the protocol or anyone who has false expectations of the purpose of the clinical trial. Nevertheless, few physicians took the time to ascertain definitively whether this was the case. They were more likely to prejudge the patient and not to offer a clinical trial as an option. When questioned, most physicians felt justified in their decisions, claiming that their considerable experience with patients resulted in a kind of "intuition." For example, one physician explained, "If a patient can't keep an appointment or follow medication instructions, he or she is unlikely to be able to comply with a trial protocol." Clearly physicians in this study do not themselves as harboring racial/ethnic bias, which would conflict with their antidiscriminatory principles and the ethical commitments of medicine (van Ryn, 2001).

Another constraint on physicians' enrollment of minority patients in clinical trials is also grounded in medical ethics but has a clear ethnic component as well. A significant percentage of the patient population was comprised of immigrants, many of whom neither spoke English nor were literate in it. Ethically, in the absence of a translator, such patients would not be candidates for a clinical trial. In reality, one patient, a man from eastern Europe, was enrolled in a clinical trial. Most, however, had translators, but in the form of family members. From the physicians' perspectives, this complicated the picture. The difficulty was explained as follows by an older physician with many years of research experience: "My patient population includes Russian, Chinese, Creole, Polish, and Hebrew speakers, but consents are only available in English. In my experience, family members are not always trustworthy or appropriate translators. They often want to protect the patient, rather than be honest with respect to the prognosis, or even the diagnosis of the disease, not to mention the details of the clinical trial protocol. If they don't want the patient to know their true status, I won't enroll them."

Taken together, these prescreening practices, whether well intentioned or not, work against the enrollment of certain categories of patients, particularly those who are not well informed prior to their arrival at the cancer center. Unfortunately, many, though by no means all, minority patients fail to meet these criteria.

This study suggests that physicians make assumptions concerning the ability of patients to understand and comply with clinical trial protocols, thereby exercising significant influence over access to these trials. The findings presented here are consistent with the relatively well-documented gatekeeping in other areas of medical treatment, specifically coronary artery bypass graft surgery rates. Hannan and others (1999, p. 68) found that "even after controlling for appropriateness and necessity for coronary bypass graft surgery in a prospective study, African-American patients had significant access problems in obtaining coronary bypass graft surgery. The problems appeared not to be related to patient refusals." A study of race and sex differences in rates of invasive cardiac procedures in U.S. hospitals found that "race and sex differentials in the rates of invasive cardiac procedures remained despite matching for the hospital of admission and controlling for other factors that influence procedure rates, suggesting that the race and sex of the patient influence the use of these procedures" (Giles and others, 1995, p. 318). Whittle, Conigliaro, Good, and Lofgren (1993, p. 621) found that "even when financial incentives are absent, whites are more likely than blacks to undergo invasive cardiac procedures. These findings suggest that social or clinical factors affect the use of these procedures differently in blacks than whites." Finally, perhaps the most definitive study of the effect of race and sex on physicians' recommendations for cardiac catheterization comes from Schulman and others (1999), who used actors to portray patients with specific characteristics in scripted interviews. The study, which included a survey of 720 physicians, concluded: "Our finding that race and sex of the patient influence the recommendations of physicians independently of other factors may suggest bias on the part of physicians or, more likely, could be the result of subconscious perceptions rather than deliberate actions or thoughts" (1999, p. 624).

Collectively, these studies suggest that medical gatekeeping continues to be practiced in such a way as to maintain differential access to cutting-edge medical care and clinical trials based on race, gender, and class. Clearly, the women and men of color in this study were willing to participate in clinical trials, provided they were treated with the respect that allowed them to trust their physicians and research nurses. However, this study supports in part the findings of others "that neither the health care system as a whole nor individual providers are fully insulated from attitudes toward race, ethnicity, and social class that are prevalent (though often unacknowledged) in the larger society" (Geiger, 2003, p. 440). As Geiger (Chapter Nine, this volume) argues:

> In sum, the evidence of differential treatment for African Americans, Hispanics, Native Americans, and Asian/Pacific Islanders is credible and robust, in studies that are appropriately controlled for such major confounding variables as insurance status, income and education, age, gender, stage and severity of disease, and presence or absence of comorbid illness. Furthermore, these studies examine the care of patients who are already in the health care system, minimizing access to care as a factor. This pattern has been found not only for such high-technology intervention as angioplasty and coronary artery bypass grafting, advanced cancer chemotherapy,

and renal transplantation but also for such routine processes as general medical and surgical procedures and the treatment of asthma, diabetes, congestive heart failure, and pneumonia.

Despite substantial progress in research substantiating claims of clinical gatekeeping, this behavior continues to create barriers to recruitment for clinical trials and cutting-edge treatment strategies. If structural barriers pertaining to poverty and medical gatekeeping inhibit access to clinical trials and cutting-edge medical treatment, why then does the conventional wisdom continue to blame the underserved minority populations for their own lack of access? Why are minority populations accused of naively believing in medical conspiracy theories and therefore refusing to participate in clinical trials? One approach to this question lies in the history of minority representation in medical experimentation.

HISTORICAL RAMIFICATIONS OF DISCRIMINATION IN MEDICINE

Any discussion of minority representation in clinical trials in the United States must be examined against a historical background of exploitation and its natural consequence: mistrust. The institution of chattel slavery in the United States created a vulnerable population, for whom consent was not a problem. Physicians took advantage of this "opportunity" to develop new surgical techniques, illustrate unusual cases, and test new pharmacological treatments (Fry, 1975; Kipple and King, 1981; Mettauer, 1840; 1847; Savitt, 1978; Sims, 1852; for further explication of this point, see Mwaria, 2001). The abolition of slavery, far from ending the more malignant forms of medical experimentation, expanded them to include other vulnerable populations: women, children, the mentally disabled, and the poor (Mwaria, 2001; Lederer, 1995).

Not all of the exploited were from characteristically vulnerable populations, nor was all medical research exploitive. Early experimental research on human subjects focused largely on the prevention of communicable diseases and nutritional disorders and can be dated back some 250 years to Lind's study of patients with scurvy. By 1887, funding for research to promote public health was provided by the U.S. government through the establishment of

NIH. However, as can be expected in any highly stratified, race-based society, not all such experimental research was benign. Given that issues of race remain charged and divisive in many corridors of American society, it is not surprising that medical conspiracy theories reflecting racial misunderstanding and mistrust frequently circulate. Legends also reflect class and status differences and thereby illustrate fears based on the expected behavior of others. Fine (1992, p. 8) opines, "The depiction of class and status differences is a regular feature of contemporary American legends, appearing within the contexts of the texts. The texts are structured as 'realist tales' and in their implicit claims to truth they reflect the class structure— both the way that it is and the way that it *should be*. These texts are fragmented reflections of social and historical circumstances."

One early medical conspiracy theory, circulating in the African American community in the late nineteenth and early twentieth centuries, reflected both race and class status: that medical students robbed the graves of blacks in order to use them for dissection (Mwaria, 2001). The legend was so common, according to folklorist Fry (1975), that the image of the "night doctor" became firmly established in the African American oral tradition. Fry herself, however, was unable to find any evidence of a demand for black bodies for medical studies or experiments during the late nineteenth and early twentieth centuries despite her comprehensive research. Perhaps the most infamous example of highly unethical medical research, based on the exploitation of poor blacks, was the Tuskegee experiment in which the U.S. government sponsored a forty-year study of the "natural history of syphilis" using African American men, mostly illiterate sharecroppers, as subjects.

Contemporary medical conspiracy legends abound and serve an important cultural purpose, not just for African Americans. They express anxieties about *others,* those with control over the fate and bodies of the disenfranchised, the marginalized, the poor. They underscore for some, whether disenfranchised or empowered, racial fears of *others* who are unknown and unknowable, whose behaviors cannot be reliably predicted. Within a context of inequality, they serve as cautionary tales. When surgeon Christiaan Barnard performed his second heart transplant at Groote Schuur Hospital in South Africa, he used the heart of a "colored" man—Clive Haupt, who was in a stroke-induced coma. Haupt's heart was placed in

Dr. Phillip Blaiberg, who was asked if he would accept the heart of a "colored" man. The operation was viewed by some in South Africa as a nod toward racial tolerance, but blacks in both South Africa and the United States saw it otherwise, as noted by journalist Chester Himes, who wrote in *Jet*'s "People Are Talking About" column: "Why the 1,600,000 colored and 11,000,000 blacks in South Africa are not jubilant over the transplanting of a colored man's heart into the body of a white South African. They fear that success of the operation may turn the entire nonwhite population into one huge spare parts bank for hearts, kidneys, livers, eyes and perhaps other parts of black bodies which white rulers may want" (1968, p. 42).

Race and class are intertwined in this complex web of mistrust. As Herek and Capitanio (1994, p. 356) have argued, "To some extent, it is perhaps inevitable that a group lacking political power will respond with suspicion when it is disproportionately affected by a feared disease." Distrust about AIDS appears to be highest in communities disproportionately affected by the epidemic (Herek and Capitanio, 1994). For African Americans, whose government countenanced slavery, racial discrimination, and a history of past medical abuses, suspicion and mistrust seem not only logical but also prudent. Legends of medical conspiracies are not entirely beyond credibility (Hopkins, 1997). They tend to fall into two distinct categories, characterized by Turner (1993) as malicious intent and benign neglect: either the government and its handmaiden, the medical community, are deliberately engaged in unethical behavior directed at African Americans, or the government/medical community is deliberately withholding vital information from African Americans as a group. In either case, blacks suffer as a result of a pattern of behavior that is essentially racist. As Scheper-Hughes (1996, p. 5) argues, "To say—as have a generation of critical interpretive anthropologists (see Comaroff, 1985; Taussig, 1991; Nash, 1979; Niehaus, 1993)—that the stories are metaphorically true, operating by means of symbolic substitutions, is not enough. In the violent everyday encounters in shanty-towns and squatter camps, the metaphors are materialized in the grotesque enactments of medical, economic, and social relations, which are experienced at the immediate level of the violated and dismembered body." I might add that the urban poor in many of America's ghettos also experience those same "violent encounters."

It would not be surprising, then, if medical legends, particularly those involving the government, were pervasive in the African American community, but to argue that they account for the racial/ethnic and gender disparities in clinical trial participation not only does a disservice to those populations; it also ignores the evidence presented earlier in this chapter that many African American and other minority patients were willing, if not eager, to participate in clinical trials. Such an argument also ignores evidence that researchers often deliberately restricted their subjects to white males. Goering, noting the reasoning researchers use to justify excluding women and minorities, argues that it is "varied and extensive, covering problems from financing and recruitment to problems with tight experimental control and subject safety" (1994, p. 186). The exclusion of women, she asserts, has been defended through the claim that "their fluctuating hormonal cycles were a confounding factor" or that they might become pregnant (p. 186). Clearly, such arguments were spurious, but the white male model had become so entrenched that Dresser (1992) reported a pilot study of the impact of obesity on breast and uterine cancers solely on men, despite the fact that women disproportionately suffer from these cancers, whether obese or not and clearly men do not get uterine cancer.

By the 1990s the white male model as sole research subject had seriously come into question. Purvis (1990) had noted that diets based on studies of men that recommend a general cholesterol reduction could be harmful for women; Cotton (1990) found that lithium treatment, with its high toxicity, greatly increased the already high risk of renal failure among African American men; Sirgio, Cook, and Modrak (1986) demonstrated that hypertensive blacks do not respond as well to beta-blockers as whites; and Zhou (1989) demonstrated that Asians have a much faster metabolism for propanolol than whites and that among Asians, a smaller percentage of the dose is inactivated by plasma protein binding. Biologists and social scientists continue to question such findings, suggesting that the pharmaceutical market may be driving the results (Duster, 2003). Nevertheless, these and other studies led ethicists to take up the call for the inclusion of women and minorities in clinical trials. As Goering (1994, p. 188) argued: "Today we must understand that women and minorities have much to gain from participation in clinical studies. As long as their participation is carefully controlled and not abused, they will be able to reap benefits that have for too long accrued almost exclusively to white men."

The pendulum has seemingly come full circle, from a period when women and minorities, as members of vulnerable populations, were used in unethical medical research to their equally unethical exclusion from the benefits of clinical studies. Race/ethnicity, gender, and income continue to have a profound but varying impact on the process of patient accrual for clinical trials.

The call for greater representation of women and minorities in clinical trials is not without problems. Goering (1994, p. 188) warns: "Acknowledging inherent differences between races and sexes may inadvertently cause a rise in racism and sexism. It may refuel the fires of the once livid nature/nurture debate, which will bring with it all the misconceptions about superior and inferior genetic abilities associated with eugenics."

It may also, as Osborne and Feit (1992, p. 277) opine, "serve only the interests of those eager to blame the disproportionate share of the burden of poverty and disease borne by minorities on inherent racial traits and genetic defects rather than on societal problems such as poverty, sub optimal health care, or a legacy of racial prejudice." Nevertheless, failure to be inclusive in clinical trials is both racist and lacking in rigor.

CONCLUSIONS

This chapter suggests how complex the resolution of this dilemma can be, for even the call for greater representation based on race/ethnicity, gender, or class can hark back to a time when these categories were used to justify exploitation. Moreover, the very hallmarks of ethical standards for clinical trial participants designed to prevent such exploitation—informed consent and protection of patient privacy—have been used as barriers to minority patient participation in clinical trials. This raises another dilemma articulated by Geiger (Chapter Nine, this volume): that "it is necessary—in medical care as in multiple other areas of American life—to count race until race no longer counts." This will require, he continues, "that all clinical records in every health facility be coded by the patient's self-reported race/ethnicity and, possibly, by primary language and indicators of social class." Some of these data are already being collected on patients participating in clinical trials, particularly trials involving radiation oncology, where photos of patients are routinely taken for treatment purposes. While such practices may encounter resistance, it must be surmounted if we are truly to monitor the impact of disparities in health status and access to health care and design methods to overcome such discrepancies.

Claims that African Americans and other minority group members are reluctant to seek medical treatment or participate in clinical trials because they believe in medical conspiracy theories or generally mistrust the medical establishment have not been borne out through empirical research. Rather, patients have been shown to be proactive participants when given the opportunity to do so and the clearly articulated support of their physicians and medical support staff. It is time to change the persistent unequal access to state-of-the-art prevention, early detection, and treatment trials for heart disease and cancer. We must abandon worn-out stereotypes of the "other" by embracing those empirical insights that show precisely where and how changes can be most effective. Among them are two pointed out by Geiger (Chapter Nine, this volume): to focus on "the rigorous monitoring of quality of care and implementation of standardized expert guidelines and evidence-based clinical practices for *all* patients in all types of health care institutions. The second approach, focused on specific disparities, . . . proposes both research and policy actions to deal with the issues of race/ethnicity, gender, and class."

This latter approach includes continued qualitative research on the intersectional nature of race, gender, and class and its impact on access to health care, particularly clinical trial participation. Communities must band together to demand a balanced and carefully considered distribution of medical resources, including access to teaching hospitals and their staff. Physicians and health care workers must receive an enlightened education that embraces rather than devalues difference. Patience, perseverance, and shared medical decision making between physicians and their patients must be valued over hierarchical decisions made on the basis of unarticulated assumptions on the part of both patients and medical personnel. Community outreach to educate patients regarding new treatments and clinical trials must be expanded, and, most important, we must demand universal health care insurance to underwrite even the possibility of equal access to health care. Finally, we must remember that the relative significance of race/ethnicity, gender, or class is neither fixed nor absolute in determining patient behavior or desire to participate in clinical trials or overall medical compliance but is rather dependent on the overall sociohistoric context and prevailing social factors. Thus, these categories should not be used to inhibit access to state-of-the-art health care.

References

Alexander, G. A., Chu, K. C., and Ho, R.C.S. "Representation of Asian Americans in Clinical Cancer Trials." *Annals of Epidemiology,* 2000, *10*(8, suppl. 1), S61–S67.

Brown, D. R., Fouad, M. N., Basen-Engquist, K., and Tortolero-Luna, G. "Recruitment and Retention of Minority Women in Cancer Screening, Prevention, and Treatment Trials." *Annals of Epidemiology,* 2000, *10*(S8), S13–S21.

Comaroff, J. *Body of Power, Spirit of Resistance.* Chicago: University of Chicago Press, 1985.

Cotton, P. "Is There Still Too Much Extrapolation from Data on Middle Aged White Men?" *Journal of the American Medical Association,* 1990, *263*(8), 1049–1050.

Dresser, R. "Wanted: Single, White Male for Medical Research." *Hastings Center Report,* 1992, *22*(1), 24–29.

Duster, T. "Medicine and People of Color Unlikely Mix—Race, Biology and Drugs." *San Francisco Chronicle,* Mar. 17, 2003. http://sfgate.com/cgi-bin/article.cgi?file=/chronicle/archive/2003/03/17/ED263680.DTL.

Fine, G. A. *Manufacturing Tales: Sex and Money in Contemporary Legends.* Knoxville: University of Tennessee Press, 1992.

Fouad, M. N., and others. "Minority Recruitment in Clinical Trials: A Conference at Tuskegee, Research and the Community." *Annals of Epidemiology,* 2000, *10*, S35–S40.

Frieden, T. R., and Karpati, A. M. "Health Disparities in New York City: A Report from the New York City Department of Health and Mental Hygiene." Dec. 2004. http://www.nyc.gov/html/doh/pdf/epi/disparities-2004.pdf.

Fry, G. M. *Nightriders in Black Folk History.* Knoxville: University of Tennessee Press, 1975.

Gamble, V. "Under the Shadow of Tuskegee: African Americans and Health Care." *American Journal of Public Health,* 1997, *87,* 1773–1778.

Geiger, H. J. "Racial and Ethnic Disparities in Diagnosis and Treatment: A Review of the Evidence and a Consideration of Causes." In B. D. Smedley, A. Y. Stith, and A. R. Nelson (eds.), *Unequal Treatment: Confronting Racial and Ethnic Disparities in Health Care.* Washington, D.C.: National Academy Press, 2003.

Giles, W. H., and others. "Race and Sex Differences in Rates of Invasive Cardiac Procedures in U.S. Hospitals: Data from the Hospital Discharge Survey." *Archives of Internal Medicine,* 1995, *155,* 318–324.

Giuliano, A. R., and others. "Participation of Minorities in Cancer Research: The Influence of Structural, Cultural, and Linguistic Factors." *Annals of Epidemiology,* 2000, *10,* S22–S34.

Goering, S. "Women and Underserved Populations: Access to Clinical Trials. " In M. G. Secundy and S. Williams (eds.), *It Just Ain't Fair: The Ethics of Health Care for African Americans.* Westport, Conn.: Praeger, 1994.

Hannan, E. L., and others. "Access to Coronary Artery Bypass Surgery by Race/Ethnicity and Gender Among Patients Who Are Appropriate for Surgery." *Medical Care,* 1999, *37*(1), 68–77.

Herek, G. M., and Capitanio, J. P. "Conspiracies, Contagion, and Compassion: Trust and Public Reactions to AIDS." *AIDS Education and Prevention,* 1994, *6*(4) 365–375.

Himes, C. "People Are Talking About. " *Jet,* Jan. 18, 1968, p. 42.

Hodge, F. S., Weinmann, S., and Roubideaux, Y. "Recruitment of American Indians and Alaska Natives into Clinical Trials." *Annals of Epidemiology,* 2000, *10,* S41–S48.

Holcombe, R. F., Jacobson, J., Li, A., and Moinpour, C. M. "Inclusion of Black Americans in Oncology Clinical Trials: The Louisiana State University Medical Center Experience." *American Journal of Clinical Oncology (CCT),* 1998, *22*(1), 18–21.

Hopkins, J. "The Conspiracy Theory: An Old Query Revisited." *Review Online: Independent Student Newspaper of the University of Delaware,* Nov. 7, 1997. http://www.review.udel.edu/archives/web-archives/ 1997_Issues/11.07.97/e3.html.

Hughes, C. K., Tsark, J. U., Kenui, C. K., and Alexander, G. A. "Cancer Research Studies in Native Hawaiians and Pacific Islanders." *Annals of Epidemiology,* 2000, *10,* S49–S60.

Kagawa-Singer, M. "Improving the Validity and Generalizability of Studies with Underserved U.S. Populations Expanding the Research Paradigm." *Annals of Epidemiology,* 2000, *10,* S92–S103.

King, D. "Multiple Jeopardy, Multiple Consciousness: The Context of a Black Feminist Ideology." In B. Guy-Sheftall (ed.), *Words of Fire: An Anthropology of African-American Feminist Thought.* New York: New Press, 1995.

Kipple, K. F., and King, V. H. *Another Dimension to the Black Diaspora: Diet, Disease and Racism.* Cambridge: Cambridge University Press, 1981.

Last, J. M. *A Dictionary of Epidemiology.* (4th ed.) New York: Oxford University Press, 2001.

Lederer, S. E. *Subjected to Science: Human Experimentation in America before the Second World War.* Baltimore: Johns Hopkins Press, 1995.

Lillie-Blanton, M., Martinez, R. M., Taylor, A. K., and Robinson, B. G. "Latina and African American Women: Continuing Disparities in Health." *International Journal of Health Services,* 1993, *23*(3), 555–584.

Mettauer, J. P. "Vesico-Vaginal Fistula." *Boston Medical and Surgical Journal,* 1840, *22,* 154–155.

Mettauer, J. P. "On Vesico Vaginal Fistula." *American Journal of Medical Sciences,* 1847, *14,* 117–121.

Mwaria, C. "Biomedical Ethics, Gender and Ethnicity: Implications for Black Feminist Anthropology." In I. McLaurin (ed.), *Black Feminist Anthropology: Theory, Politics, Praxis, and Poetics.* New Brunswick, N.J.: Rutgers University Press, 2001.

Nash, J. *We Eat the Mines, and the Mines Eat Us.* New York: Columbia University Press, 1979.

National Institutes of Health." NIH Guidelines on the Inclusion of Women and Minorities as Subjects in Clinical Research." *Federal Register,* 1994, Pt. VIII 59FR.

Niehaus, I. "Coins for Blood and Blood for Coins: Toward a Genealogy of Sacrifice in the Transvaal Lowveld." Paper presented at the Meeting of the Society for South African Anthropology, Johannesburg, 1993.

Novick, A., "Noncompliance in Clinical Trials: I. Subjects." *AIDS Public Policy Journal,* 1990, *5*(2), 94–96.

Osborne, N., and Feit, M. D. "The Use of Race in Medical Research." *Journal of the American Medical Association,* 1992, *267*(2), 275–279.

Parsons, S., Simmons, W., Shinhoster, F., and Kilburn, J. "A Test of the Grapevine: An Empirical Examination of Conspiracy Theories among African Americans." *Sociological Spectrum,* 1999, *19,* 201–222.

Purvis, J. D. "Cancer Clinical Trials. A Case for Collaboration." *Cancer,* May 15, 1990, pp. 2391–2393.

Roberson, N. L. "Clinical Trial Participation: Viewpoints from Racial/ Ethnic Groups." *Cancer Supplement,* 1994, *74*(9) 2687–2691.

Savitt, T. L. *Medicine and Slavery: The Diseases and Healthcare of Blacks in Antebellum Virginia.* Urbana: University of Illinois Press, 1978.

Scheper-Hughes, N. "Theft of Life: The Globalization of Organ Stealing Rumours." *Anthropology Today,* 1996, *12*(3), 3–11.

Schulman, K. A., and others. "The Effect of Race and Sex on Physicians' Recommendations for Cardiac Catheterization." *New England Journal of Medicine,* 1999, *340*(8), 618–626.

Shavers-Hornaday, V., Lynch, C. F., Burmeister, L. F., and Torner, J. C. "Why Are African Americans Under-Represented in Medical Research Studies? Impediments to Participation." *Ethnicity and Health,* 1997, *2*(1/2), 31–45.

Sims, J. M. "On the Treatment of Vesico-Vaginal Fistula. " *American Journal of Medical Sciences,* Jan. 1852.

Sirgio, M. A., Cook, C. A., and Modrak, J. B. "Hypertensive Therapy in Blacks: Significance of Pathophysiologic Observations." *Journal of Clinical Hypertension,* 1986, *1,* 1–6.

Stone, P. H., and others. "Influence of Race, Sex and Age on Management of Unstable Angina and Non-Q-Wave Myocardial Infarction." *Journal of the American Medical Association,* 1996, *275*(14), 1104–1112.

Swanson, M. G., and Ward, A. J. "Recruiting Minorities into Clinical Trials: Toward a Participant-Friendly System." *Journal of the National Cancer Institute,* 1995, *87*(23), 1747–1759.

Taussig, M. *Nervous System.* New York: Routledge, 1991.

Turner, P. A. *I Heard It Through the Grapevine: Rumor in African-American Culture.* Berkeley: University of California Press, 1993.

U.S. Bureau of the Census. *Statistical Abstract of the United States.* Washington, D.C.: U.S. Government Printing Office, 2000.

van Ryn, M. "The Implications of Social Cognition Research and Theory for the Provider Contribution to Race/Ethnicity Disparities in Health Care." Washington, D.C.: Physicians for Human Rights, 2001.

Whittle, J., Conigliaro, J., Good, C. B., and Lofgren, R. "Racial Differences in the Use of Invasive Cardiovascular Procedures in the Department of Veterans Affairs Medical System." *New England Journal of Medicine,* 1993, *329*(9), 621–627.

Zhou, H. H. "Racial Differences in Drug Response—Altered Sensitivity to and Clearance of Propanolol in Men of Chinese Descent as Compared to American Whites." *New England Journal of Medicine,* 1989, *320*(9), 565–570.

CHAPTER ELEVEN

WHOSE HEALTH? WHOSE JUSTICE?

Examining Quality of Care and Forms of Advocacy for Women Diagnosed with Breast Cancer

Mary K. Anglin

What are the studies being conducted to protect our future? Is poverty a carcinogen? Please help us (my community) to understand the research and what it means. Let the community be included in decisions that affect our lives. I meet more and more African American women under the age of 40 being diagnosed with breast cancer. How do I save my sisters, our families, and our communities? (Holly, 2002).

Along with other breast cancer activists testifying before the California Legislature's Joint Hearing on Breast Cancer and the Environment in 2002, Karen Holly presented her life story as further evidence for the argument that conventional approaches to breast cancer risk do not account for that state's high rates of incidence. Particularly noteworthy was Holly's insistence on social context. She viewed her own experience with metastatic breast cancer as a reflection of the relationship among economics, race, environment, disease, and mortality. This chapter draws its inspiration from activists like the late Karen Holly and engages public health and anthropological literatures, in conjunction with qualitative interviews and participant observation from ongoing research (2001 to the present) in northern California, to consider the kinds of questions she raised.

In the broadest sense, such a consideration would entail analysis of the extent to which, and the means by which, social class, ethnicity, race, and gender collectively shape differences in quality of life for women diagnosed with breast cancer, in addition to breast cancer incidence and mortality rates. Given the limits of contemporary biomedical research on breast cancer, as Holly well understood, such questions cannot be readily answered. Rather, they constitute a call for new approaches to breast cancer research and for policies that reflect the diversity of women living and dying with this disease. Accordingly, in this chapter, I discuss the notion of health disparities used by public health researchers and policymakers to depict the vulnerability of poor people and persons of color to adverse health outcomes, as well as debates in the epidemiological literature concerning racial/ethnic differences in breast cancer incidence and mortality. I then move to a discussion of findings from ongoing qualitative research on the varied experiences of breast cancer diagnosis and treatment reported by low-income women and women of color living in California.

For Holly and many of the other respondents in the qualitative study, such questions are necessarily connected to issues of advocacy and forms of popular, as well as scholarly, representation. Much of the current understanding of breast cancer as social phenomenon, not simply personal crisis, and of advocacy and activism related to this disease comes from analyses of predominantly white, middle-class women responding to what they have termed an "epidemic of breast cancer," in addition to specific problems stemming from their own diagnoses and subsequent encounters with medical treatment (Anglin, 1997, 1998; Batt, 1994; Brenner, 2000; Casamayou, 2001; Kaufert, 1998; Klawiter, 1999; Leopold, 1999; Soffa, 1994). In effect, the national breast cancer movement has taken the stance of knowledgeable consumers advocating on their own behalf for improvements in diagnostic procedures and treatments, more sophisticated clinical research, greater access to experimental therapies, and, to greater and lesser degrees, research on the link between environmental pollutants and breast cancer.

However well intentioned or broadly claimed, such efforts reflect the concerns of a constituency whose privileged position affords them increased access to the medical system and greater reliance on technological medicine, with its benefits and its potential for harm. Thus positioned, the national movement is unable to address the contexts of treatment and prospects for survival for women who live without disposable incomes and private insurance; who deal with health care systems that are, at best, unresponsive to differences of race, ethnicity, culture, and class; and those whose priorities speak as much to the concerns of families and communities as to their own health statuses. In a thoughtful examination of breast cancer activism, Brenner noted, "It is not enough for organizations to advocate on issues affecting underserved women. *A breast cancer movement that actually reflects the diversity of those who are affected by breast cancer must represent the entire range of issues that affect all women*" (2000, pp. 347–348, emphasis in original). Yet even here, there remains the possibility of representing low-income women and women of color as persons with pressing health problems but not necessarily as strategists and activists in their own right.

Morgen reaches conclusions comparable to those of Brenner in a history of the U.S. women's health movement from 1969 to 1990. She notes that "dreams of diversity often collided in the clinics with dilemmas over difference" due to variance in the definitions of sisterhood and the limitations of North American feminism in contending with structural dimensions of racism and the political, as well as economic, underpinnings of class (Morgen 2002, p. 207; see also King, 1995). In the wake of breast cancer activism of the 1990s and 2000s, dilemmas over difference are related to definitions of social justice and the question of whether authority resides in formally defined expertise, professionalism, and large-scale organizations or in experience, identification with particular communities, and locally negotiated agendas. It is noteworthy but not surprising, then, that Holly (2002) used her testimony before the California legislature as an opportunity to describe the efforts of African American women, including herself, "to empower my community and other communities to be responsible and advocate for themselves with reference to health care issues." Besides seeking better health policies and legislation, that kind of advocacy focuses attention on the problems of low-income neighborhoods and communities of color in districts known for high levels of environmental contamination, legacies of industrial profiteering, and governmental disregard.

Accordingly, while the primary aim of this chapter is to depict the range of women's experiences of health care and the social context of diagnosis and care for breast cancer, I also offer a preliminary argument about the implications of differences in social location for models of illness and health and efforts related to advocacy. The first step along this route is an examination of breast cancer through the lens of health disparities. As noted earlier, the notion of disparities enables researchers, policymakers, and the public to assess differential susceptibilities to, and outcomes from, diseases, including breast cancer. It also provides a framework for making, or disputing, allegations concerning the health effects of racial/ethnic, gendered, and class-based discrimination in the United States and for claiming health as a civil right (Perez, 2001).

ACCOUNTING FOR BREAST CANCER INCIDENCE AND MORTALITY

According to the National Cancer Institute (n.d.), the concept of health disparities refers to "differences in the incidence, prevalence, mortality, and burden of cancer and related adverse health conditions that exist among specific population groups in the United States." The Center to Reduce Health Disparities, also part of NCI, moves this discussion further by presenting health disparities as evidence that "*the Nation's 'broken health care system is failing people with cancer.'* The system is broken when there is a disconnect or gap between cancer research and cancer care delivery" (NCI, 2004, emphasis added). From this vantage point, adverse cancer outcomes are attributed to structural problems within the system of health care in the United States, more specifically the inability of that system to address the needs of diverse population groups.

The Institute of Medicine's *Unequal Treatment: Confronting Racial and Ethnic Disparities in Health Care* (Smedley, Stith, and Nelson, 2003), puts forth an even stronger argument. That study reaches the conclusion that not only is there overwhelming evidence of disparities in the quality of health care and consequently the health outcomes for racial and ethnic minorities, but that such disparities carry societal as well as personal costs (see also Karpati and others, 2004). The Institute of Medicine further argues that a priority of the United States should be the development of strategies to reduce health disparities and—consistent with Holly's concern about the exposure of communities of color to the risk factors of poverty and racism—that these strategies must address relationships of inequity extending beyond the provision of health care.

The effectiveness of such an undertaking rests on the creation of new theoretical perspectives and methodologies capable of comprehensively documenting health disparities in racial and ethnic minority populations and investigating their root causes. However, the absence of a national cancer database, and more specifically a database that characterizes the impact of cancer in ethnic minority and medically underserved populations, means that reported differences in cancer incidence and mortality attributable to cancer in all likelihood underestimate the magnitude of social inequities (Haynes and Smedley, 1999). Little is known about how different populations come to have an excess burden of cancer, or how to develop and evaluate effective cancer control strategies with respect to these populations (Haynes and Smedley, 1999). Breast cancer serves as a case in point.

Reviewing the literature on breast cancer in ethnic minority and medically underserved communities, Shinagawa (2000) reports that the incidence of breast cancer was 12.5 percent higher among European American women, in comparison with African American women, while breast cancer mortality among African American women exceeded mortality rates for European American women by 44 percent (see also Wingo and others, 1998). More recent data from the American Cancer Society (2003a, 2003b) revise this, albeit slightly. Breast cancer incidence rates in 2003 are reported to be 140.9 per 100,000 population for European American women and 121.7 per 100,000 population for African American women, with 211,300 new cases of invasive breast cancer diagnosed that year among all U.S. women. While breast cancer mortality rates declined by 2.3 percent per year between 1990 and 2000, 39,800 U.S. women were expected to die from breast cancer in 2003. Moreover, African American women continue to experience significantly higher rates of mortality from breast cancer: 35.9 compared to 27.2 per 100,000 among European American women, or an excess of 31.9 percent.

In 2003, breast cancer incidence among women defined as Asian or Pacific Islanders was reported to be 97.2 per 100,000, and the mortality rate was 12.5 per 100,000. For women of Hispanic descent, the rate of breast cancer incidence was 89.8 per 100,000, while mortality from breast cancer was reported as 17.9 per 100,000 (American Cancer Society, 2003a). To the notion that rates of breast cancer incidence and mortality are apparently lower among Latinas and women defined as Asian or Pacific Islanders, relative to African American and European American women, Shinagawa (2000) offers an important caveat. The aggregation of women of heterogeneous ethnic groups, nationalities, and immigrant statuses under purportedly stable racial/ethnic categories could, in fact, serve to obscure differential risks within population subgroups (see also Kagawa-Singer, 2000). However, without meaningful information on the respective populations, this question cannot be addressed. Furthermore, the concern Shinagawa raised has relevance for epidemiological research on other populations, whose heterogeneity is similarly concealed through the use of unidimensional markers of race and ethnicity.

Three additional themes emerge from this brief report of breast cancer incidence and mortality rates. First and foremost, despite increased attention to breast cancer in the past decade and a half, too many women continue to be diagnosed with and die from this disease, second only to lung cancer as the cause of cancer deaths among women in the United States. Furthermore, the relationships among race, ethnicity, age, and incidence of invasive disease cannot be fully assessed because of limitations in current cancer surveillance systems, including the Surveillance, Epidemiology and End Results, which serves as the closest approximation to a national database. Given the failure of cancer registries in the United States to routinely collect socioeconomic data, analyses of the relationship between social class and breast cancer incidence (or mortality) are, at best, speculative (Isaacs and Schroeder, 2004; Krieger and Fee, 1994; Krieger and others, 1999; Navarro, 1990). Finally, and especially pertinent to this discussion, not enough is known about why low-income women and women of color who are diagnosed with breast cancer fare so badly.

One could certainly argue that black-white disparities in cancer mortality, including breast cancer mortality, are well documented

(Brawley and Freeman, 1999). Regarding the lower rates of survival from breast cancer and poor health outcomes experienced by African American women, public health and clinical researchers have investigated a variety of hypotheses, including involvement in mammography screening, with the expectation that women from particular racial/ethnic and socioeconomic groups would be under-represented in preventive screening programs; delayed diagnoses (and therefore later stage of disease at diagnosis); differences in tumor biology, leading to more aggressive forms of breast cancer; fatalism, along with other cultural values that theoretically militate against involvement in cancer treatment (or cancer screening, for that matter); and the possibility that socioeconomic factors account for observed racial/ethnic differences in stage at diagnosis, treatment, and mortality.

Yet what emerges from this body of literature is a complicated, at times contradictory, picture. For example, if in the 1980s African American women were less likely to receive mammography screening than European American women, the trend had reversed by the early 1990s (Makuc, Breen, and Freud, 1999). In 2003, African American women's mammography screening rates, reported at the national level, continued to be higher than those reported for white women (American Cancer Society, 2003a, 2003b). However, as Breen (2002) points out, it is hardly enough to emphasize participation in mammography screening as a form of secondary prevention, if low-income women and women of color then face difficulties with respect to receiving test results, gaining access to follow-up services, or having regular health providers to assist them with treatment decision making.

Similarly, delayed breast cancer diagnoses can be the end result of a variety of factors, often working in concert: insurance status, employment or unemployment (insofar as limited financial resources or job seeking may limit access to care), closures or relocations of inner-city hospitals, and even physicians' responses to low-income and racial/ethnic minority patients (Mandelblatt, Yabroff, and Kerner, 1999; Bradley, Given, and Roberts, 2002; Roetzheim and others, 1999; Wojcik, Spinks, and Optenberg, 1998; Rice, 1987; van Ryn and Burke, 2000; Taira and others, 1997; Chapter Ten, this volume). In other words, delays in breast cancer diagnoses are not simply attributable to problematic health behaviors, such as reluctance to report symptoms or failure to meet scheduled appointments, as some of the literature suggests (Howard, Penchansky, and Brown, 1998). What some researchers characterize as evidence of fatalism (Lannin and others, 1998; Mayo, Ulreda, and Parker, 2001; Ramirez and others, 2000), for example, is interpreted by other researchers as pragmatism on the part of low-income and ethnic minority women about the availability (and quality) of health care services (Chavez and others, 1997). Still others argue that research findings on fatalism indicate pervasive problems in survey methodologies, particularly with respect to conceptualizations of cultural values and practices (Passick and others, 2001; Ashing-Giwa, 1999; Kagawa-Singer, 2000, 2001).

That African American women experience lower rates of survival, irrespective of stage at diagnosis (American Cancer Society, 2003b), suggests that racial disparities in mortality might be due to differences in tumor biology (tumor size, tumor grade, estrogen receptor status, and the presence or absence of oncogenes) indicative of more aggressive forms of breast cancer, or alternatively that such disparities point to differences in the quality and availability of health care. The findings concerning racial/ethnic differences in tumor biology and prognostic indicators are equivocal. While some researchers have found evidence of an independent association between ethnicity/race and tumor biology (for example, Chen and others, 1994; Porter and others, 2004), others suggest that the limitations of research methodology do not allow a comprehensive examination of racial variations in breast cancer biology (Bacquet and Commiskey, 2000). At the same time, there are studies, including those of considerable scope and methodological sophistication, whose findings argue that perceived differences in tumor biology are attributable to socioeconomic status rather than race/ethnicity (Miller, Hankey, and Thomas, 2002; see also Adams, White, and Forman, 2004; Gordon, 2003; Gordon and others, 1992; Krieger and others, 1999).

The issue of whether African American women receive appropriate treatment for breast cancer has prompted further examination of minimum expected therapies in relation to stage of disease (Breen and others, 1999), as well as the possibility of racial bias in health care facilities (Farley and others, 2001; Mandelblatt, Yabroff, and Kerner, 1999). Within the public health literature, there continues to be disagreement over the extent to which socio-economic factors might themselves account for the persistence of health disparities and the significance of racial/ethnic discrimination in determining health policies, institutional practices, and, ultimately, substandard forms of treatment (Bradley, Given, and Roberts, 2002; Haynes and Smedley, 1999; Smedley, Stith, and Nelson, 2003; Miller, Hankey, and Thomas, 2002; Perez, 2001; Shinagawa, 2000).

In sum, biomedical research on disparities in breast cancer incidence and mortality suggests that there is utility in examining the status of being medically underserved as a socially produced outcome, not simply a measure of distance from idealized levels of health care services or a reflection of the heightened vulnerability of specific constituencies to personal crises, health related and otherwise.[1] Problematic health outcomes and high rates of mortality from breast cancer, in other words, can be viewed as the end results of social processes operating through the intersections of gender, class, race, ethnicity, and community. From this vantage point, it becomes possible to move the discussion of disparities still further, toward new methodological approaches and, ultimately, broad-based policies addressing the differential experience of health and illness as aspects of structural violence (Smedley, Stith, and Nelson, 2003; Mullings and Wali, 2000; Lock and Kaufert, 1998). That, as Holly's testimony (2002) indicates, is one of the steps we must take.

HEALTH DISPARITIES AND SOCIAL JUSTICE: ETHNOGRAPHIC FINDINGS

Women's narratives about their experiences of diagnosis and initial treatment for breast cancer provide one opportunity to pursue such an approach. In place of assumptions about a global sisterhood, the narratives allow us to consider gender as part of a web of relationships that constitute social location and cultural identities and explore salient dimensions of social location as they shape the contexts of diagnosis, treatment, and illness.

The basis for this discussion are recent findings from ongoing ethnographic research (an initial ethnographic study, 1992–2000, and the current study, 2001 to the present) in urban northern California, a part of the United States notable for its alarmingly high rates of breast cancer. My initial research examined breast cancer activism as an emerging phenomenon that drew its strength from 1990s models of AIDS activism, the longer history of women's health activism, and the contexts of rising rates of incidence and public concern about this disease (Anglin, 1997, 1998).[2]

In conjunction with the ongoing exploration of women's cancer activism, the current work (2001–2004) documents the health care experiences of women of color, as well as low-income women, who have been diagnosed with breast cancer. Fifty-eight semi-structured interviews, derived from a convenience sample, have been completed to date. Among these are thirty-seven interviews conducted with women of color, the majority of whom are African American, as well as with low-income women of different races and ethnicities diagnosed with breast cancer. My research entails participant observation in a variety of public settings: the meetings of community groups, breast cancer organizations, and local task forces; city and regional conferences on health (the health of particular constituencies, health problems of significance to the city and region, and questions of health equity); public health programs (women's health clinics, town hall meetings, and other forms of outreach); and academic symposia on breast cancer.

EXPERIENCES WITH DIAGNOSIS AND TREATMENT

The question that prompts this exploration is not that of formal access to health services, but rather the variance in diagnostic procedures and breast cancer treatment provided to women in different social locations and the implications of such differences for quality of life, morbidity, and ultimately survival. From a legal standpoint, all Californians are ensured timely access to breast cancer screening and treatment. The National Breast Cancer and Cervical Cancer Mortality Prevention Act of 1990 authorized the Centers for Disease Control (CDC) to provide breast and cervical cancer screening services to underserved women. Even before the enactment of federal legislation, California laws required private insurers and Medi-Cal, the state's version of Medicaid, to cover the costs of mammography. Similarly, California laws anticipated the passage of the federal Breast and Cervical Cancer Treatment Act of 2000, which extended Medicaid coverage to uninsured women diagnosed through the CDC program, in establishing a state program to provide breast cancer treatment for uninsured and underinsured women with incomes at or below 200 percent of the poverty line.

The following discussion draws on a sample of the interviews conducted to date. The interviews have been purposively selected to illustrate how issues related to the quality and form of health care vary within subsets of the study population. Of the study participants diagnosed with breast cancer, 65 percent (twenty-four) are African American, 14 percent (five) are Asian/Pacific Islander, 14 percent (five) are European or European American, 5 percent (two) are Latina, and 3 percent (one) are Native American. In addition, 14 percent (five) of study participants who defined themselves as African American or European American noted that their families of origin include Native American (predominantly Cherokee) ancestors. The majority (56 percent) of study participants reported an annual household income of less than $30,000, with 36 percent reporting incomes of less than $20,000 per year;[3] 28 percent reported household incomes from $30,000 to $50,000 per year, and 17 percent reported household incomes of more than $50,000 per year.[4]

The interviews of two women recently or temporarily housed—in other words, lacking access to housing apart from the temporary assistance of urban programs or kin networks—are reflective of the experiences reported by approximately 10 percent of the participants in this study. These interviews were selected to indicate the variance in health strategies and treatment experiences for homeless women, a population group whose characteristics are too often oversimplified. Similarly, three interviews were selected to illustrate problems in obtaining a breast cancer diagnosis for women with health care resources (health insurance or membership in a health maintenance organization) and for those whose only form of health care is that provided through the state of California. The purpose here is to illustrate the ways in which themes may vary for specific, intentional subsets of the population. By way of contrast, several of the narratives presented here illustrate encounters with providers whose care is described by study participants as exemplary and might constitute standards of care that should be made available to all citizens, regardless of their ability to pay.

Access to mammography screening does not, in itself, prevent breast cancer. This is an argument long made by breast cancer activists advocating better diagnostic technologies, along with alternative approaches to risk for this disease. As one study participant, the daughter of European immigrants and in her mid-sixties when she was diagnosed with breast cancer, learned, mammography is less effective at detecting individual cases of breast cancer than in screening population groups for disease: "I only found this out last year. A girl that I used to work with for years, she went in for her mammogram every year. They never found anything. And all of a sudden, she felt a lump. She went in. They took another mammogram, and couldn't find anything. The doctor felt the lump. They took a biopsy, and she has just had two breasts removed and the chemo and the radiation. The mammogram did not show anything. . . . I thought if you had a mammogram, and the mammogram was clear, you were clear" (interview 13). In her own case, she realized, she had been "very lucky" that the mammogram did reveal a suspicious area that proved, on biopsy, to be a small cancerous tumor.

Another respondent, an African American woman in her forties at the time of her diagnosis, spoke passionately about the women she knew to be left out of screening programs and educational campaigns about breast cancer: "I see a lot of homeless women down there, a lot of women that stays in the shelter. They don't have that type of stuff." She knew about this from her own experience of delayed diagnosis and health care providers indifferent to her health care concerns. Much like the women she described, she had been "in addiction and you know using drugs, you don't take care of your health problems, do you?" Even so, she sought care for the breast lump she had discovered: "Oh, well, I went to the doctor. The doctor examined me and I told him I had lumps. He did a breast examination, and he said, 'Oh, it's not a hard mass.' He knocked on the desk like 'knock, knock.' 'As long as it's not hard like that, I wouldn't worry about it." And so I went on for years and years. And it's not; it wasn't only him. I told like two or three other doctors after that" (interview 3).

Not until five years later, when she told her drug rehabilitation counselor about the painful mass in her breast, did this woman receive a thorough examination and the appropriate diagnostic tests (mammography, sonogram, and surgical biopsy). The drug rehabilitation counselor made an appointment at the breast clinic in the public hospital and accompanied her there. "But [the counselor] went along with me. And she said, 'Explain it to them like you explained it to me.' Because [the doctor] asked questions like, 'How long have they been there?' and 'Is it one or two or three or how many lumps?' At this point we had two." The biopsy revealed that the two breast masses, 3.0 and 1.5 centimeters in size, were malignant and that the breast cancer had spread to three lymph nodes. After years of being told not to worry about the lumps in her breast, this respondent was, in her words, stunned by the news that she had breast cancer and that she would have to undergo mastectomy followed by chemotherapy. The support of the drug rehabilitation counselor made it possible to follow the recommended treatment regimen. Otherwise, she noted, "I probably wouldn't have showed up knowing I'm going to lose a part of my body, you know. Because I'm scared, even to the fact I'm in shock. Right?"

For other study participants, particularly those with health insurance, the issue was not so much that of receiving regular screening but of having access to test results and treatment recommendations. In one instance, a woman who was herself an HIV counselor at a community health clinic, found that her doctor was unwilling to communicate the results from her mammogram: "I went to a doctor that a coworker recommended. And I had a bad experience with him. He tells me to have a mammogram. When I had my mammogram done, it was, I think, five days, maybe a week gone through and he didn't say anything. He calls me at work at a quarter to five on a Friday and tells me . . . 'I have your mammogram and it doesn't look good.' I said, 'What do you mean, 'it doesn't look good'?" (interview 48).

The doctor refused to provide further information about her case. As he explained, he was about to leave for a vacation and did not have the time to discuss the findings or their implications (the need for further testing and the possibility of a cancer diagnosis). But rather than accept his advice to "make an appointment in two weeks," the respondent kept pressing until, finally, the doctor agreed to send a copy of the report. "Because, here, all my coworkers saw me just blah and start crying. And they were all telling me, 'Why don't you fax it?'" With the help of a coworker, she located another doctor at a well-regarded breast health clinic, made an appointment for the following week, and found out, when a surgical biopsy was performed shortly after, that she had stage two breast cancer. As difficult as it was to receive the news of her diagnosis, she was relieved to find that the doctors at the second hospital were "wonderful, very caring" and that she received comprehensive treatment for her breast cancer. The experience taught her to "be alert. Look at your body and make sure that you . . . I don't know. Some Hispanic people, I guess, some of us have been brought up that our bodies are too personal. If you are looking too much at your body, what are you doing? We have to look at our bodies. Make sure our bodies are still the same." Equally important to this respondent was moving on to doctors who gave immediate attention to her health problem and trustworthy advice about treatment options (see Wright, Holcombe, and Salmon, 2004).

Yet it is not easy to change doctors or seek second opinions, as a number of respondents found. Doing so requires health insurance, membership in a health maintenance organization, access to financial resources sufficient to pay for costly consultations, and the ability to pursue treatment through different health care facilities. In the previous example, the study participant was able to move from one hospital system to another without financial repercussion, precisely because of the kind of health insurance she had. Furthermore, self-advocacy of this sort requires proficiency in English, and more specifically the terminology used by health care systems and providers in the United States, or the services of a translator or other intermediary. Such resources are unavailable to many Latinas in California.

That language differences influence the kind of health care one receives was a major theme in the interviews conducted with ethnic Chinese women. One study participant, who emigrated from Hong Kong twenty-five years ago with her husband and children, noted first that her own experience of diagnosis and treatment was exceptional: "Because maybe I can speak a little bit, some English, to a limit. So, I can communicate with people, even though I speak slowly or I have my accent. I have that Chinese language accent. But I still can communicate—can use my own way to try to make other people understand me. So that part has really helped myself. Whatever I need or I request, my chemotherapy doctor, my surgeon doctor, or even my nurse, everybody treated me very nicely. Then, I feel very fortunate that I don't have discrimination" (interview 39).

But working part time as a cancer navigator in a public hospital, she has found that many of the Chinese patients, for whom she serves as translator, are frustrated by what they perceive to be inattentiveness and substandard treatment from health care providers: "That's why one of my patients just called me today. She is in the hospital today and she cannot communicate with the nurse what she wants to ask. She just leaves the message on my phone, then tells me to call the nurse and ask the nurse the questions. . . . Then, some Chinese patients they do feel discrimination, because the language problem, the language barrier, then the attitude from all different clinics."

If it is difficult to understand the actions of nurses and doctors, there is little opportunity to ask about the nature of the diagnosis, the recommended form of surgery, or whether adjuvant therapy will be needed. One certainly cannot discuss the experience of pain or anxiety. Rather, the patient waits for the translator in order to decipher what has just happened or what to expect.

In the words of another study participant, who emigrated from mainland China sixteen years ago and spoke to me through a Cantonese translator, "They [the doctors] just tell me to 'go to this room, this room.' I don't really know what they're doing" (interview 14). All of her interactions with oncologists, surgeons, resident physicians, social workers, and hospital administrators—the last with respect to financial information and eligibility for state and federal programs—are mediated by the one cancer navigator fluent in Cantonese and Mandarin, the primary dialects spoken by ethnic Chinese populations in northern California. She observed, "Without a translator, I will go through a lot of channels with no direction." It is not surprising that several times during this interview, the respondent commented about the importance of establishing "universal medicine, for the whole nation" so that no one feels excluded or worries about being able to pay for the health care she needs to survive.

This issue most obviously pertains to women who do not meet eligibility criteria for the federal and state programs providing breast cancer screening and treatment to the medically underserved and who do not have private insurance. However, it is also a concern voiced even by those women eligible for breast cancer treatment but whose access to care is terminated with the completion of the recommended treatment regimen. In the absence of universal health coverage, one study participant discussed the value of Medi-Cal in ensuring higher quality, as well as the availability, of health care services. Compared to those without health insurance, for whom the only option is to find public hospitals contracting with the state of California to provide breast health services to under- and uninsured women, Medi-Cal recipients have a degree of choice in determining where they receive health care. The respondent, who described herself as "Heinz 57" but noted that her social security card lists her as Cherokee, had been homeless for a number of years when she discovered her breast lump. Having lost access to Social Security Disability Income (SSDI) as a result of changes in eligibility requirements, she sought the help of a lawyer to protect her Medi-Cal eligibility. "My attorney said, 'Look, you guys screwed up. You're going to leave the Medi-Cal or we're going to file a lawsuit because she's going to have chemotherapy and you can't take the medical insurance minimum'" (interview 56). The threat of a lawsuit was sufficient for her to maintain coverage through Medi-Cal. That did not, of course, make it any easier to undergo chemotherapy while living as a single woman on the street. Indeed, she deferred some aspects of her treatment for breast cancer—radiotherapy, for example—because it was difficult to plan regular appointments. "You don't know where you're going to be from one day to the next."

Study participants who received health care through health maintenance organizations (HMOs) expressed different kinds of concerns with respect to diagnosis and treatment for breast cancer. For these respondents, as for those with private insurance, breast cancer screening was routinized as part of the annual health examination given to women who were forty years of age or older. However, as the following examples illustrate, one place where differential experiences of diagnosis and treatment emerge is in follow-up on suspicious findings from screening mammograms or lumps that women have found through self (as opposed to clinical) breast examination.

In many instances, respondents described this aspect of their encounters with health providers in very positive terms. For example, an African American woman, diagnosed with breast cancer in her forties, described being treated "like a queen. I don't know how a queen is treated but I could imagine. They treated me good, oh yeah" (interview 4). This respondent appreciated the thoroughness of her doctors, who took extra time in reviewing her mammogram. They first contacted her former provider, who was part of the same HMO but located in a different city, to obtain copies of earlier mammograms for comparative purposes. Following that analysis, they ordered a surgical biopsy just to be certain that "a tiny, tiny spot" on the X-ray was not indicative of a cancerous lesion. When a biopsy showed this to be breast cancer, "three doctors" told her that she needed a mastectomy because of the size of the tumor. Even so, the surgeon was willing "to go in one more time" to see if it was possible to eradicate all of the cancerous tissue through a lumpectomy. "So I still have my breast. And I feel good," despite having to undergo chemotherapy and radiation.

Other study participants, however, had problematic interactions with health care providers and with the HMO system itself. A respondent, who referred to herself as "African American, if that's what they're going by this season," and who had been a city bus driver prior to being diagnosed with breast cancer, provides a good example. As part of her yearly examination, she had been screened for breast cancer and was called back for a second mammogram. When the second X-ray also indicated a suspicious finding, the doctors ordered an ultrasound. Although a nurse practitioner told the respondent that this was only a cyst, she was not convinced. "Well, you know, when somebody tells you not to worry about it, that's when you begin to worry" (interview 38). Several months later, she returned to the physician because the lump had become painful and she wanted it removed. The doctor declined, saying, "It's not bothering you." Six months later, she succeeded in making an appointment with a different doctor, who did perform a biopsy. However, the procedure was poorly done, and the respondent subsequently developed a massive infection in the breast: "This started leaking. And I called them and told them. And that's when they prescribed something else. Well, when I went back to the doctor, he said, 'Oh, you've got an infection.' And the infection eventually led to the mastectomy because it never cleared up. So I went back. No, before I went back for the second time, they're calling me on the phone and telling me, 'Your test results are in. You have breast cancer.'"

During the second appointment, the respondent was told to have a double mastectomy, a procedure with which she was completely unfamiliar. By removing both breasts, the doctor explained, he would be able to treat the stage two disease in her left breast, and she would have no need to "worry about it [the cancer] coming in the other breast."

The respondent left that doctor's office determined to get a second opinion but soon learned that the fees associated with consulting doctors outside the HMO system were prohibitively expensive. Accordingly, she sought the advice of a physician in a different facility but within the HMO. "He never unfolded his arms. And he never examined me. And he said, 'Well, what did the first doctor tell you?' And I told him. He said, 'Well, then, that's what it is.'" Frustrated but determined to find a caring as well as competent doctor, she called once more to the administrative offices of the HMO. She located a physician who took her case seriously and hospitalized her for nine days to take care of the uncontrolled infection in her breast. Moreover, the doctor apologized to her because the infection left him no alternative but to perform a mastectomy. The respondent commented, "My surgeon, if I could hoist him up on a pedestal, I would. Because he really took time to not only tell me and my old man, but my daughter" about her breast cancer diagnosis and the course of treatment that would be necessary. After eleven months of wrangling with health care providers and the HMO itself, this woman's concerns about her body and her treatment for breast cancer were finally taken into consideration. Yet three years after the interview and more than two years since the completion of chemotherapy, she still contends with the disabling effects of that treatment and has not been able to return to her job.

Awareness of Sociocultural and Economic Factors Affecting Treatment

The schematic rendering of data from a small number of qualitative interviews is at best suggestive of an argument about the social relations in which breast cancer diagnosis and treatment are embedded. Nonetheless, in the narratives described, study respondents offer commentaries about the sociocultural and economic factors that shaped their experiences of health care. With gender as the frame of reference for their commentaries, they discuss the significance of race, ethnicity, formal education, language differences, technical understanding of biomedical terminology, family and community knowledge regarding particular diseases, sources and differences in income, private health insurance, Medicaid/Medi-Cal, access to housing, age, body size, family support, comorbidities (including, but not limited to, drug addictions), their ideas about health and treatment of the body, and the cultural beliefs (often stereotypes) of health care providers. These aspects of social location and identity worked conjointly in determining whether respondents received timely diagnoses, information on the range of treatment options and involvement in decision making about treatment, competently or poorly performed surgical procedures, and answers to their questions about breast cancer.

Returning to the arguments put forth by Shinagawa (2000) and the Institute of Medicine's Committee on Cancer Research Among Minorities and the Medically Underserved (Smedley, Stith, and Nelson, 2003), a more comprehensive understanding of health disparities would incorporate an examination of social location and cultural identity, not as prognostic factors to be considered separately but rather as mutually constitutive processes. Thus, in the examples, there were considerable differences in the experience of breast cancer diagnosis and treatment for two women who had lived on the streets and dealt with long-term drug addictions. As each woman explained, educational background affected how well she was able to navigate systems of health care. In one instance, the respondent had completed the sixth grade and referred to her limited reading skills, while the other respondent described her reliance on technical skills acquired through two years in college. There is also the issue of what Rapp (1993) has referred to as scientific literacy, which, in this instance, encompasses knowledge about diagnostic procedures, standards of care for diseases like breast cancer, the laws of individual states and the federal government regarding access to care for citizens with little or no income, and ways to assess the health care facilities and other resources available to the poor. Insofar as one of the respondents had greater knowledge of the health care system and diagnostic procedures, she was more successful in seeking care and more determined to follow a difficult treatment regimen, even while living as a homeless woman with an addiction.

That an encounter with the local office of a nationally based HMO was described by one woman as "a horror story come on" (interview 38) and by another as being treated "like a queen" (interview 4) could be a reflection of many factors. The horror story of the former might be attributed to miscommunication or the random encounter of a patient with providers so overworked that they failed to respond appropriately to her health care needs. In this comparison, both women were African American, with comparable educations (one and two years of college, respectively). The woman who had experienced considerable difficulty offered her own conjecture: "I don't know. I've just found a lot of people to be rude thinking. I don't know if they feel that because I'm a large woman, that they have to press hard [in a physical examination]. Or, if it's because of my race, that they don't think we have feelings" (interview 38). As was the case for many of the women interviewed in this study, the various sources of employment available, including, for a time, the dream job in a high-technology firm, provided what was considered to be a desirable health care option: membership in the HMO. Nevertheless, as a working-class woman who was used to an arduous work schedule and functioning as the primary support for her family, the respondent was not willing to accept the indifference of the health care facility or what she perceived as substandard care on the part of the call nurses and the first two physicians assigned to her case.

The relationship among employment, health insurance, and disability informs this account and many other narratives provided by study participants. For women who are self-employed or engaged in informal economic activities, breast cancer diagnoses and the disabling dimensions of treatment carry devastating consequences for household economies, adding to the enormity of their concerns. Being in treatment in many instances leads to a precipitous drop in income. For example, one respondent indicated that her income had dropped by 63 percent in the year following her diagnosis and treatment for metastatic disease. It could also mean the loss of income altogether and, where possible, dependence on the resources of family members. Those who hold jobs with wage contracts and disability policies might not face such dire prospects immediately, but, as several respondents noted, nonetheless feel the pressure of returning to work within specified time limits. And for women with physically demanding work, the aftermath of surgery or chemotherapy can mean, in some instances, that they are unable to return to their former occupations and the promise of continued health insurance.

Because breast cancer is not in itself regarded as disabling, eligibility for SSDI is restricted to women currently in treatment for advanced disease. Not surprisingly, a number of study participants regarded the interview as an opportunity to advocate change in disability policies and for universal health coverage. This was the case for the Cantonese respondent quoted earlier on the difficulty of receiving health care mediated (or not) by translators. This respondent was unable to return to her former work as a seamstress in a sewing factory, since her arm had been weakened by surgery (the lymph node dissection that is part of diagnostic procedures). While she remained the sole source of economic support for her household, she knew that her disability income would be terminated when she completed the adjuvant therapies. Put another way, her experience of breast cancer treatment and its aftermath was shaped by socioeconomic factors operating in conjunction with gendered expectations and ethnicity or, as Kagawa-Singer (2000) would say, distance from the European American norms of (economic) autonomy and individualism that are embedded in biomedical practice.

The narrative provided by the community health worker suggests the importance of locating analyses of cultural beliefs and practices within the broader context of women's lives. This respondent viewed the interview as an opportunity to comment on both her cultural heritage and her life experiences. As a Latina of a particular generation, she had been taught to regard her body as private and intimate, not to be spoken of publicly. Yet because she was a health educator with supportive colleagues and a woman living with breast cancer, she recognized the need to be "alert on my body" and to "stay and fight it" rather than "run from the problem." Thus, she participated in the interview as an aspect of her advocacy on behalf of other women, and Latinas in particular, dealing with breast cancer. "Well, you know, I really love what you are doing. I only wish that I was informed of all this, before my breast cancer. Because, when I was diagnosed with it, I didn't even know . . . nothing, really, about it. Now that I have gone through it, my intentions are to try to help as many people as I can" (interview 48).

In addition, she had been instrumental in the planning and organization of a (temporary) women's health clinic and breast cancer town hall meeting that were to be held in a predominantly working-class, multicultural neighborhood. Sadly, she died from breast cancer just months before the clinic and meeting were convened.

THE NEED FOR ADVOCACY

Few of the women interviewed in this study, apart from those explicitly identified with breast cancer organizations, were familiar with breast cancer activism or organizations addressing women's health as matters of policy and grassroots advocacy. Yet almost all of the respondents spoke at length about ways of better addressing the needs of women in circumstances similar to their own. As they noted, this might entail rewriting breast cancer educational materials so that homeless women and poor women recognized themselves as part of the audience. Such material would stand in dramatic contrast to ads featuring affluent women and messages that are not readily understood because of limited literacy or language differences. It might require different forms of outreach. "So I mean it's a lot, it's hard work getting the message to a lot of women, a lot of us women that need more programs. . . . Places where they can walk in and find out this information. You know, and know that this place is there. A lot of women may pass by it but then, too, a lot of women's going to stop and go in" (interview 3).

It could also mean developing new kinds of networks around the concerns of specific constituencies. As the respondent's own narrative makes evident and in the light of Breen's findings (2002), such informational strategies must be connected to medical programs tailored for low-income women in order to be effective.

Several respondents were engaged in building local-national ties through conferences specifically oriented toward communities of color, for example, the Sister to Sister Network, through which "they all share information on what they do and how they do things to get people to become educated and show us how we can build our support network" (interview 4). Still others worked within the context of their own lives, for example, incorporating information about breast cancer into the weekly women's group at a drug treatment facility: "It just dawned on me, [there are] all these women here and breast cancer [awareness] month," which could serve as the impetus for inviting speakers to the facility and for the staff to incorporate scientific literacy into programs of experiential learning (interview 56). Others went to support groups with the idea of sharing the knowledge they had learned the hard way, so that other women would not face similar prospects. "God, there's so much that I learned because I didn't know anything about breast cancer. And I'm still learning" (interview 38). In short, just as their commentaries suggest some of the myriad ways that health disparities are produced and experienced, so also have the women participating in this study depicted various means for addressing health as a civil right.

These contributions are crucial, Crenshaw notes, and not only because of what she has described as the limited value or the "trickle-down effects" of mainstream feminism (2004). Here Crenshaw points to the failure of mainstream feminism to acknowledge the simultaneity of race and gender hierarchies or their implications for the daily lives and political practice of women of color. The consequence is that mainstream feminist discourse and activist practices adopt a unidimensional, even assimilationist character in operating as if experiences of inequality (and their remedy) are fundamentally the same for all women (see also Brenner, 2000; Morgen, 2002). Yet as King's work demonstrates, African American women have historically drawn on their encounters with multiple jeopardy, or forms of discrimination operating conjointly, to advance comprehensive and thus especially useful approaches to social justice (1995). By arguing that cancer is political, Lorde (1980, 1988) similarly calls attention to racialized and classed, as well as gendered, practices of medicine in the United States that privilege certain constituencies over others and, even in instances of privilege, provide forms of health care linked as much to profitability as efficacy. In ways that resonate with Holly's testimony,

Lorde (1988, p. 126) addresses the fact that so many people of color engage in the daily business of living, "all carrying within our bodies the seeds of a destruction not of our choosing." Resisting destruction necessitates simultaneous engagement on many fronts, as both women understood. "Battling racism and battling hetero-sexism and battling apartheid share the same urgency inside me as battling cancer. None of these struggles are ever easy, and even the smallest victory is never to be taken for granted" (Lorde, 1988, pp. 116–117).

If health disparities, or the differential distribution of prob-lematic health outcomes, are usefully viewed as aspects of structural violence operating through the intersections of gender, race, and class, then there are indeed many forms of struggle to consider. Women's narratives about diagnosis, treatment, and living or dying with breast cancer provide an opportunity to examine the social contexts that engender health disparities and move the discussion forward, toward their prevention. That would be no small victory.

Notes

I gratefully acknowledge the helpful comments of the editors and the par-ticipants in the Working Conference on Gender, Race, Class and Health. Funding for this research was provided by the College of Arts and Sci-ences, University of Kentucky. Finally, and most important, this research would not have been possible without the involvement of public health workers, community activists, and the women who volunteered to talk about their experiences of breast cancer.

1. In this respect, it is useful to examine the controversy surrounding different drafts of the first "National Health Disparities Report," man-dated by Public Law 106–129 and issued by the Department of Health and Human Services (http://www.ahrq.gov/qual/nhdr03/ndhrsum03.htm). The Special Investigations Division of the Minority Staff of the U.S. House of Representatives Committee on Government Reform found that the Department of Health and Human Services edited the findings developed by a panel of scientific experts on health disparities in the United States. The effect of the revision was to argue, in contrast with the conclusions reached by the scientific panel, that there are no systematic or structural reasons for the disproportionate burden of illness and premature death observed in U.S. racial/ethnic minority and poor populations (see U.S. House of Representatives Committee, 2004). In response to the congressional report and criti-

cal commentary by various members of the scientific community, the Department of Health and Human Services released the original report written by the scientific panel.

2. That fieldwork investigated the means through which women with breast cancer organized themselves, as well as the threefold purpose of their activism: to address the problems of their own health (a critical issue for many of the early activists, who were dealing with metastatic breast cancer), call attention to the limits of current diagnostic techniques and forms of treatment, and alter discourse—biomedical as well as popular—on risk factors for breast cancer and primary prevention of the disease. The focal points of field research in the 1990s were two women's cancer organizations—representative of the initial development of breast cancer activism in the form of small, predominantly white, middle-class grassroots groups—and, to a lesser extent, the orchestration of national networks oriented toward mainstream political, as well as biomedical, advocacy.

3. Two study participants reported zero funding. One of these persons was allocated state funding, which was used to reimburse the relatives who provided her housing. The other person was in a drug treatment facility, which received state funding on her behalf.

4. Because a major concern of the study was to examine the quality and range of health care provided to women of color, the study included women of color with varying income levels.

References

Adams, J., White, M., and Forman, D. "Are There Socioeconomic Gradients in Stage and Grade of Breast Cancer at Diagnosis? Cross Sectional Analysis of UK Cancer Registry Data." *British Medical Journal.* 2004, *329*, 142. http://doi:10.1136/bmj.38114.679387.AE.

American Cancer Society. *Breast Cancer Facts and Figures, 2003–2004.* Atlanta: American Cancer Society, 2003a.

American Cancer Society. *Cancer Facts and Figures for African Americans, 2003–2004.* Atlanta: American Cancer Society 2003b.

Anglin, M. K. "Working from the Inside Out: Implications of Breast Cancer Activism for the Policies and Practices of Biomedicine." *Social Science and Medicine,* 1997, *44,* 1403–1415.

Anglin, M. K. "Dismantling the Master's House: Cancer Activists, Discourses of Prevention, and Environmental Justice." *Identities: Global Studies in Culture and Power,* 1998, *5,* 183–218.

Ashing-Gina, K. "Health Behavior Change Models and Their Socio-Cultural Relevance for Breast Cancer Screening in African American Women." *Women and Health,* 1999, *28,* 53–71.

Bacquet, C. R., and Commiskey, P. "Socioeconomic Factors and Breast Carcinoma in Multicultural Women." *Cancer*, 2000, *88*(suppl.), 1256–1264.

Batt, S. *Patient No More: The Politics of Breast Cancer.* Charlottetown, P.E.I., Canada: Gynergy Books, 1994.

Bradley, C. J., Given, C. W., and Roberts, C. "Race, Socioeconomic Status, and Breast Cancer." *Journal of the National Cancer Institute*, 2002, *94*, 490–496.

Brawley, O. W., and Freeman, H. P. "Races and Outcomes: Is This the End of the Beginning for Minority Health Research?" *Journal of the National Cancer Institute*, 1999, *91*, 1908–1909.

Breen, N. "Social Discrimination and Health: Gender, Race, and Class in the United States." In G. Sen, A. George, and P. Ostlin (eds.), *Engendering International Health: The Challenge of Equity.* Cambridge, Mass.: MIT Press, 2002.

Breen, N., and others. "The Relationship of Socio-Economic Status and Access to Minimum Expected Therapy Among Female Breast Cancer Patients in the National Cancer Institute Black-White Cancer Survival Study." *Ethnicity and Disease*, 1999, *9*, 111–125.

Brenner, B. A. "Sister Support: Women Create a Breast Cancer Movement." In A. S. Kasper and S. J. Ferguson (eds.), *Breast Cancer: Society Shapes an Epidemic.* New York: St. Martin's Press, 2000.

Casamayou, M. H. *The Politics of Breast Cancer.* Washington, D.C.: Georgetown University Press, 2001.

Chavez, L. R., and others. "The Influence of Fatalism on Self-Reported Use of Papanicolau Smears." *American Journal of Preventive Medicine*, 1997, *13*, 418–424.

Chen, V. W., and others. "Histological Characteristics of Breast Carcinoma in Blacks and Whites." *Cancer Epidemiology Biomarkers and Prevention*, 1994, *3*, 127–135.

Crenshaw, K. "Mapping the Margins: Intersectionality, Identity Politics, and Violence Against Women of Color." 2004. http://www.hsph. harvard.edu/grhf/WoC/feminisms/crenshaw.html.

Farley, J. H., and others. "Equal Care Ensures Equal Survival for African American Women with Cervical Carcinoma." *Cancer*, 2001, *91*, 869–873.

Gordon, N. H. "Socioeconomic Factors and Breast Cancer in Black and White Americans." *Cancer and Metastasis Reviews*, 2003, *22*, 55–65.

Gordon, N. H., and others. "Socioeconomic Factors and Race in Breast Cancer Recurrence and Survival." *American Journal of Epidemiology*, 1992, *135*, 609–618.

Haynes, M. A., and Smedley, B. D. (eds.). *The Unequal Burden of Cancer: An Assessment of NIH Research and Programs for Ethnic Minorities and the Medically Underserved.* Washington, D.C.: National Academy Press, 1999.

Holly, K. Testimony, Joint Informational Hearing on Breast Cancer and the Environment, Senate Health and Human Services Committee and Assembly Health Committee, Sacramento, Calif., Oct. 23, 2002. http://www.breastcancerfund.org/environment_hearing_holly.htm.

Howard, D. L., Penchansky, R., and Brown, M. B. "Disaggregating the Effects of Race on Breast Cancer Survival." *Family Medicine,* 1998, *30,* 228–235.

Isaacs, S., and Schroeder, S. "Class—The Ignored Determinant of the Nation's Health." *New England Journal of Medicine,* 2004, *351,* 1137–1142.

Kagawa-Singer, M. "Improving the Validity and Generalizability of Studies with Underserved U.S. Populations Expanding the Research Paradigm." *Annals of Epidemiology,* 2000, *10,* (supp.) S92–S103.

Kagawa-Singer, M. "From Genes to Social Science: Impact of the Simplistic Interpretation of Race, Ethnicity, and Culture on Cancer Outcome." *Cancer,* 2001, *9*(S1), 226–232.

Karpati, A., and others. *Health Disparities in New York City.* New York: New York City Department of Health and Mental Hygiene, 2004.

Kaufert, P. A. "Women, Resistance, and the Breast Cancer Movement." In M. Lock and P. A. Kaufert (eds.), *Pragmatic Women and Body Politics.* Cambridge: Cambridge University Press, 1998.

King, D. K. "Multiple Jeopardy, Multiple Consciousness: The Context of a Black Feminist Ideology." In B. Guy-Sheftall (ed.), *Words of Fire: An Anthology of African-American Feminist Thought.* New York: New Press, 1995.

Klawiter, M. "Racing for the Cure, Walking Women and Toxic Touring: Mapping Cultures of Action Within the Bay Area Terrain of Breast Cancer." *Social Problems,* 1999, *46,* 104–126.

Krieger, N., and Fee, E. "Social Class: The Missing Link in U.S. Health Data." *International Journal of Health Services,* 1994, *24,* 25–44.

Krieger, N., and others. "Social Class, Race/Ethnicity, and Incidence of Breast, Cervix, Colon, Lung, and Prostate Cancer Among Asian, Black, Hispanic, and White Residents of the San Francisco Bay Area, 1988–92 (United States)." *Cancer Causes and Control,* 1999, *10,* 525–537.

Lannin, D. R., and others. "Influence of Socioeconomic and Cultural Factors on Racial Differences in Late-Stage Presentation of Breast Cancer." *Journal of the American Medical Association,* 1998, *279,* 1801–1807.

Leopold, E. *A Darker Ribbon: Breast Cancer, Women, and Their Doctors in the Twentieth Century.* Boston: Beacon Press, 1999.

Lock, M., and Kaufert, P. (eds.). *Pragmatic Women and Body Politics.* Cambridge: Cambridge University Press, 1998.

Lorde, A. *The Cancer Journals.* Argyle, N.Y.: Spinsters, 1980.

Lorde, A. *A Burst of Light.* Ithaca, N.Y.: Firebrand Books, 1988.

Makuc, D. M., Breen, N., and Freud, V. "Low Income, Race, and the Use of Mammography." *Health Services Research,* 1999, *34,* 229–239.

Mandelblatt, J. S., Yabroff, Y. R., and Kerner, J. F. "Equitable Access to Cancer Services: A Review of Barriers to Care." *Cancer,* 1999, *86,* 2378–2390.

Mayo, R. M., Ulreda, J. R., and Parker, V. G. "Importance of Fatalism in Understanding Mammography Screening in Rural Elderly Women." *Journal of Women and Aging,* 2001, *13,* 57–72.

Miller, B. A., Hankey, B. F., and Thomas, T. L. "Impact of Sociodemographic Factors, Hormone Receptor Status, and Tumor Grade on Ethnic Differences in Tumor Stage and Size for Breast Cancer in U.S. Women." *American Journal of Epidemiology,* 2002, *155,* 534–545.

Morgen, S. *Into Our Own Hands: The Women's Health Movement in the United States, 1969–1990.* New Brunswick, N.J.: Rutgers University Press, 2002.

Mullings, L., and Wali, A. *Stress and Resilience: The Social Context of Reproduction in Central Harlem.* Norwell, Mass.: Kluwer, 2000.

National Cancer Institute. "Cancer Health Disparities: Fact Sheet. 2004. http://www.cancer.gov.

National Cancer Institute, Center to Reduce Health Disparities. "Why do Racial and Ethnic Disparities Exist?" n.d. http://crchd.nci.nih.gov/chd/racial_ethnic_disparities.html.

Navarro, V. "Race or Class versus Race and Class: Mortality Differentials in the U.S." *Lancet,* 1990, *336,* 1238–1240.

Passick, R., and others. "Quality of Data in Multiethnic Health Surveys." *Public Health Reports,* 2001, *116*(S1), 223–243.

Perez, T. E. "Health and Civil Rights." *Cancer,* 2001, *91*(S1), 217–220.

Porter, P. L., and others. "Racial Differences in the Expression of Cell Cycle-Regulatory Proteins in Breast Carcinoma." *Cancer,* 2004, *100,* 2533–2542.

Ramirez, A. G., and others. "Hispanic Women's Breast and Cervical Cancer Knowledge, Attitudes, and Screening Behaviors." *American Journal of Health Promotion,* 2000, *14,* 292–300.

Rapp, R. "Accounting for Amniocentesis." In S. Lindenbaum and M. Lock (eds.), *Knowledge, Power, and Practice: The Anthropology of Medicine and Everyday Life.* Berkeley: University of California Press, 1993.

Rice, M. F. "Inner-City Hospital Closures/Relocations: Race, Income Status, and Legal Issues." *Social Science and Medicine,* 1987, *24,* 889–896.

Roetzheim, R. G., and others. "Effects of Health Insurance and Race on Early Detection of Cancer." *Journal of the National Cancer Institute,* 1999, *91,* 1409–1415.

Shinagawa, S. M. "The Excess Burden of Breast Carcinoma in Minority and Medically Underserved Communities: Application, Research, and Redressing Institutional Racism." *Cancer,* 2000, *88*(S5), 1217–1223.

Smedley, B. D., Stith, A. Y., and Nelson, A. R. (eds.). *Unequal Treatment: Confronting Racial and Ethnic Disparities in Health Care.* Washington, D.C.: National Academy Press, 2003.

Soffa, V. *The Journey Beyond Breast Cancer: From the Personal to the Political.* Rochester, Vt.: Healing Arts Press, 1994.

Taira D. A., and others. "The Relationship Between Patient Income and Physician Discussion of Risk Behaviors." *Journal of the American Medical Association,* 1997, *278,* 1412–1417.

U.S. House of Representatives. Committee on Government Reform. Minority Staff. *A Case Study in Politics and Science: Changes to the National Healthcare Disparities Report.* Washington, D.C.: U.S. Government Office, Jan. 2004. http://www.reform.house.gov/min.

van Ryn, M., and Burke, J. "The Effect of Patient Race and Socio-Economic Status on Physicians' Perceptions of Patients." *Social Science and Medicine,* 2000, *50,* 813–828.

Wingo P. A., and others. "Cancer Incidence and Mortality, 1973–1995: A Report Card for the U.S." *Cancer,* 1998, *82,* 1197–1207.

Wojcik, B. E., Spinks, M. K., and Optenberg, S. A. "Breast Carcinoma Survival Analysis for African American and White Women in an Equal-Access Health Care System." *Cancer,* 1998, *82,* 1310–1318.

Wright, E., Holcombe, C., and Salmon, P. "Doctors' Communication of Trust, Care, and Respect in Breast Cancer: Qualitative Study." *British Medical Journal,* 2004, *328,* 864–868.

PART FIVE

DISRUPTING INEQUALITY

CHAPTER TWELVE

RESISTANCE AND RESILIENCE

The Sojourner Syndrome and the Social Context of Reproduction in Central Harlem

Leith Mullings

Isabella Baumfree was born into slavery in the area of Ulster County, New York, in the late 1790s. Sold away from her parents and her one remaining sibling at the age of nine, she was enslaved for almost thirty years in extremely difficult conditions before being liberated by the New York State Emancipation Act of 1827. During slavery, she was sexually abused and physically assaulted. Some of her children were sold into bondage. In 1843, she assumed the name Sojourner Truth and began to travel across the country as an abolitionist itinerant preacher, promoting the idea of black freedom to inspire northern whites to oppose the legality of slavery. She worked closely with leading abolitionists and became involved in the early women's rights movement. Her personal story of suffering and her courageous determination to overcome adversity awed and inspired thousands of people. Her name became identified with the strength and resilience of African American women who, like her, have faced numerous obstacles to personal and collective advancement.

The story of Sojourner Truth has become an important symbol of both the constraints and activism characterizing the lives of African

American women. It conveys a message about the interaction of race, class, and gender, as well as the dialectic of oppression, resilience, and resistance. Named for Sojourner Truth, the Sojourner Syndrome offers an interpretive framework designed to provide a broader understanding of why African American women and men die younger and, as compared to whites, have higher rates of morbidity and mortality for most diseases. It incorporates an intersectional approach, which emphasizes the necessity of examining how race, class, and gender operate in the lives of African American women and how they interact to produce health effects.

The intersectional lens refocuses our perspective on health and illness in several important ways. It invites us to understand race, class, and gender as relational concepts: not as attributes of people of color, the dispossessed, or women but as historically created relationships of differential distribution of resources, privilege, and power, of advantage and disadvantage. Attention to the historical and contemporary processes by which populations are sorted into hierarchical groups with different degrees of access to the resources of society shifts our analysis to racism rather than race, toward gender subordination as well as sex as biology, and to resource distribution as the larger context that constrains and enables what appears as voluntary lifestyle choices.

The intersectional approach also requires that we interrogate the manner in which these axes of stratification intersect. It emphasizes the ways in which race, class, and gender are not additive but rather interlocking, interactive, and relational categories, "multiplicative" (King, 1988, p. 42), "simultaneous" (Andersen and Collins, 1995, p. ii), "mutually constituted" (Brodkin, 2000, p. 240), and characterized by "the articulation of multiple oppressions" (Brewer, 1993, p. 13). It seeks to understand how they interrelate at a given historical moment and, in the study of health disparities, structure vulnerability and resilience. Finally, this framework also recognizes the many forms of resistance (for example, Collins, 1991) or "transformative work" (Mullings, 1995) that are generated by black women's location at the intersection of class, race, and gender. In this chapter, I use an intersectionality framework to discuss research on infant mortality and reproductive health among African American women in Harlem, New York.

REPRODUCTION IN HARLEM

The Harlem Birth Right project explored the meaning of inequality in the everyday lives of women in Harlem by investigating the ways in which class, race, and gender interact in specific situations to condition health and to produce such consequences as elevated morbidity and mortality.[1] This approach contrasted sharply with research attributing racial disparities in disease to race as biology or culture, or both (see Chapter One). Funded by the Division of Reproductive Health in the National Center for Chronic Disease Control and Prevention, this research was one of several projects designed to shed light on the meanings of the epidemiological studies demonstrating that black women have problematic birth outcomes regardless of their socioeconomic position, that they fare worse than white women at every economic level, and that even college-educated African American women have twice the infant mortality rate of college-educated white women (Schoendorf and others, 1992).

The initial research was carried out in Harlem from 1993 through 1997 by an interdisciplinary team of researchers.[2] Central Harlem, a predominantly African American community of approximately 100,000, is located in northern Manhattan. Although significantly shaped by segregation and discrimination, Harlem has always been a vibrant social, political, and cultural axis for African Americans of all classes and is home to historic institutions, families with many years of residence, and, at the time of the research, a small but stable middle and professional class.

Harlem has historically been subject to cycles of fluorescence and decline. During the past quarter of a century, Harlem, along with the rest of New York City, has been deeply affected by the processes of global economic restructuring reflected in the shift from an industrial-based economy to one based on the information and service sectors (Mollenkopf and Castells, 1991; Sassen, 1991; Smith, 1997). The core elements of globalization—the relocation of domestic jobs overseas, significant cuts in social services, privatization of publicly funded institutions, repeal of union agreements about benefits and work conditions, and the abandonment of the state's responsibility to assist the disadvantaged—have had significant adverse effects on many Harlem residents. During the

1980s, New York City lost 33 percent of its manufacturing jobs (Mollenkopf and Castells, 1991). The financial and economic crisis of the mid-1970s intensified an already initiated process of disinvestment. Government investment in urban public transportation, infrastructure, social services, and housing declined.

As these recent global processes unfolded, they interacted with longstanding patterns of race and gender discrimination. As a result of the civil rights movement and subsequent legislation, there has been a significant expansion of the black middle class in the past three decades (U.S. Bureau of the Census, 1997). However, the distribution of occupations is disproportionately concentrated in the public sphere and social service sectors of the economy—the areas most affected by government disinvestment. For workers, the consequences of the elimination of tens of thousands of manufacturing jobs as national and international corporations pulled up stakes to pursue higher profits in other countries were particularly devastating. In Harlem, job losses were reflected in an official unemployment rate of 15.8 percent by 1990, twice that of New York City. At the time we did this research, approximately 60 percent of residents sixteen years and older were not in the labor force (New York City Department of City Planning, 1990), taking into account those who dropped out of the labor force and joblessness among teens, and more than one-third of all households had incomes below the federal poverty level (Citizens' Committee for Children, 1999; New York City Department of City Planning, 1990). After 1974, as public investment in housing collapsed, city-owned buildings and parks were abandoned. Harlem residents were subject to significant levels of housing displacement (Fullilove, 1996), and infant mortality rates were more than twice that of New York City as a whole (Health and Hospitals Corporation, 1991).

METHODOLOGY

The research design included participant observation, individual case studies, focus groups, an ethnographic questionnaire, and a strategy of community participation.[3] Teams of two ethnographers spent three to four months at each of ten representative neighborhood and workplace sites. The three neighborhood sites reflected different levels of income, types of housing, and rates of infant mortality; the work sites, which included informal sector workers as well as service, clerical, and professional workers, were selected to reflect the occupational categories in which African American women were found nationally as well as locally. At each site, ethnographers participated in daily activities and neighborhood events, observed behavior and organizational patterns, and interviewed study participants, incorporating such traditional ethnographic tools as network analysis, life histories, and genealogies. In addition, twenty-two women (longitudinal case studies) were followed over the course of a year or more. Maintaining consistent contact with study participants over two years allowed researchers to observe individuals over time. As Susser (1996) notes, surveys and interviews tend to reify identities, such as "unemployed" or "homeless," as they appear at one point in time rather than presenting the continuum of employment, unemployment, and employment or the process of doubling up, homelessness, and displacement. The research team held eleven focus groups on topics such as housing, women who head households, budget cuts, culture, men, and youth. An open-ended interview, the Ethnographic Questionnaire (EQ), on a range of subjects including work, family, environment, and health was administered to eighty-three randomly selected women in Central Harlem. For each research strategy, study participants were sampled from diverse social strata, including variation by level of education, occupation, and income.[4] Structured participation and collaboration of community residents was a key aspect of the research. We held open community meetings at various points during the research to discuss the study, answer questions, and solicit advice. Throughout the project, the Community Advisory Board met quarterly to advise the research team on all aspects of the research and review findings. A series of community dialogue groups (CDGs) were convened to discuss specific aspects of the research, such as site selection and questionnaire topics.

During the data analysis phase of the research, physiological evidence that women who experience more prenatal stress have significantly higher rates of adverse birth outcomes became available. Because "potential mediators of these relationships remain unexplained" (Rini and others, 1999, pp. 333–334), at the request of the

Centers for Disease Control, the research findings were reported in the framework of the "social organization of stress" (Dressler, 1991, p. 1). The project, then, analyzed the ways in which resource inequality, institutionalized racism, and gender discrimination together structure access to such resources as employment, housing, recreation, health care, and supportive relationships, as well as how women confront these constraints. Ironically, both the class, race, and gender hierarchies and women's attempts to address these conditions may be potential sources of stress and chronic strain that could have implications for health and disease. The following discussion provides some representative examples of the full findings, which are reported in Mullings and Wali (2001).

ENVIRONMENT AND HOUSING

During the course of the research, Harlem was at the beginning of a significant transition characterized simultaneously by investment in high-end housing and new retail establishments by the private sector and increased neglect by the city and the state governments, reflected in budget cuts and cutbacks in services. Between 1970 and 1990, the number of available housing units in Harlem had declined by 27.1 percent, as housing stock was abandoned or neglected by the city, as well as by private landlords (New York City Department of City Planning, 1990).

The need for shelter in the face of poor housing and housing scarcity was a severe problem for both low- and middle-stratum women and affected many areas of their lives as they engaged in long-term struggles to resolve housing problems. Efforts to obtain, retain, and maintain adequate shelter often seemed to dominate the lives of our low-income participants. While middle-income women had more money to spend on housing, their resources were often insufficient to completely offset the stressors caused by lack of affordable quality housing. All women were confronted with significant housing problems that stemmed primarily from the neglect of both private property owners and the city, which acquires buildings when landlords default on city property taxes. Among EQ respondents, 64 percent reported that getting repairs done was a problem, and that complaint was relatively consistent at all levels of education. Residents of all socioeconomic groups expressed the view that the poor condition of housing in Harlem was a consequence of discriminatory practices on the part of individual landlords as well as governmental bodies. Eighty-three percent of EQ respondents believed that discrimination affected their housing (with no significant variation by level of education). Housing problems had implications for many other aspects of women's lives, and struggles to resolve housing problems appeared to expose them to long-term stressors. Fully 50 percent of the long-term participants in the study were engaged in some efforts to resolve housing problems.

Poor housing has been linked with a variety of health issues (Health and Hospitals Corporation, 1991; Wallace and Wallace, 1990; Fullilove, 1996), but for pregnant women, both the need for extra space associated with an additional child and the day-to-day physical strain associated with housing problems appeared to be a significant source of stress and chronic strain. Seven of the eleven pregnant women in the longitudinal sample experienced housing problems, including being forced to move from badly maintained apartments, being evicted during their pregnancy, struggling with landlords over repairs, and looking for a new apartment because of growing space needs. Not only did housing cause problems for women, but pregnancy often created or accelerated housing problems, impelling women to act on this issue while struggling on other fronts during pregnancy.

Broader aspects of the environment, including the lack of quality retail and grocery stores, the neglect of public spaces such as parks, and the problem of pollution, affected poor women more directly and immediately but also affected women across socioeconomic strata. In addition to a large sewage treatment plant and a sanitation transfer station, six of the city's bus depots are located in Harlem and are significant sources of airborne pollutants. A recent study linking pollutants in the air to lower birth weights in Upper Manhattan and the Bronx (Perera and others, 2003) becomes even more ominous in the light of a recent report (Nicholas and others, 2005) of a 28.5 percent prevalence rate of childhood asthma in Central Harlem, which is four times the national estimate of 7 percent and one of the highest rates ever documented for an American neighborhood. In addition, there were more than eighteen hundred vacant lots in Harlem, which were potential sources of rodent infestation. Furthermore, during the years we conducted research, no major supermarkets were located in Central Harlem, so women had to expend significant time and energy to obtain quality food and other retail items.

Despite the salient environmental sources of potential stress, many positive aspects of the environment may have served as protective factors and mitigated some of the stressors and strains. These included the presence of a large variety of spiritual and faith institutions—churches, mosques, and other spiritual and cultural activities. Among respondents to the EQ, 94 percent described various faith institutions as a positive aspect of the community. Perhaps even more significant was respondents' view of the perceived cultural, historical, and social advantage of living in a black community: 99 percent of EQ respondents cited living in a black community as a positive aspect of their environment. One resident of Striver's Row, a block of elegant brownstones, described the benefits of living in Harlem: "First of all . . . the warm sense of your neighbors. Harlem is like . . . a little town. You know people in a block. . . . They . . . see me every day and I . . . go to work and come home and feel more comfortable." Another brownstone owner who worked in publishing commented on "a lot of the cultural things that are available. We went to see black filmmakers and black music in Aaron Davis Hall. You know, things that would not be available to us elsewhere in the city unless it's Black History Month are available up here all the time. A lot of cultural things that we have access to, which I enjoy."

It was particularly notable that middle-stratum participants, by choosing to live in Harlem, appeared to be willing to exchange one set of stressors for another. They were willing to live under conditions of systematic neglect and higher levels of poverty in exchange for the protective features offered by living in a black community, including a more limited exposure to racism (as discussed below).

Women used both individual and collective strategies in their myriad attempts to procure, maintain, and hold onto adequate shelter for themselves and their families and to improve their housing and neighborhood conditions. These strategies ranged from daily actions such as house cleaning (particularly difficult in a deteriorating environment) to organized struggles for more long-term solutions. One recourse women employed was to take landlords to housing court for neglecting repairs. Almost 40 percent of the respondents to the EQ had been to housing court, and over two-thirds of those had represented themselves without the benefit of a lawyer. Others worked with block associations, tenant organizations, and a wide range of community groups.

Individually and collectively, across social strata, women were active participants in efforts to improve the quality of public space in Harlem: requesting the removal of garbage and the cleanup of vacant lots, planting flowers, turning vacant lots into community gardens or organizing against "environmental racism." What distinguished these efforts and organizations from those in more affluent white areas of New York was the high level of frustration residents reported about the lack of cooperation on the part of city and state agencies, which residents perceived to be based on discriminatory practices. All of these interventions of "transformative work" (Mullings, 1995, p. 133)—efforts to address and transform the constraints that confronted them in the domains of work, household, and community—required considerable energy, effort, and time and became a significant stressor in their lives. Despite this, respondents to the EQ reported that good things resulted from participating in community organizations—for example, "you get to see an important change . . . in our neighborhoods, learn to work with each other . . . you feel like you are not alone."

The negative environmental and housing conditions that structured study participants' daily lives as a result of residential segregation and discrimination—such as the poor physical condition of buildings, the interweave of decay and renovation, poor access to public telephones, the lack of quality retail and grocery stores, environmental toxins, and the city's reluctance to provide adequate public services such as sanitation and rodent control—affected poor women directly and immediately but also affected the quality of life for middle-stratum women who lived in the neighborhood. However, across the board, respondents also reported the mitigating features of the positive aspects of living in a black community: a comfortable social environment, a respite from everyday racism, the close relationships between neighbors, and the presence of cultural and faith institutions all compete with the negative factors. The positive and negative characteristics of environments, and the diverse ways in which environment acts as both a source of acute stress and chronic strain and a site of protective resources, interacted in complex ways.

EMPLOYMENT

The interaction of hierarchies of race, class, and gender was clearly evident in women's attempts to obtain and secure adequate income and benefits. On the national level in 1990, though approximately one-fifth of African American women in the labor force were in managerial and specialty professions, most were concentrated in service, technical, clerical, and laborer occupations (Bennett, 1995). As Krieger and her colleagues (1994) note in assessing the impact of race and class on black women, numerous studies have established that the economic return for the same level of education is lower for blacks than it is for whites; that within the same occupation, blacks are likely to find themselves in lower-paying and lower-status positions; that black poor are much poorer than white poor; that many black women are segregated in menial, low-paying, dead-end, insecure jobs; and that there are significant pressures on high-achieving black career women. These historical patterns of race and class discrimination are exacerbated by the flight of industry to other countries in search of profits, resulting in a consequent loss of manufacturing and blue-collar jobs and accompanied by a drop in wages and benefits. Low-income women in Harlem were subject to a continuum of employment and unemployment that severely affected their income security and access to work-related benefits. The study participants found themselves at various times having to piece together income from a number of sources, losing access to benefits, or struggling to maintain benefits and searching for new jobs.

The description of Ms. Barnes, compiled from our field notes, provides a sense of these efforts:

> Ms. Barnes, a longitudinal participant, is a twenty-seven-year-old mother of five children who lives in public housing. Her history demonstrates the ways women move serially through employment, informal work, training, and the search for new employment. She was employed at the fast-food establishment but left during the course of the study because of conflicts with her supervisor. She

began selling Tupperware and working at a day care center during the day. Four days a week she also worked the night shift at a bar on 125th Street that was owned by a family friend. She would go to work at 11 P.M. and work until the early hours of the morning. She also received supplemental income through a public assistance program, although this income stopped when her income from the bar was reported. At the same time, she was taking general equivalency diploma classes and registered for training for certification to become a home health aide. This training was free for those on public assistance, and Ms. Barnes had been on the waiting list. She was finally called after she had been technically removed from public assistance. Ms. Barnes had begun the program and purchased the uniform when the program was defunded because of budget cuts. She had attended several sessions and taken a series of tests on which her lowest score was 80 percent. Despite all these efforts, Ms. Barnes was frequently short of money. In 1994, her children did not attend the first day of school because she felt she did not have appropriate clothes for them and by the end of the study we lost contact with her because her phone was cut off.

Ms. Barnes had invested time and money to improve her employment opportunities, only to lose any return on that investment because of budget cuts. She was fairly typical of our low-income study participants, almost all of whom worked hard at a variety of strategies to secure income. Women who were employed at low-income jobs could suddenly become unemployed.

In order to feed and clothe themselves and their children, households developed flexible strategies for garnering resources. The ethnographic research revealed a picture very different from the traditional one suggesting that women receiving state subsidies do not work outside the home. Among low-income participants, households' strategies included piecing together resources garnered from state subsidies; work in the formal, informal, and underground sectors; use of private food pantries and charities; and private transfers in the form of services, information, and resources from relatives and friends. People created work from such activities as deejaying, flower arrangement, kitchen planning, baby-sitting, hair care, and vending all manner of goods. Household strategies frequently included education for one or more members of the household, often at a public college facility. Contrary to popular media representation, all of our longitudinal study participants had worked at some point during their lives. Among respondents to the survey, virtually all (96 percent) of those reporting themselves as currently unemployed had held paid jobs in the past.

Although our middle-income participants may have long periods of employment, they too faced income and employment insecurity. As a consequence of historic patterns of race and gender occupational segregation, African American women are disproportionately concentrated in the public sector: in 1990, slightly more than 26 percent of African American women in the labor market worked in the public sector (Burbridge, 1994; see also Bernhardt, Dresser, and Hill, 2000), which, for example, has historically included twice as many African American women as white women working as clerical workers (King, 1993). The fact that 85 percent of professional African American women worked in three major sectors dominated by government and nonprofit employment (health, social service, and education) (Burbridge, 1994) combines with the current cuts in federal and state spending, downsizing, and privatization to help explain the vulnerability of the African American middle class.

The specter of downward mobility and fragility of status were consistent concerns. A remark by Mr. R., a young professional at the office site, was fairly typical: "Those of us making $40,000 plus can become poor in a month." Indeed, during the course of the fieldwork, the office site was shut down, and all employees were dismissed. Several middle-stratum participants worked at sites subject to downsizing and elimination. They frequently described the tension resulting from unpredictability and uncertainty surrounding jobs in the public and service delivery sectors. Ms. S., an administrator of a hospital scheduled for cuts, observed: "It's a lot of stress, and I find that with my staff there are a lot of call-ins, hypertension . . . people are out sick . . . injuries on the job . . . working under stress is very difficult when you're trying to provide service that has to do with taking care of another person." In the same hospital, a nurse commented about the possibilities of privatization: "Buyouts mean that they fire you and give you enough money to buy a cup of coffee and a newspaper so that you can look for another job."

The research team selected sites for study based on the national census data on occupation in which African American women work. It was particularly remarkable that during the course of the fieldwork, all work sites studied by the ethnographers (with the exception of the fast-food restaurant) were affected by downsizing, modification, budget curtailment, or outright elimination. Given this, it was not surprising that 72 percent of the respondents to the survey reported that they lived from paycheck to paycheck. When their responses were examined according to educational level, no significant differences were found.

African American professional women we interviewed often worked in a situation of resource scarcity and the poor physical environment that resulted from chronic underfunding and lack of resources. For example, at the large public hospital, the media frequently reported on the lack of basic supplies, such as wheelchairs and stretchers, cleaning supplies, detergents, mops, and brooms. Doctors and nurses reported that frequently toilet paper and delivery gowns were not available. In addition, African American women professionals often reported that they did not get the service and respect accorded their male counterparts.

At the social service sites, where a major part of the work involved interacting with customers or clients, these interactions could be tense or conflictive and a source of chronic strain, as service providers attempted to cope with clients who were deeply stressed by chaotic economic conditions. This was particularly true when the providers had limited resources to offer services to low-income clientele experiencing escalating pressure from strained and diminished incomes, lack of opportunities, and punitive policies generated by budget cuts in federal, state, and city social welfare programs. The legal services director of a large legal services provider reported that in addition to the normal stressors of litigation, and the fact that "there were enormous caseloads with voluminous, challenging work," the lawyers experienced stress because their clients were poor. Lawyers described how difficult it could be to try their cases properly. Their clients might fail to keep appointments because they were often juggling several serious problems at the same time and might be involved in addressing another equally difficult problem.

However, here too there are complex relationships between the protective aspects of the job and the difficulties that stem from discrimination. Middle-stratum participants reported that working with African American personnel was often positive compared to experiences of discrimination they had encountered in job settings outside of Harlem. A young professional couple stated that they worked around white people all day and that this could be very stressful: their perceptions of stressors ranged from white colleagues wanting to discuss every crime African Americans are accused of committing to the use of the "n" word in their presence. The wife reported that during the trial of a group of young black men who were accused of assaulting and raping a young white woman in Central Park (a crime for which they were later exonerated after spending fifteen years in jail), she wore a personal radio to screen out insensitive comments from white people.

Race and gender shape class in that a disproportionate share of the poor are black women (Crenshaw, 1995), and race and gender, as numerous studies have demonstrated, also influence the way they experience poverty. For low-income women in our study, the lack of access to adequate income from jobs, instability of work, lack of employment, and precarious access to benefits added a great deal of stress, uncertainty, and unpredictability to their lives. Assessing the direct impact of these stresses and strains on health must take into account both constraints on access to health care itself and, perhaps more important, the stress that results from efforts to piece together meager income, get access to benefits, and care for children.

Middle-income women also faced income and employment insecurity. In addition to the structural constraints of race, class, and gender that limit their position in the occupational structure, their concentration in the public and service sectors of the economy not only produced certain unique sources of stress and chronic strain but also made them vulnerable to job loss and income insecurity. We studied middle-income women at an office, a public hospital, and social service and legal services sites. During the three years of the study, the office was eliminated, and thirty-seven people were put out of work, and the hospital and legal services sites were subject to significant downsizing. Middle-stratum African American women may experience unique sources of stress in managerial and professional occupations. Adding to the stress that may stem from well-documented constraints of discrimination based on race and gender in those positions, race and gender may

interact to produce conditions in which professional women sometimes experience conflictive tensions between their status in the
occupational and class hierarchy, on one hand, and race and gender solidarity, on the other. Furthermore, in situations where scarce
resources and persistent discrimination structured the daily experiences of both the providers and the clients, providers seemed to
incur additional burdens of stress while trying to mitigate the
impact of resource scarcity on their clients.

KINSHIP

As women carried out these subsistence and caretaking responsibilities, family and social support networks, involving both men and
women, played an important part in their lives. Since slavery,
African Americans have constructed households, families, and support networks, but the ways in which they have been able to do
so have been constrained by the inequalities of class, race, and gender. Prior to the 1950s the typical African American household
consisted of two parents, with the father or both parents working
(Gutman, 1976). However, deindustrialization and the consequent
disproportionately high levels of unemployment (Wilson, 1996)—
as well as the expansion of the prison-industrial complex, largely
based on racial discrimination in policing and sentencing and
selective enforcement of laws (Mullings, 2003)—have resulted in
a shortage of what sociologist William Julius Wilson has called
"marriageable men" and an increase in women raising children
without support from men. This phenomenon affects African
American women across social strata, and in Central Harlem at the
time of the research, approximately two-thirds of all households
with children under age eighteen were described as headed by
women (New York City Department of City Planning, 1990).

However, contrary to the theme of family deterioration that per-
vades the scholarly, policy, and popular literature, the researchers
found that although economic conditions severely strained support systems, people perceived family to be important and were
involved in a variety of flexible support systems. Almost all the
respondents to the survey (95 percent) commented on the importance of family ties, and overall, 90 percent of women reported
that family relationships were most important to them. Despite

popular perceptions concerning the absence of men, the researchers observed that women related to men in a variety of roles, including through their own consanguineal networks.

The ethnographic research revealed the fluid and dynamic nature of family and support networks, the continuing importance of consanguineal kinship, variety and flexibility of residential arrangements, the significance of nonblood kin, and the importance of women-centered networks. These women-centered support systems occurred across social strata, but there were also important differences in the ways in which support systems were recruited and functioned among low-income, as compared to middle-stratum, women.

Clearly, there were differences in access to financial, informational, and other resources. However strong a support system, it cannot offset the consequences of scarcity, though it may serve important functions in mitigating those effects. Middle-stratum women, though their networks included both family and friends, were more likely than low-income women to recruit support systems in which friends were more important than family. That friends may be dominant in middle-class support networks may have implications for African American women during their reproductive years. While middle-stratum women may have greater material resources for child care (although our case studies demonstrated frequently these were not adequate), because family members are less likely to be coresident and may be less available to them because of distance, mobility, or conflicting obligations, they may have fewer family resources. To the extent that middle-stratum women deem it inappropriate to call on friends for certain types of help with infant and child care, they may find themselves in difficult circumstances. In contrast, low-income women may rely primarily on families but find that in the context of resource scarcity generated by worsening economic conditions, all family members have less to give, there is little to exchange, and networks are fragile.

In all cases, across social strata, women are responsible for recruiting and servicing support networks. Anthropologists have described this activity as "kinwork" (di Leonardo, 1984), noting that, unlike housework and child care, it is generally unlabeled. While our study participants reported positive experiences with family and support systems, they also reported constraints. These may vary among social strata. Among EQ respondents, the higher the level of education, the more frequently family was reported as a major source of stress. This might be explained by the heterogeneity of African American middle-stratum families: our middle-stratum study participants were frequently the only ones in their family to attain middle-class status. Recent studies suggest that a "tend-and-befriend" response may be an adaptive female response to stress (Taylor and others, 2000) and that low-income women who traditionally use large social networks were more strongly affected by strategies affecting others in their network and had higher illness levels (Williams and Lawler, 2001). While the social support networks we documented are an important "resistance resource" (Antonovsky, 1979), in conditions of class, race, and gender inequality, kinwork may be simultaneously stressful and protective. Hence, the responsibilities of household headship and organizing support networks may help to explain some of the health vulnerabilities of African American women across socioeconomic strata.

THE SOJOURNER SYNDROME

In order to incorporate and conceptualize the multiplicative effects of class, race, and gender on health, as well as to integrate a history of resistance and allow exploration of agency, we developed a framework we termed the *Sojourner Syndrome* (Mullings, 2000). The model is inspired by "John Henryism" (James, 1994) in that it represents a behavioral strategy which has important health consequences. John Henry was a legendary "steel-driving" man who was known among late-nineteenth-century railroad and tunnel workers for his strength and endurance. In a contest of man against new technology, John Henry and his nine-pound hammer were pitted against a mechanical steam drill. In a close race, John Henry emerged victorious but moments later died from physical and mental exhaustion. John Henryism, a framework developed by Sherman James, describes high-effort coping or a strong behavioral predisposition to cope actively with psychosocial environment stressors. James hypothesizes that this tendency interacts with low socioeconomic status to influence the health of African Americans, particularly the incidence of hypertension.[5]

The Sojourner Syndrome may represent a more gendered form of John Henryism. The message of intersecting and overlapping gendered notions of responsibility is found in the symbol of Sojourner Truth.[6] In a speech that underscores the memorable phrase "Ain't I a Woman," Sojourner Truth dramatically depicts the various responsibilities of African American women carried out in circumstances characterized by racial and gender oppression:

> That man over there says that women need to be helped into carriages, and lifted over ditches, and to have the best place everywhere. Nobody ever helps me into carriages, or over mud-puddles, or gives me any best place, and ain't I a woman? Look at me! Look at my arm. I have ploughed, and planted and gathered into barns, and no man could head me! And ain't I a woman? I could work as hard as much and eat as much as a man—when I could get it—and bear the lash as well! And ain't I a woman? I have borne thirteen children, and seen them most all sold off to slavery, and when I cried out with my mother's grief, none but Jesus heard me! And ain't I a woman? [cited in Rossi, 1973, p. 428].

The story of Sojourner Truth has become emblematic of the lives of African American women. Like John Henry, Sojourner Truth is a larger-than-life legend and assumes extraordinary role responsibilities. Her account embodies the findings of the research: the assumption of economic, household, and community responsibilities, which are expressed in family headships; working outside the home (like a man); and the constant need to address community empowerment—often carried out in conditions made difficult by discrimination and scarce resources. In addition, the model of Sojourner Truth speaks to the contradiction between ideal models of gender and the lives of black women: exclusion from the protections of private patriarchy offered to white women by the concepts of womanhood, motherhood, and femininity; the experience of being silenced; and last, but not least, the loss of children. Exploration of the consequences of these intersecting responsibilities that exist for African American women across class may give us insight into the way race, class, and gender structure constraints and choices, and therefore risk, for black women.

The Sojourner Syndrome expresses the combined effects and joint influence of race, gender, and class in structuring risk for

African American women. Elevated risk is also observed for the college educated among these women because of their simultaneous exposure to both racism and sexism. This framework may help to clarify the mechanism by which race mediates both gender and class status. First, the consequences of race and gender—of being a black woman—contribute to the instability of class status. Hence we saw this vulnerability in the middle-stratum women in our study, whose employment situation was frequently precarious due to restructuring or downsizing in the public sector. Furthermore, race dilutes the protections of class. For example, middle-stratum black women may have attained the achievements necessary for middle-class status, but they continue to suffer job and occupational discrimination; they are less likely to marry and more likely to become single heads of households because of the shortage of "marriageable men," as a consequence of disproportionate unemployment and the prison-industrial complex. For middle-class women in the study who moved to a black community to avoid racism, their class advantage was diluted by the structural discrimination and neglect to which black communities are subject. All these factors have the potential to become sources of stress and chronic strain.

It is also important to consider the interaction of race, class, and gender discrimination on the one hand with agency and resistance on the other (see Karlsen and Nazroo, 2002). As many scholars have pointed out, there is also a liberatory potential that emerges from the sites of race, gender, and class subordination. The Sojourner Syndrome—which speaks not only to the structural constraints that have implications for illness but also to what people do about them—represents a strategy for fostering the reproduction and continuity of the black community. The usual roles historically assumed by African American women have allowed African Americans to survive through four hundred years of slavery, Jim Crow segregation, discrimination, and postindustrial redundancy. During slavery, when the family was illegal, African American women's assumption of motherhood and nurturance responsibilities facilitated the rearing of children. After emancipation, when married white women generally did not work outside the home, African American women's work outside the home as domestics and laundresses allowed the family to subsist when wage discrimination against black men and women did not permit a family wage. Throughout, African American women's individual and collective efforts on behalf of their community have facilitated group survival. In other words, the Sojourner Syndrome is a survival strategy, which may have both short-term and long-term benefits. But it has many costs, and among them are health consequences.

After the completion of the research reported here, Wadhwa and colleagues (2001) described physiological mechanisms by which hormones released during episodes of acute stress and chronic strain can initiate early labor. Furthermore, they found that these alterations during pregnancy may heighten maternal susceptibility to infections, suggesting that stress may be implicated in early onset of labor, as well as lowered resistance to infections, which may itself contribute to early onset of labor. Since that time, several studies have supported the link between stress and adverse birth outcomes of low-birth-weight and preterm delivery (see Coussons-Reide, Okun, and Simms, 2003, for a review of literature on the relevance of prenatal stress to pregnancy and infant development). The Harlem research underscored the importance of examining the social conditions that produce biological processes that may render populations more susceptible to exposure. While race may not be biological, racism has biological consequences.

SUMMARY, DISCUSSION, AND REFLECTIONS

The Sojourner Syndrome is a metaphoric model intended to speak not only to a public health audience but to the subjects of our research, African American women, about their lived experience. It allows the recognition and naming of issues that are frequently unlabeled. It is an attempt as well to bridge the gap between critical medical anthropology and public health models by demonstrating the ways in which the intersections of race, class, and gender hierarchies are embodied (Krieger, 1999).

Although it is applicable to specific women, the Sojourner Syndrome speaks not to individual risk but to the relationships among groups defined by their positions in race, class, and gender hierarchies. It suggests that the intersections of racism and sexism in the lives of low-income and middle-income African American women cannot be wholly understood by looking separately at the risk factors of race, class, and gender. In this sense, it challenges the concept of individual risk, which has the potential to move the emphasis from social reform to personal behavior (see Alcabes, 2003), as well as research emphasizing dysfunctional cultural and individual behaviors that produce recommendations for what many policymakers consider to be "manageable" interventions in the lives of the subjects. Instead, by directing attention to the structural constraints and the ways in which people resist them, it points to the need for large-scale changes that provide access to employment, shelter, education, and health care.

Short-term public health interventions must focus on measures that support building resources for Harlem residents but, in doing so, confront the multiple sources of strain women face. These include the ways gender inequity, racial discrimination, and class inequality impose limitations on access to health care and, more important, on secure jobs, adequate housing, nutrition, child care, a safe and healthy environment, and social services—all of which are necessary for good health.

In the early 1990s, it became clear that Harlem had structural problems so profound that a more integrated and systemic approach on the part of the government was required to enhance the quality of everyday life for residents of the neighborhood. In 1992, based on extensive research, we developed a proposal calling for the establishment of an "Opportunity Zone" for Central Harlem—"targeted area[s] in which impediments to employment, education, health and housing are minimized in order to develop healthy, adequately educated citizens" (Mullings and Susser, 1992, p. 59). The proposal, which included specific recommendations for employment strategies to increase the number and variety of jobs available to residents of Central Harlem, community health centers, creative public schooling, affordable housing, and community empowerment strategies,[7] differed from traditional interventions in taking an integrated approach to addressing systemic inequalities and encouraging full participation of residents in developing intervention programs.

Public health interventions must also build on and support the protective mechanisms, community assets, and community organizations that community residents have developed. Harlem, in particular, has a wide range of grassroots and community organizations and institutions that work under difficult conditions to render valuable services to the community. Long-term interventions must direct attention to such major structural changes as a living wage and full employment, restoration of full civil rights for former prisoners who have completed their terms of incarceration, free quality public education for all, and universal health care. While in today's political climate, these proposals may seem unrealistic, such a direction, which redefines the rights of citizens and legal residents, and what they have to a right to expect from their society and their government, could benefit the entire U.S. population.

One of the greatest victories of Sojourner Truth was her ability to convince some in the white majority that their future was directly linked with the status of oppressed African Americans. She understood the continuities among racial discrimination, class exploitation, and gender subordination and that the enslavement of 4 million African Americans had a negative social, economic, and political impact on millions more who were white. The civil rights struggle of the 1950s and 1960s ended legal segregation, but it also enhanced and expanded democracy for labor, women, the elderly, the disabled, new immigrants, Latinos, Asians, Native Americans, gays, and lesbians. A generation later, when 45 million Americans—white, black, Latino, and Asian—lack health insurance and millions more are outside the paid labor force, perhaps we should keep in mind the connections between communities like Harlem and the rest of America. What happens to African Americans frequently presages emerging conditions for millions of other Americans who are not racialized. The elimination of stable employment in the formal economy for Harlem residents in the 1980s and 1990s is now taking place in many white middle- and working-class communities throughout the United States as a result of outsourcing jobs abroad. The number of households headed by women is now increasing in all ethnic and class groups in most industrialized and developing countries (Castells, 2004). As Sojourner Truth proclaimed, we are all interconnected in the struggle to achieve our full potential.

Notes

I am greatly indebted to Alaka Wali, my coauthor for *Stress and Resilience: The Social Context of Reproduction in Harlem,* from which much of this chapter is drawn. I also thank my coeditor, Amy Schulz, and the other conference participants, Sister Scholars, and Manning Marable, for their helpful comments on the chapter. Finally, I am very grateful to the graduate students who assisted me with the preparation of this chapter: Santa Cruz Hughes, Andrea Morrell, and Katrina Scott. This chapter was originally published in *Transforming Anthropology*, 2005, *13*(2), 79–91. I thank the editors of the American Anthropology Association and the University of California Press for permission to reprint this article.

1. This section is largely drawn from Mullings and Wali (2001).
2. The coprincipal investigators were Leith Mullings, an anthropologist; Diane McLean, an epidemiologist; and Janet Mitchell, a neonatologist. Alaka Wali, an anthropologist, served as the senior ethnographer. Denise Oliver, Sabiyha Prince, Sayida Self, Deborah Thomas, and Patricia Tovar, anthropology graduate students at the time of the research, were involved in ethnographic and other research activities. The research was funded in part by the Centers for Disease Control and Prevention under contract 200–92–0664 to the New York Urban League.
3. The methodology is fully described in Mullings and others (2001).
4. Though in keeping with Centers for Disease Control and Prevention use in other studies, social strata were used to include variation by level of education, occupation, and income, it became evident during the research that these criteria could not be conflated because they may have varying degrees of salience with respect to other social factors. In this study, *middle stratum* is generally used to refer to people in professional and managerial occupations or with some degree of income security, or with a postsecondary education that could lead to professional careers.
5. However, the Sojourner Syndrome differs in emphasis from John Henryism in significant ways. While John Henryism tends to be an individual measure, the Sojourner Syndrome emphasizes structural relationships of race, class, and gender. In addition, the Sojourner Syndrome explicitly incorporates an element of historical patterns of activism and resistance.
6. I use the term *symbol* advisedly as there are two versions of Sojourner Truth's famous speech and some controversy about which version is accurate.
7. The proposed "Opportunity Zone" contrasted with the more traditional enterprise or empowerment zone in several important ways. In an enterprise zone, the operative principle is suspension of taxes and laws for businesses that locate there. An opportunity zone, as we envisioned it, is predicated on "investing in people to actualize their potential for productive contributions to society" (Mullings and Susser, 1992, p. 59), and involves residents of the community in a proactive role in fashioning policy.

References

Alcabes, P. "Epidemiologists Need to Shatter the Myth of a Risk-Free Life." *Chronicle of Higher Education,* May 23, 2003, pp. 11–12.

Andersen, M. L., and Collins, P. H. "Preface." In M. L. Anderson and P. H. Collins (eds.), *Race, Class and Gender: An Anthology.* Belmont, Calif.: Wadsworth, 1995.

Antonovsky, A. *Health, Stress, and Coping.* San Francisco: Jossey-Bass, 1979.

Bennett, C. *The Black Population in the United States: March 1993 and 1994.* Washington, D.C.: U.S. Government Printing Office, 1995.

Bernhardt, A., Dresser, L., and Hill, C. *Why Privatizing Government Services Would Hurt Women Workers.* Washington, D.C.: Institute for Women's Policy Research, Oct. 2000.

Brewer, R. M. "Theorizing Race, Class and Gender: The New Scholarship of Black Feminist Intellectuals and Black Women's Labor." In S. M. James and A.P.A. Busia (eds.), *Theorizing Black Feminisms: The Visionary Pragmatism of Black Women.* New York: Routledge, 1993.

Brodkin, K. "Global Capitalism: What's Race Got to Do with It?" *American Ethnologist,* 2000, *27*(2), 237–256.

Burbridge, L. C. "The Reliance of African American Women on Government and Third Sector Employment." *American Economic Review,* 1994, *84,* 103–107.

Castells, M. *The Power of Identity: The Information Age: Economy, Society, and Culture.* Cambridge, Mass.: Blackwell, 2004

Citizens' Committee for Children. *Keeping Track of New York City's Children: A Citizen's Committee for Children Status Report.* New York: Citizens' Committee for Children, 1999.

Collins, P. H. *Black Feminist Thought: Knowledge, Consciousness, and the Politics of Empowerment.* New York: Routledge, 1991.

Coussons-Reide, M., Okun, M., and Simms, S. "The Psychoneuroimmunology of Pregnancy." *Journal of Reproductive and Infant Psychology,* 2003, *21*(2), 103–112.

Crenshaw, K. "Mapping the Margins: Intersectionality, Identity Politics, and Violence Against Women of Color." In K. Crenshaw, N. Gotanda, G. Peller, and K. Thomas (eds.), *Critical Race Theory.* New York: New Press, 1995.

di Leonardo, M. *The Varieties of Ethnic Experience: Kinship, Class and Gender Among California Italian-Americans.* Ithaca, N.Y.: Cornell University Press, 1984.

Dressler, W. W. *Stress and Adaptation in the Context of Culture: Depression in a Southern Black Community.* Albany: State University of New York Press, 1991.

Fullilove, M. T. "Psychiatric Implications of Displacement: Contributions from the Psychology of Place." *American Journal of Psychiatry,* 1996, *153,* 1516–1522.

Gutman, H. *The Black Family in Slavery and Freedom, 1750–1925.* New York: Pantheon, 1976.

Health and Hospitals Corporation. *A Summary Examination of Excess Mortality in Central Harlem and New York City.* New York: Office of Strategic Planning, 1991.

James, S. A. "John Henryism and the Health of African Americans." *Culture, Medicine and Psychiatry,* 1994, *18,* 163–182.

Karlsen S., and Nazroo, J. "Agency and Structure: The Impact of Ethnic Identity and Racism on the Health of Ethnic Minority People." *Sociology of Health and Illness,* 2002, *24*(1), 1–20.

King, D. "Multiple Jeopardy, Multiple Consciousness: The Context of a Black Feminist Ideology." *Signs: Journal of Women in Culture and Society,* 1988, *14,* 42–72.

King, M. C. "Black Women's Breakthrough into Clerical Work: An Occupational Tipping Model." *Journal of Economic Issues,* 1993, *27,* 1097–1125.

Krieger, N. "Embodying Inequality: A Review of Concepts, Measures, and Methods for Studying Health Consequences of Discrimination." *International Journal of Health Services,* 1999, *29*(2), 295–352.

Krieger, N., and others. "Racism, Sexism and Social Class: Implications for Studies of Health, Disease and Well-Being." *American Journal of Preventative Medicine,* 1994, *9*(6 suppl.), 82–122.

Mollenkopf, J., and Castells, M. (eds.). *Dual City: Restructuring New York.* New York: Russell Sage, 1991.

Mullings, L. "Households Headed by Women: The Politics of Race, Class, and Gender." In F. Ginsburg and R. Rapp (eds.), *Conceiving the New World Order: The Global Politics of Reproduction.* Berkeley: University of California Press, 1995.

Mullings, L. "African-American Women Making Themselves: Notes on the Role of Black Feminist Research." *Souls: A Critical Journal of Black Politics, Culture, and Society,* 2000, *2*(4), 18–29.

Mullings, L. "Losing Ground: Harlem, the War on Drugs, and the Prison Industrial Complex." *Souls: A Critical Journal of Black Politics, Culture, and Society,* 2003, *5*(2), 1–21.

Mullings, L., and Susser, I. "Harlem Research and Development: An Analysis of Unequal Opportunity in Central Harlem and Recommendations for an Opportunity Zone." New York: Graduate Center, City University of New York, 1992.

Mullings, L., and Wali, A. *Stress and Resilience: The Social Context of Reproduction in Central Harlem.* New York: Kluwer Academic/Plenum, 2001.

Mullings, L., and others. "Qualitative Methodologies and Community Participation in Examining Reproductive Experiences: The Harlem Birth Right Project." *Maternal and Child Health Journal,* 2001, *5*(2), 85–93.

New York City Department of City Planning. *Persons 16 Years and Over by Labor Force Status and Sex, New York City, Boroughs and Community Districts.* New York: Department of City Planning, 1990.

Nicholas, S. W., and others. "Addressing the Childhood Asthma Crisis in Harlem: The Harlem Children's Zone Asthma Initiative." *American Journal of Public Health,* 2005, *95*(2), 245–249.

Perera, F. P., and others. "Effects of Transplacental Exposure to Environmental Pollutants on Birth Outcomes in a Multiethnic Population." *Environmental Health Perspectives,* 2003, *111*(2), 201–205.

Rini, C., and others. "Psychological Adaptation and Birth Outcomes: The Role of Personal Resources, Stress, and Sociocultural Context in Pregnancy." *Health Psychology,* 1999, *18,* 333–345.

Rossi, A. (ed.). *The Feminist Papers.* New York: Bantam, 1973.

Sassen, S. *The Global City: New York, London, Tokyo.* Princeton, N.J.: Princeton University Press, 1991.

Schoendorf, K. C., and others. "Mortality Among Infants of Blacks as Compared to White College-Educated Parents." *New England Journal of Medicine,* 1992, *326,* 1522–1526.

Smith, N. *The New Urban Frontier: Gentrification and the Revanchist City.* New York: Routledge, 1997.

Susser, I. "The Construction of Poverty and Homelessness in U.S. Cities." *Annual Review of Anthropology,* 1996, *25,* 411–435.

Taylor, S. E., and others. "Biobehavorial Responses to Stress in Females: Tend-and-Befriend, Not Fight-or-Flight." *Psychological Review,* 2000, *107*(3), 411–429.

U.S. Bureau of the Census. *Surveys of Minority- and Women-Owned Business Enterprises.* Washington, D.C.: Government Printing Office, 1997.

Wadhwa, P. D., and others. "Stress and Preterm Birth: Neuroendocrine, Immune/Inflammatory, and Vascular Mechanisms." *Maternal and Child Health Journal,* 2001, *5*(2), 119–125.

Wallace, R., and Wallace, D. "Origins of Public Health Collapse in New York City: The Dynamics of Planned Shrinkage, Contagious Urban Decay and Social Disintegration." *Bulletin of the New York Academy of Medicine,* 1990, *66,* 391–434.

Williams, D., and Lawler, K. "Stress and Illness in Low-Income Women: The Roles of Hardiness, John Henryism, and Race." *Women and Health,* 2001, *32*(4), 61–75.

Wilson, W. J. *When Work Disappears: The Work of the New Urban Poor.* New York: Knopf, 1996.

CHAPTER THIRTEEN

INTERSECTIONS OF RACE, CLASS, AND GENDER IN PUBLIC HEALTH INTERVENTIONS

Amy J. Schulz, Nicholas Freudenberg, Jessie Daniels

In recent years, scholars, practitioners, and activists have produced voluminous new evidence documenting the contributions of racial, socioeconomic, and gender inequalities to the disparities in health observed in the United States and elsewhere. While recording these differences is an important first step, progress toward the international goal of "health for all" requires moving beyond documentation to action. If we are to achieve greater social and health equity, we must better understand the social, cultural, and political processes that produce disparities in health. Only then will we be able to act effectively to reverse or mitigate those processes.

In this chapter, we present two case studies in which we examine gender, race, and class in the social production of unequal health. We use these case studies to consider the potential for scholars, activists, community members, and practitioners to intervene to promote greater equity in health. The first case study examines the social context within which young men of color in New York City experience heightened risk of HIV, substance abuse, and incarceration. It describes the development of a targeted intervention

(REAL MEN) designed to mitigate those processes. The second case describes the Mothers of East Los Angeles, a group of women and families who for the past twenty years have actively mobilized to resist a variety of environmental threats to health in their neighborhoods. These case studies highlight the dynamic interplay of gender, race, and class within the two local contexts—New York City and East Los Angeles—as they shape the conditions of people's lives and contribute to the stark inequalities in health that now characterize the United States.

INTERSECTIONAL ANALYSIS AND HEALTH

Our analysis emerges from several distinct bodies of literature. First, public health researchers have documented persistent relationships between social inequalities and health: people who have fewer economic resources, and those who command less social or political power, have poorer health. These relationships hold across multiple health outcomes and persist over time, even as the major causes of death have undergone a transition from infectious to chronic diseases (Link and Phelan, 1995; House and Williams, 2000). In other words, social and economic inequalities produce inequities in both length and quality of life. How they do so and what opportunities exist for disrupting, resisting, or reversing those processes to create more equal life circumstances are less well understood. Moreover, while inequalities of race, class, and gender are endemic in the United States, the specific processes through which these inequalities are produced and sustained unfold within local contexts, varying geographically as well as historically (Almaguer, 1994; Buck, 2001; Stoler, 1995).

Second, beginning in the 1980s and inspired by the social movements of the 1960s and 1970s, African American and Latino feminist activists and scholars developed a critique of social analyses that focused on any single system of oppression—that is, race, or class, or gender. They argued that such an approach limits our understanding of the ways that these categories intersect to create and maintain inequities. Central to this intersectionality theory is the tenet that racism and sexism, as well as other forms of oppression such as homophobia, ageism, and ableism, operate as mutually reinforcing systems of inequality (Collins, 1990; Combahee River Collective, 1983; Stockdill, 2003). Furthermore, intersectional theory views race, gender, and class not as fixed and discrete categories or as properties of individuals but as social constructs that both reflect and reinforce unequal relationships between classes, racial groups, and genders (Daniels, 1997; Ferber, 1998; Omi and Winant, 1994). Within health, this approach posits that one cannot understand or reduce racial or gender disparities in health without examining the ways that institutionalized racism intersects with gender and class to shape educational and economic opportunities, risk of imprisonment and associated health risks, and opportunities to promote health and well-being. Since these unequal and mutually reinforcing social relationships play a major role in creating the unique patterns of ill health that characterize the United States today, they become an important arena for intervention to improve population health (House and Williams, 2000).

The third source for our analysis here is the literature on the evaluation of public health interventions. Health practitioners and officials judge their efforts by their success in reducing illness and death. Most interventions address a single health condition, work on one level of social organization, and focus on short-term improvements. Another strand of intervention, however, links health and social justice and depends on the force of social movements and political mobilizations to make broader changes in living conditions (Brown and others, 2004; Johnston, Larana, and Gusfield, 1994). In the United States in the past five decades, the labor, civil rights, women's, environmental, and gay and lesbian movements have all contributed to improved health and reductions in health disparities based on class, gender, or race.

In the two case studies, we use insights from these three bodies of literature as a lens to examine the potential of intersectional analyses to inform action to promote health and reduce disparities. Although both cases unfold in large urban areas—New York City and East Los Angeles—they differ on multiple other dimensions, including the gender and ethnicity of participants, the health issues of concern, and the roles of residents, professionals, and related social movements. In each, we examine the interplay between locally produced symbolic and material resources and differently positioned social actors in reinforcing or challenging interlocking inequality shaped by class, gender, and race. In each, we illuminate not only the processes that perpetuate inequalities and ill health but also potential strategies toward improved health and greater health equity.

RETURNING EDUCATED AFRICAN AMERICAN, LATINO, AND LOW-INCOME MEN TO ENRICH NEIGHBORHOODS

Health professionals in consultation with community members developed Returning Educated African American, Latino and Low-Income Men to Enrich Neighborhoods (REAL MEN) as a short-term health intervention for young men leaving jail and returning to their communities. Its founders analyzed the ways that social constructions of masculinity, race, and class shaped the lives of young men of color in New York City; the strategies they developed to survive; and the ways that life circumstances not only conspired to push young men into the path of HIV infection, violence, substance abuse, and incarceration but also created opportunities for transformation.

REAL MEN seeks to increase young men's chances of economic and social stability, and thus better health, by linking them to employment and educational opportunities on their release from jail. The program also seeks to engage participants in a critical examination of how dominant social constructions of masculinity and race influence not only the contexts that they encounter but also their own actions and health risks. In providing opportunities for young men to analyze these social processes, REAL MEN hopes to help them identify within their life circumstances and communities tools and opportunities that may enhance their chances of staying out of jail and protect their own health and the well-being of people they care about.

STRUCTURING PATHWAYS TO HEALTH AND DISEASE IN NEW YORK CITY

In the past three decades, criminal justice, poverty, and educational policies have dramatically diminished the life opportunities available to low-income urban young people of color. Disinvestment in public education, large class sizes, and poorly trained teachers contribute to high dropout rates: as a result, fewer than half the young people now entering high school in New York City graduate (Gootman, 2004). Over the past decade, New York State has transferred almost $1 billion from public higher education to building, staffing, and filling prisons (Correctional Association, 2004). As a result of the loss of manufacturing jobs, poor educational preparation, and other factors, half a million men of African descent in New York City lack jobs (Levitan, 2003), and these limited employment opportunities lead many young men into the illegal economy, selling drugs or engaging in other criminal activity.

Easy availability of drugs and alcohol and limited availability of effective prevention and treatment programs in low-income communities contribute to high rates of substance abuse. New York City's emphasis on aggressive policing, "zero tolerance" for low-level crime (Ayers, Ayers, Dorhn, and Jackson, 2001), and incarceration prior to sentencing (Jacobsen, 2001) increase the likelihood that young men who sell or use drugs will be arrested and incarcerated. Black and Latino young men are the primary targets of the criminal justice system through institutionalized practices of racial discrimination that include racial profiling, street sweeps, "buy and bust" operations, and other drug enforcement strategies that disproportionately affect low-income communities of color (Miller, 1996). Although African Americans and Latinos make up roughly 30 percent of the population of New York State, the prison population is 94 percent Latino or of African descent (New York State Division of Criminal Justice Services, 2004). Representations of young men of color in tabloid newspapers, television, movies, music, and videos promulgate racialized images of violent, misogynist, and selfish males—images that influence teachers, health providers, police, and corrections officers as well as young men themselves (Males, 1996; George, 1998).

These life circumstances influence the health of young men of color both directly and indirectly. Young men who have been in jail or prison have higher rates of HIV and other sexually transmitted infections (STIs) than comparable nonjailed populations (Malow and others, 1997), primarily due to unprotected heterosexual contact before and after incarceration. HIV infection and drug use increase significantly between adolescence and early adulthood, among both incarcerated and general populations (Staton and others, 1999; Stiffman, Dore, Cunningham, and Earls, 1995). Most young men leave jail, prison, or juvenile detention without exposure to effective HIV prevention programs or linkages to community services (Freudenberg, 2001).[1] A majority of those leaving jail are rearrested within a year of release, creating a revolving door that serves to increase HIV infection and drug use by further disrupting the lives of these young men, their partners, and their communities (LeBlanc, 2003).

As in the past, African American and Latino communities have mobilized to resist and reverse the processes creating these inequalities. These include efforts to achieve more equitable funding and smaller class size for New York City public schools, drop New York State's punitive drug laws, protest police racial profiling or abuse, end race-based job discrimination, and promote youth employment (Campaign for Fiscal Equity, 2004; Drop the Rock, 2004). While these mobilizations are essential to redress the inequities that place young men at risk, they do not, for the most part, meet the needs of young men already caught up in the criminal justice system, or address the specific physical and mental health concerns that may prevent young men from participating in social action.

GENDER, RACE, AND CLASS AND THE FOUNDATIONS OF REAL MEN

REAL MEN is grounded in an analysis of how social constructions of masculinity, race, and class create unequal life opportunities, provide frameworks young men use to negotiate within the context of those inequalities, and combine to create unequal opportunities for health. It recognizes that young men often leave jail with a commitment to changing their lives but that those intentions are often overwhelmed by the social, economic, and political contexts they encounter after release. Macrolevel factors (such as systematic racism, blocked educational opportunities, and media representations of young men of color as violent or misogynist), community-level factors (such as social support networks and educational opportunities), and microlevel factors (such as family disruptions and interactions with peer networks) shape young men's lives following release from jail and their chances for financial and social stability, substance use, HIV and other sexually transmitted infections, and for being victims or perpetrators of violence.

In contrast to the majority of public health programs that have attempted to take on issues of HIV infection, substance abuse, mental health, or violence among incarcerated men, REAL MEN was developed to address selected aspects of broader life circumstances and dynamics of race, class, and gender that can perpetuate or protect against health risks. Specifically, working in conjunction with community organizations, young men participating in the program are linked to high school, general equivalency diploma, literacy, and job readiness programs in their communities. As appropriate, they are also connected to local providers of substance abuse as well as physical and mental health services in an effort to support their transition back to the community. In addition to helping young men plan for release and make connections to community resources, REAL MEN offers them an opportunity to engage in a critical examination of masculinity and racial/ethnic identities and to explore how these social concepts influence health by, for example, influencing both social context and actions taken within those contexts.

The curriculum for this latter component of REAL MEN was developed by program staff in consultation with young men in the community.[2] It builds on a body of research that suggests that gendered conceptions of risk, trust, and power profoundly affect health and health behavior (see, for example, Aronson, Whitehead, and Baber, 2003; DiClemente and others, 2004). Furthermore, the intervention uses growing evidence that some components of racial identity, such as ethnic pride, may help reduce the degree to which psychosocial assaults of racism are injurious to adolescents' mental health, self-esteem, and academic achievement (see Chapter Six, this volume) and may also reduce drug use or sexual risk behavior (Belgrave, 2002; Brook and others, 1998; Harvey and Hill, 2004; Johnson, 2002).

Based on these sources, REAL MEN planners hypothesized a number of pathways through which conceptions of masculinity may shape decisions made by young men as they are leaving jail. For example, the belief that manhood requires multiple sexual partners or having sex when high may increase the vulnerability of young men and their partners to HIV, unwanted pregnancies, and other adverse outcomes. Young men who believe that they will be perceived by their peers as "less manly" for taking action to protect their health and the health of their partners may be less likely to do so. The use of violence or coercion in relationships may also be linked to conceptions of masculinity that emphasize male power. Taking risks, and exhibiting an absence of fear in the face of risks, is promoted through both mainstream and alternative culture as a desirable characteristic of men (Canada, 1998) and may influence young men's willingness to engage in risky behaviors.

In a series of workshops offered in jail and after release, young men are encouraged to consider their options related to drugs, relationships, sex, criminal activity, and jail. In role plays, discussions of popular films and hip-hop lyrics, and group exercises, participants examine their own and media notions of manhood. In all sessions, participants develop and consider alternative responses to situations they are likely to encounter with friends, sexual partners, employers, and family. REAL MEN also offers activities designed to reinforce racial pride and solidarity in order to bolster young men's protection against the injurious effects of racism, foster attitudes and behaviors that promote community well-being, and motivate young men to plan a better future. Following release from jail, participants spend two full days in more group sessions, sign up for educational and employment services at Friends of Island Academy, the program's community sponsor, and attend sessions with their parents or partners.

While evaluation data for REAL MEN are not yet available, experience to date indicates that it is possible to engage young men in a critical examination of masculinity. The challenges of offering programs for young men leaving jail are daunting; they include implementation of programs in facilities where security and control trump rehabilitation; competition for young men's postrelease attention and time with girlfriends, families, peers, and street life; a glamorized popular culture that offers some of the little economic opportunity in the neighborhood; development of activities that deliver core messages consistently yet with enough flexibility to accommodate young men's complex scheduling needs; and ensuring that the project's community partner finds the resources it needs to offer crucial educational and employment services in a time of shrinking public resources.

Interventions such as REAL MEN illustrate both the potentials and limits of targeted efforts grounded in an intersectional analysis to promote health and health equity. Such efforts can be an important point of intervention to reduce or alleviate the harmful effects of structural inequalities on the health of young men as they leave the prison system. While by themselves they do not address the underlying processes that create health inequalities in the first place, in conjunction with broader social movements for change, they can contribute to social justice and health equity.

The Mothers of East Los Angeles

The Madres del Este de Los Angeles (MELA) was founded in 1984 by a group of Mexican American women and families living on Los Angeles's east side.[3] MELA's mission statement suggests a group identity forged at the intersection of ethnicity, class, and gender: "Not economically rich—but culturally wealthy; not politically powerful—but socially conscious; not mainstream educated—but armed with the knowledge, commitment and determination that only a mother can possess."

With roots in Saul Alinsky's Industrial Areas Foundation, the Chicano movement of the 1960s (Hernandez, 1980; Marin, 1991), and women's volunteer organizing efforts with local Catholic churches (Pardo, 1998), MELA grew into a network that at its peak included more than four hundred families and mobilized over thirty-five hundred people. Over a twenty-year period, MELA successfully organized to address a series of controversial issues related to the environment and health in East Los Angeles neighborhoods. They mobilized successful efforts to block construction of a state prison in their community (1986), halt an oil pipeline that would have passed under a junior high school (1987), prevent the construction of a toxic waste incinerator in their neighborhood (1987), and stop a chemical company from building a plant to treat cyanide and other hazardous wastes across the street from a local high school (1989) (Pardo, 1998; Freudenberg, 2004). Establishing ties to a variety of environmental groups nationally, MELA was active in local, state, and national environmental coalitions; collaborated with universities to study environmental causes of children's health problems; and worked on water conservation, lead poisoning awareness, and graffiti abatement programs.

The goal that guided these far-reaching activities clearly linked environmental issues to political influence and well-being: "To promote the environmental, political, and educational awareness, advancement, and well-being of the Latino population within (but not limited to) the East Los Angeles community" (http://clnet.sscnet.ucla.edu/community/intercambios/melasi/). In the following paragraphs we examine historical and contemporary intersections of race, class, and gender as these have produced inequalities and shaped the health, well-being, and political activism of those involved with MELA.

STRUCTURING PATHWAYS TO HEALTH AND DISEASE IN EAST LOS ANGELES

Longstanding political disenfranchisement and racist residential and employment policies have placed communities of color in jobs and residential neighborhoods in which they experience greater exposure to environmental toxins (for example, garment sweatshops, deteriorated housing in older urban areas) and limited access to the political and economic resources necessary to influence zoning or enforce environmental regulations (Brugge and Goble, 2002; Taylor, 2002). As a result, Mexican American, American Indian, and African American communities have experienced disproportionate exposure to toxic wastes, noxious land uses, and air pollutants (Bullard, 2000; Camacho and Cuesta-Camacho, 1998; Maantay, 2002; Shepherd, Northridge, Prakash, and Stover, 2002; Taylor, 2002).

East Los Angeles is no exception, and class and race oppression created the particular health and social problems that MELA organized to address over two decades: prisons, toxic waste incinerators, and oil pipelines under schools. Although it had initially been a predominantly Jewish community, increasing numbers of Mexican Americans had located in East LA by the 1940s. As in many other urban neighborhoods in the years after World War II (Wilson, 1987; Sugrue, 1996), when white and middle-class residents left East LA, employment opportunities and services such as banks and grocery stores soon followed (Pardo, 1998). Mexican Americans remained in East LA as housing discrimination enforced by racist covenants and police harassment limited their movement into neighboring areas whose residents were predominantly white (Escobedo, 1979; Pardo, 1998).[4]

The vulnerability of East LA residents to unwanted local land uses was evident following World War II when five freeways were constructed through East LA, uprooting thousands of residents, contributing noise and pollution, and shaping the political consciousness of community members (Escobedo, 1979). In her ethnography of MELA, Pardo notes "all but one of the core activists [of MELA] shared the experience of losing a home and having to relocate to make way for a freeway" (1998, p. 72). This shared economic and political vulnerability of the community contributed to a political consciousness oriented toward social justice. Pardo quotes MELA activist Juana Gutierez as saying: "One of the things that really upsets me is injustice, and we have seen a lot of that in our community. Especially before, because I believe our people used to be less aware, we didn't assert ourselves as much. In the 1950s they put up the freeways, and just like that they gave us notice that we had to move" (1998, p. 73).

Living conditions within the community and prevailing stereotypes about its predominantly Mexican American population shaped outsiders' perceptions of the neighborhood. These perceptions made the neighborhood a target for undesirable projects and discrimination and limited residents' political influence. These same conditions contributed to the emergence of a sense of shared racial and class identity, political consciousness, and collective mobilization that led eventually to the development of MELA.

GENDER, RACE, CLASS, AND THE FOUNDATIONS OF COMMUNITY MOBILIZATION

The history of community activism within East Los Angeles predates MELA by several decades. In the late 1940s, community residents worked with a field organizer for the Industrial Areas Foundation (IAF) to create the Community Service Organization (CSO). In East LA, the CSO organized "house meetings" that engaged both men and women in the development of mobilization strategies for more than a decade. By the 1950s, residents of East LA were mobilizing around poor city services, voter registration, police brutality, and inadequate infrastructure and housing discrimination (Rose, 1994; Pardo, 1998).

In the 1960s, the Chicano movement, which was active in East Los Angeles, emphasized development of Mexican American leadership (Acuña, 1984; Muñoz, 1989; Taylor, 2002). Movement goals included fostering a positive Chicano identity, fighting against racism, and promoting equal rights (Acuña, 1984; García, 1986; Romo, 1983). Hernandez (1980) notes that while both women and men were active in the movement, men held the majority of the leadership positions. As with many other social movements of the time, there is some evidence that gender frameworks were actively used to discourage women from leadership positions. For example, women activists who challenged men's leadership roles were subject to labeling as "women's libbers and lesbians"—explicitly gendered labeling intended to be pejorative, thus trivializing women and the issues they raised (Marin, 1991; Pardo, 1998).

In the 1970s, the United Neighborhood Organization (UNO) emerged in East Los Angeles, cosponsored by the Catholic church and with organizers trained by Saul Alinsky's IAF (Ortiz, 1984). UNO was grounded in theological perspectives that incorporated both personal faith and the transformation of society toward the goal of social justice (Ortiz, 1984). The first president of UNO, Gloria Chavez, began her community activities through the PTA and her children's school activities, eventually translating those skills into organizing for social justice (Pardo, 1998).

Although each of these social justice movements differed somewhat in its emphasis (on class, Chicano identity, liberation theology), each offered opportunities for participants to develop organizing skills and a shared political consciousness that valued participation toward the goal of social justice or equality. Many of the women who became active in MELA had histories of working with one or more of these organizations and developed leadership skills as well as networks with other community activists through those experiences (Pardo, 1998).

Intersections of gender, race, and class shaped educational and employment opportunities as well as community activism. Opportunities for employment for Mexican American men in East Los Angeles were primarily in physically demanding positions (Pardo, 1998). Many women did not work outside the home, due to a combination of the poor quality of jobs available to women with their educational backgrounds, their desire to devote time to their families, and their partners' ability to earn sufficient income to support the households. While men often returned home following long and physically exhausting workdays, women's activities as church volunteers, as well as many of their histories in CSO, the Chicano movement, and UNO, provided organizing and fundraising skills that transferred readily to organizing around other community issues. Furthermore, at-home mothers were often the only community members available to attend daytime public hearings regarding land use and environmental issues (Rysavy, 1998).

In addition to the opportunities to participate in community organizing afforded by their gendered family, work, and community locations, MELA activists appealed directly to women as mothers. For example, Elsa Lopez, MELASI program director, described recruiting women, saying, "We ask them, 'Are you ready to defend and protect your family?'" (Rysavy, 1998).[5] Women also used maternal frames to influence policymakers, claiming the moral force that can be marshaled through the symbolism of motherhood and the protection of children and simultaneously defusing efforts to discredit them with stigmatizing portrayals of women activists. Even as they used their identities as mothers to promote their organizing efforts, women were acutely aware that their activism sometimes tested more traditional gender frameworks (Pardo, 1998). Thus, although they drew on frameworks of motherhood in their mobilizing efforts, women nonetheless engaged in critiques that challenged stereotypical gendered categories.

MELA activists also recognized that intersecting images of race, gender, and class contributed to the environmental health threats that they experienced. Film and media representations of East LA as a dangerous and deteriorated community with gangs of young Mexican American men fed negative and stereotyped images. Such representations rendered invisible the long-term residents who were working to stabilize the community and raise their children in it, and fostered outsiders' perceptions that there was little in the community worth protecting from, say, a prison or an incinerator (Pardo, 1998). The women of MELA recognized that these symbolic representations played an important role in shaping decisions that threatened the health of their communities, and worked skillfully to challenge portrayals of their community as graffiti-filled and gang-ridden. By posing counterimages of stable working-class families committed to education and community and by working with local policy makers to curtail film crews' continued production of negative imagery (Acuña, 1984; Pardo, 1998), MELA resisted the perpetuation of social inequalities that compromised the health of East LA residents.

TRANSFORMATION AND HEALTH

Thus, the women of MELA confronted local environmental threats imposed by racial and class inequalities. In their roles as workers, mothers, and residents, they developed organizing skills, became involved, and assumed leadership in collective efforts to promote healthful conditions in their community. In these efforts, women recognized the power of racialized and gendered representations in creating or reinforcing social inequalities, as well as their potential to promote social justice.

MELA's strategies both emerged from and sought to transform the racial, economic, and gendered inequalities that shaped their lives. Racial segregation, redlining, relocation, and removal to make way for freeway expansion; class, race, and gender discrimination in employment; and the gendered nature of child rearing in the latter part of the twentieth century influenced women's opportunities for community activism. Identities, political skills, and analyses of class, race, and gender inequalities were further shaped by the interplay of community mobilizations and broader social movements of the 1950s and beyond. Acting on the basis of those identities and analyses, women within MELA influenced both the life conditions and symbolic representations of their communities to promote health.

PROMOTING EQUITY IN HEALTH: POTENTIALS AND LIMITATIONS OF INTERSECTIONAL ANALYSES

How can the intersectional analyses illustrated in these case histories inform efforts to improve health and reduce health inequities? We identify several themes that illustrate both potentials and limitations of intersectional analyses in efforts to understand the underpinnings of health inequalities and develop effective strategies to promote greater equality.

RACE, CLASS, AND GENDER SHAPE MATERIAL CONDITIONS AND SYMBOLIC REPRESENTATIONS

By looking at the combined impact of class, race, and gender on health, scholars and activists can develop a more comprehensive understanding of the complex social processes that influence well-being. The case histories show how the social categories of class, race, and gender affect health through two linked pathways: the material conditions that structure opportunities for health and disease and the symbolic representations that influence consciousness, political mobilization, and policy. The cases also demonstrate the potential for intervention through these two pathways.

In the New York case, material conditions limited job and educational opportunities, pushed young men into the illegal economy, and put them at risk of substance abuse, HIV infection, violence, and incarceration. In East Los Angeles, these material conditions exposed families to toxic substances, reduced opportunities for income, and segregated Mexican Americans into resource-poor neighborhoods. In each community, through processes that unfolded locally, these living conditions worsened the health of community residents. Any investigation of these communities that used only a single lens of class, race, or gender would miss the powerful synergy of the three in creating the inequities in health that characterize America today.

The case histories also show how symbolic representations of class, race, and gender have real consequences for health. In New York City, media portrayals of young men of color contributed to policy decisions that redirected funds from schools to jails. Public perceptions of young men of color limited their access to social support from caring adults, increased their isolation, and sometimes made young men themselves feel they had to live up to these negative images. Together, these class, race, and gender perceptions reinforced and amplified the adverse health consequences of deteriorating living conditions.

In East Los Angeles, symbolic representations of the community reflected racialized, classed, and gendered images, such as gangs of dangerous young Mexican American men. These stereotypical images, promoted by the film industry, influenced outsiders' perceptions of the neighborhood and contributed to the political and economic disenfranchisement of the community. These in turn played a role in the loss of retail and other services within East Los Angeles and numerous efforts to locate noxious facilities in these neighborhoods.

THE TRANSFORMATIVE POWER OF INTERSECTIONAL ANALYSES

The case studies also show how expanding the scope of analysis from class, race, or gender alone, and from properties of individuals to concepts that illuminate social relationships, can create new opportunities for intervention. REAL MEN helps participants consider multiple identities—as partners, friends, fathers, family providers, and people responsible for their community and ethnic group. By exploring the contradictions within these identities and the discrepancy between young men's aspirations and their life circumstances, REAL MEN seeks to mobilize young men for personal and community transformation. Selecting release from jail as the point of intervention, REAL MEN moved beyond many more narrowly focused HIV/AIDS prevention efforts to help young men expand their limited educational and employment opportunities and cope more effectively with a hostile policy and economic environment that put them in the path of HIV infection and substance abuse. Postulating that prevalent conceptions of masculinity could amplify the risk in this environment, they sought to connect young men to organizations and individuals that could help them overcome barriers to school and work while engaging them in a critical structural examination of race and gender. By intervening at a critical point in the lives of young men whose health is actively threatened by the social context in which they exist, REAL MEN may help them better protect their own health and the health of their partners and communities.

The second case study also illustrates how a blended class, race, and gender analysis can reveal opportunities for intervention.

Throughout its twenty-year history, MELA effectively used community mobilization, social protest, and conflict strategies to contest decisions about the siting of a variety of environmental health hazards in their communities. These decisions reflected broader economic and political inequalities, and by focusing on social justice for women, low-income communities, and Mexican Americans, as well as on health, MELA was able to mobilize wider constituencies than may have been possible with an appeal to any single category. As in REAL MEN, the personal experiences of oppression, dislocation, and injustice sparked resistance and proactive engagement in the community. In MELA, these shared experiences contributed to a sense of collective identity, critical analysis of socially structured inequalities, and the development of effective community mobilization skills. Women's location within the community as housewives, activists, mothers, and church volunteers provided an additional pillar for sustained local mobilization.

Working with existing political structures, as well as through informal networks, MELA resisted and sought to transform images of their communities as part of a larger struggle to challenge the perpetuation of inequalities. At a more personal level, they also effectively used the legitimacy attached to social roles as mothers concerned with family and community to sustain their efforts for change, while at the same time critiquing and expanding those frameworks through their activism.

NEW ACTORS AND NEW SETTINGS FOR ACTION

Another benefit of examining the multiple pathways that contribute to ill health and disparities in health is that such analyses can bring new actors into change efforts and identify additional settings for intervention activities. Among the actors involved in both case studies are individuals and their families, health professionals, community organizations, social movement members, and public officials. Settings for action include institutions like jails, schools, and service providers; mass and community media; public spaces such as streets; and government events like public hearings or court cases.

In both REAL MEN and MELA, the intervention instigators framed the problem in such a way that actors could enter the activities through multiple routes: as individuals concerned about their own or their families' health, as activists wanting to fight injustice or improve their neighborhood, or as service providers wanting to do their jobs better, for example. By defining the initial problem as one that affected individuals and families in their class, gender, and racial categories and by addressing both health and social justice, the planners invited people to decide for themselves the mix of motivations that would move them to action. This approach contrasts sharply with many traditional public health programs that use health professionals' definition of a specific disease or risk behavior as the starting point for intervention.

In East Los Angeles, social movements were a dominant presence in MELA's activities. The Chicano, community justice, environmental, women's, and prisoners' rights movements all contributed to specific actions and provided opportunities for integration with campaigns on other community issues as well as integration with regional and national efforts. In REAL MEN, the civil rights, educational equity, and prison reform movements were part of the context, raising public awareness of the social justice issues and serving as visible role models for young men in jail. Despite these differences, social movements played a key role in both cases. They focused attention on the underlying class, race, and gender inequalities; linked limited local efforts to broader regional and national mobilizations; inspired hope; and forced public officials to consider the consequences of inaction. In MELA, the social movements provided concrete support for many activities, while in REAL MEN, they provided a more symbolic representation of an alternative to a future of oppression.

FROM ANALYSIS TO ACTION: THE LIMITS OF LOCAL INTERVENTIONS

While the case studies illustrate the potential for intersectional analyses to inform local intervention efforts, they also illuminate the limits of these efforts. As we have noted, inequalities in health reflect underlying social structures that have long sorted people by class, race, and gender and exposed them to unequal living conditions and social environments that amplify disease for those lacking in political power. Obviously, no single health intervention or political action can reverse generations or a lifetime of exposure to health-damaging forces. In different ways, both MELA and REAL MEN are relatively modest interventions and can expect only modest impact. REAL MEN, for example, does not by itself seek to transform the structured social inequalities that affect health. But fortunately, REAL MEN does not exist in a vacuum. Ongoing social mobilizations in New York City seek to change punitive drug laws, modify jail reentry practices, and shift public resources from incarceration back to education. At a minimum, programs like REAL MEN offer some young men tools and options that they can use to improve their chances for survival and perhaps ultimately to contribute to the broader changes necessary for health equity. Similarly, MELA has not directly addressed racially motivated residential segregation, unequal employment opportunities, punitive immigration policies, or the underfunding of public education—all factors that maintain inequality and produce ill health. But it has mobilized thousands of people for action, activated neighborhoods, and blocked several health-damaging facilities. Like UNO, the Chicano movement, and the CSOs that preceded the emergence of MELA, it also laid the groundwork for future mobilizations with the potential for broader change.

By comparing the outcomes of interventions like REAL MEN and MELA to those of other more limited public health programs and to our larger vision of health and social justice for all, we can set limited, achievable goals that also embody optimism about the future. Finally, by linking health and social justice and by tackling the full range of oppression and potential for transformation embodied in class, race, and gender, activists and scholars can help to create new opportunities for improving well-being and reducing inequalities in health.

Notes

1. Jails incarcerate those detained but not convicted, those convicted and sentenced to less than a year, and some parole violators. Prisons house people convicted and sentenced to more than a year. Juvenile detention facilities lock up those defined as juveniles, often for offenses that would not be considered criminal if they were of the age of majority. In New York State, those under age sixteen are classified as juveniles. REAL MEN serves only adolescents incarcerated in jails.
2. The titles of the group sessions are: "Staying Free, Staying Healthy," "Being a Man in Today's World," "Sex in the Risk Zone," "My People,

My Pride/Mi Gente, Mi Orgullo," "Drugs in Your Life," and "Getting the Information You Need to Stay Free and Healthy."

3. We thank Mary Pardo for her permission to draw on material from Pardo (1998) for the case study of Mothers of East Los Angeles.

4. Racial covenants limit the use of property to members of a specified race or forbid the sale of property to nonwhites. Covenants were often included in property titles from the period following the Civil War to 1948, when the U.S. Supreme Court ruled them unconstitutional (Ramos, 2001).

5. Mothers of East Los Angeles–San Isabel spun off from the original MELA.

References

Acuña, R. F. *Community Under Siege: A Chronicle of Chicanos East of the Los Angeles River.* Los Angeles: Chicano Studies Research Center, University of California, 1984.

Almaguer, T. *Racial Fault Lines: The Historical Origins of White Supremacy in California.* Berkeley: University of California Press, 1994.

Aronson, R. E., Whitehead, T. L., and Baber, W. L. "Challenges to Masculine Transformation Among Urban Low-Income African American Males." *American Journal of Public Health,* 2003, *93,* 732–741.

Ayers, R., Ayers, W., Dorhn, B., and Jackson, J. (eds.). *Zero Tolerance: Resisting the Drive for Punishment.* New York: New Press, 2001.

Belgrave, F. Z. "Relational Theory and Cultural Enhancement Interventions for African American Adolescent Girls." *Public Health Reports,* 2002, *117*(suppl. 1), S76–S81.

Brook, J. S., and others. "Drug Use Among African Americans: Ethnic Identity as a Protective Factor." *Psychology Reports,* 1998, *83*(3 pt. 2), 1427–1446.

Brown, P., and others. "Embodied Health Movements: New Approaches to Social Movements in Health." *Sociology of Health and Illness,* 2004, *26*(1), 50–80.

Brugge, D., and Goble, R. "History of Uranium Mining and the Navajo People." *American Journal of Public Health,* 2002, *92*(9), 1410–1418.

Buck, P. D. *Worked to the Bone: Race, Class, Power and Privilege in Kentucky.* New York: Monthly Review Press, 2001.

Bullard, R. *Dumping in Dixie: Race, Class and Environmental Equality.* Boulder, Colo.: Westview, 2000.

Camacho, D. E., and Cuesta-Camacho, D. E. (eds.). *Environmental Injustices, Political Struggles: Race, Class, and the Environment.* Durham, N.C.: Duke University Press, 1998.

"Campaign for Fiscal Equity." June 25, 2004. http://www.cfequity.org/nshome.htm.

Canada, G. *Reaching Up for Manhood: Transforming the Lives of Boys in America.* Boston: Beacon Press, 1998.

Collins, P. Hill. *Black Feminist Thought: Knowledge, Consciousness and the Politics of Empowerment.* Boston: Unwin Hyman, 1990.

Combahee River Collective. "The Combahee River Collective Statement." In B. Smith (ed.), *Home Girls: A Black Feminist Anthology.* New York: Kitchen Table Women of Color Press, 1983.

Correctional Association of New York. "New York State of Mind? Higher Education vs. Prison Funding in the Empire State, 1988–1998." June 25, 2004. http://www.cjcj.org/pubs/ny/nysompr.html.

Daniels, J. *White Lies: Race, Class, Gender and Sexuality in White Supremacist Discourse.* New York: Routledge, 1997.

DiClemente, R. J., and others. "Efficacy of an HIV Prevention Intervention for African American Adolescent Girls: A Randomized Controlled Trial." *Journal of the American Medical Association,* 2004, *292,* 171–179.

"Drop the Rock." June 25, 2004. http://www.droptherock.org/.

Escobedo, R. *Boyle Heights Community Plan.* Los Angeles: Department of City Planning, 1979.

Ferber, A. L. *White Man Falling: Race, Gender and White Supremacy.* Lanham, Md.: Rowman & Littlefield, 1998.

Freudenberg, N. "Jails, Prisons and the Health of Urban Populations: Review of the Impact of the Correctional System on Community Health." *Journal of Urban Health,* 2001, *78,* 214–240.

Freudenberg, N. "Community Capacity for Environmental Health Promotion: Determinants and Implications for Practice." *Health Education and Behavior,* 2004, *31*(4), 472–490.

García, J., "Forjando Ciudad: The Development of a Chicano Political Community in East Los Angeles." Unpublished doctoral dissertation, University of California, Riverside, 1986.

George, N. *Hiphopamerica.* New York: Viking, 1998.

Gootman, E. "City Creates New Paths to a Diploma." *New York Times,* May 29, 2004, p. B1.

Harvey, A. R., and Hill, R. B. "Africentric Youth and Family Rites of Passage Program: Promoting Resilience Among At-Risk African American Youth." *Social Work,* 2004, *49*(1), 65–74.

Hernandez, P. "Lives of Chicana Activists: The Chicano Student Movement in the United States." In M. Mora and A. R. Del Castillo (eds.), *Mexican Women in the United States.* Los Angeles: Chicano Studies Research Center, University of California, 1980.

House, J. S., and Williams, D. R. "Understanding and Reducing Socioeconomic and Racial/Ethnic Disparities in Health." In B. D. Smedley and S. L. Syme (eds.), *Promoting Health: Intervention Strategies from Social and Behavioral Research*. Washington D.C.: National Academy Press, 2000.

Jacobson, M. "From the 'Back' to the 'Front': The Changing Character of Punishment in New York City." In J. Mollenkopk and K. Emerson (eds.), *Rethinking the Urban Agenda: Reinvigorating the Liberal Tradition in New York City and Urban America*. New York: Century Foundation Press, 2001.

Johnson, R. L. "The Relationships Among Racial Identity, Self Esteem, Sociodemographics, and Health Promoting Lifestyles." *Research and Theory for Nursing Practice*, 2002, *16*(3), 193–207.

Johnston, H., Larana, E., and Gusfield, J. R., Jr. (eds.). *New Social Movements: From Ideology to Identity*. Philadelphia: Temple University Press, 1994.

LeBlanc, A. *Random Families: Love Drugs, Trouble and Coming of Age in the Bronx*. New York: Scribner, 2003.

Levitan, M. *A Crisis of Black Male Employment, Unemployment and Joblessness in New York City*. New York: Community Service Society, 2003.

Link, B. G., and Phelan, J. "Social Conditions as Fundamental Causes of Disease." *Journal of Health and Social Behavior*, 1995, *36*(extra issue), 80–94.

Maantay, J. "Zoning, Equity, and Public Health." *American Journal of Public Health*, 2001, 91, 1033–1041.

Males, M. *The Scapegoat Generation: America's War on Adolescents*. Monroe, Me.: Common Courage Press, 1996.

Malow, R. M., and others. "Psychosocial Predictors of HIV Risk Among Adolescent Offenders Who Abuse Drugs." *Psychiatric Services*, 1997, *48*, 185–187.

Marin, M. V. *Social Protest in an Urban Barrio: A Study of the Chicano Movement, 1966–1974*. New York: University Press of America, 1991.

Miller, J. *Search and Destroy: African American Males in the Criminal Justice System*. Cambridge: Cambridge University Press, 1996.

Muñoz, C. *Youth, Identity, Power: The Chicano Movement*. London: Verso Press, 1989.

New York State Division of Criminal Justice Services. 2004. www.criminal justice.state.ny.us/crimenet/ojsa/cjdata.htm.

Omi, M., and Winant, H. *Racial Formation in the United States: From the 1960s to the 1990s*. (2nd ed.) New York: Routledge, 1994.

Ortiz, I. D. "Chicano Urban Politics and the Politics of Reform in the Seventies." *Western Political Quarterly*, 1984, *37*(4), 565–577.

Pardo, M. S. *Mexican American Women as Activists: Identity and Resistance in Two Los Angeles Communities*. Philadelphia: Temple University Press, 1998.

Ramos, C. "The Educational Legacy of Racially Restrictive Covenants: Their Long Term Impact on Mexican Americans." *4 Scholar: St. Mary's Law Review on Minority Issues,* 2001, pp. 149–184.

Romo, R. *East Los Angeles: History of a Barrio.* Austin: University of Texas Press, 1983.

Rose, M. "Gender and Civic Activism in Mexican American Barrios in California: The Community Service Organization 1947–1962." In J. Meyerowitz (ed.), *Not June Cleaver: Women and Gender in Postwar America.* Philadelphia: Temple University Press, 1994.

Rysavy, T. "Mothers for Eco-Justice." 1998. http://www.yesmagazine.com/6RxforEarth/rysavy.htm.

Shepherd, P., Northridge, M. E., Prakash, S., and Stover, G. N. "Advancing Environmental Justice through Community Based Participatory Research. "*Environmental Health Perspectives,* 2002, *10*(suppl. 2), 139–140.

Staton, M., and others. "Risky Sex Behavior and Substance Use Among Young Adults." *Health and Social Work,* 1999, *24,* 147–154.

Stiffman, A. R., Dore, P., Cunningham, R. M., and Earls, F. "Person and Environment in HIV Risk Behavior Change Between Adolescence and Early Adulthood." *Health Education and Behavior,* 1995, *22,* 211–226.

Stockdill, B. C. *Activism Against AIDS: At the Intersections of Equality, Race, Gender and Class.* Boulder, Colo.: Lynne Rienner, 2003.

Stoler, A. L. *Race and the Education of Desire: Foucault's History of Sexuality and the Colonial Order of Things.* Durham, N.C.: Duke University Press, 1995.

Sugrue, T. J. *The Origins of the Urban Crisis: Race and Inequality in Postwar Detroit.* Princeton, N.J.: Princeton University Press, 1996.

Taylor, D. "The Influence of Race, Class and Gender on Activism and the Development of Environmental Discourses." Seattle, Wash.: U.S. Forest Service, 2002. http://www.fs.fed.us/pnw/pubs/gtr534.pdf.

Wilson, W. J. *The Truly Disadvantaged: The Inner City, the Underclass and Public Policy.* Chicago: University of Chicago Press, 1987.

CHAPTER FOURTEEN

MOVEMENT-GROUNDED THEORY

Intersectional Analysis of Health Inequities in the United States

Sandi Morgen

Throughout the twentieth century, grassroots activists from a variety of social movements, including civil rights, women's, and labor movements, challenged injustices in the U.S. health care system. These activists drew on and contributed to a critical analysis of the health care system, recognizing and challenging the complex ways that racism, sexism, homophobia, and class inequalities together helped to produce differential health status as well as unequal access to and treatment in the health care system. By the 1990s, racial, ethnic, and gender inequities in health were officially recognized by influential health policymakers, including major federal agencies responsible for health policy.

In this chapter, I have two related aims. First, I examine the important, but neglected, role that grassroots activists played in promoting attention to health disparities. I argue that movement-grounded theory helped elaborate an intersectional analysis of health inequalities. The mainstream health policy discussion of health "disparities," while catalyzed by scholars and activists who use intersectional theory, works almost exclusively within the positivist biomedical paradigm. In the final section of the chapter I compare two recent health policy reports on racial/ethnic health disparities that illuminate differences between intersectional and positivist biomedical paradigms. I suggest that concerted action is necessary to remedy unequal health and health care by race, gender, and class and that health policymakers will be most effective if they recognize the value of research from these different approaches.

This chapter is based on over two decades of research on the women's health movement, which played an important role in developing intersectional analyses of women's health.[1] My research began in the late 1970s, when I conducted two years of fieldwork in a women's health clinic in the northeastern United States. I then returned to research on the movement in the 1990s. I interviewed forty-five women's health activists from more than twenty-five national and regional advocacy organizations and women's clinics; conducted a survey of clinics and advocacy organizations in 1990; and pored over archival materials from and about the movement. In addition, to examine the differences between the positivist biomedical and intersectional analyses of health disparities, I compared two recent reports on racial disparities in health care, one published by the Institute of Medicine and the other by the National Black Women's Health Project (NBWHP) in collaboration with the Congressional Black Caucus Health Brain Trust and the U.S. Senate Black Legislative Staff Caucus.

WOMEN'S HEALTH MOVEMENT IN THE UNITED STATES

The women's health movement emerged in the late 1960s in a context that spawned movements of women, African Americans, Latinos, Native Americans, gays and lesbians, and others. Groups of women across the country organized to reclaim control over their bodies, reproductive lives, and health care. Their activities, political strategies, and organizations were diverse. Some focused on producing information about women's bodies and health care, seeking to empower women as health consumers. An example is the influential book *Our Bodies, Ourselves,* which provided accessible health information based on medical research and women's own experiences of their bodies and health care (Boston Women's Health Book Collective, 1973, 1984).

Other activists organized women-controlled health clinics or informational and referral services (Morgen, 2002). Clinics generally provided women's reproductive health care, often including abortion, family planning, routine gynecology, and sometimes alternative birthing services. They constituted alternative models of health care delivery and organizational bases from which activists worked to change mainstream medical care. Advocacy groups formed to challenge national, state, and local health policy. They took aim at a host of issues, exposing the dangers, for example, of oral contraceptives (Seaman, 1969), diethylstilbestrol, and intrauterine devices, each of which had been found to cause serious iatrogenic health problems. They criticized pharmaceutical companies for prioritizing profits over women's health and health regulatory agencies (such as the Food and Drug Administration) for failing to protect women from poorly tested drugs and medical devices or testing without securing informed consent (Corea, 1977; Dreifus, 1977). On issues ranging from the illegality (and then inaccessibility) of abortion, to concerns about contraception, medical school admission practices, and the virtual epidemic of unnecessary hysterectomies and one-step mastectomies, to a widespread exclusion of women health care consumers from health policy decision making, health movement activists wrote books and articles, held press conferences, staged demonstrations, conducted and disseminated their own research, and founded organizations to monitor and influence national health policy.

While a comprehensive examination of the movement is beyond the reach of this chapter, it was (and is) national in scope and has had a significant impact on women's health care and on health policy (Fried, 1990; Morgen, 2002; Norsigian, 1994; Ruzek, 1978; Silliman, Fried, Ross, and Gutierrez, 2004; Weisman, 1998). While many organizations did not survive the extensive backlash from the New Right, the antiabortion movement, and the policies of the Reagan and Bush administrations in the 1980s, others did, and they successfully helped to change women's health care in important ways. In addition to providing alternative services and promoting health advocacy and activism, the movement developed political analyses of gender inequality in the health care system; mistreatment of women by physicians and other health care providers and health care institutions; the overmedicalization of women's lives and the subjugation of women by the predominantly white, male medical establishment; the exclusion of women and people of color from powerful positions in health care delivery and policy; the use of women, the poor, and communities of color for medical experimentation and training without their effective consent; the failure of the health care system to address the most basic causes of poor health, especially among the poor; and the ways the market-based health care delivery and research institutions prioritized profits for doctors, pharmaceutical companies, hospitals, and others over the needs of women.

From the movement's earliest days, some women of color argued, in print and in organizational contexts, that the health issues affecting women of color and poor women necessitated an analysis that differed from what was being articulated by the predominantly white movement's analysis of gender and sexism. Racism and economic inequality, they argued, also created significant obstacles to reproductive rights and access to high-quality health (Cade, 1970; Combahee River Collective, 1983; Davis, 1990; Smith, 1995; White, 1990). Intersectional analyses of women's health were nurtured primarily in the work of women of color who explored gender as it intersected with race, ethnicity, class, and sexuality.

For example, Frances Beale, a founding member of the Student Nonviolent Coordinating Committee's Black Women's Liberation Committee, wrote an important article arguing that women of color faced "double jeopardy" as a result of being black and female (1970). Arguing that capitalism, sexism, and racism together affected the health of women of color, she pointed to the disproportionate number of women of color who had been sterilized, often without their knowledge or informed consent. Beale criticized both the eugenicist actions of the health care system and the predominantly white women's health movement for failing to include sterilization abuse alongside abortion in the reproductive rights movement.

Women in the Puerto Rican nationalist group The Young Lords Party also developed a more inclusive reproductive rights analysis than was then extant in the movement, calling for access to voluntary birth control and safe and affordable abortions; reform of the public health care system to increase access and quality of primary health care for the poor; free day care; and an end to poverty (Nelson, 2001). Historian Jennifer Nelson credits the organization for developing an intersectional analysis in the early

1970s, long before their colleagues in most other racial justice or women's organizations did: "While many early-1970s New Left politicos singularly identified with racial oppression, gender oppression, or oppression by sexual identity, YLP women were able to construct a politics that took into account race, class and gender oppression. An inclusive reproductive rights agenda that addressed the needs of women of different identity positions was the result" (Nelson, 2001, p. 175).

These are two examples of early insights about the importance of understanding the specificities, differences, convergences, and other interrelationships among gender, race, ethnicity, class, and sexuality. While the language of movement publications may have differed somewhat from the language found in academic publications, it is important to recognize the fundamentally similar assumptions and insights between these earlier movement-grounded and current iterations of feminist intersectional analysis. Theory is often a complex coproduction by various social actors, including, in this case, academics, health practitioners and researchers, and social movement activists, all of whom seek understanding from their different vantage points and for different reasons. Nevertheless, activists rarely get credit for their roles in the development of theory, especially in fields dominated by scientific discourses.

Intersectional theory argues that gender, race, ethnicity, sexuality, and class are mutually constitutive; that they intersect in the lived experiences of those who occupy and negotiate different social locations in systems of power in the health care system and in the larger society; and that health inequalities are produced by racism, gender inequality, and class relations (for example, Anzaldua, 1990; Bair and Cayleff, 1993; Collins, 1990; Davis, 1990; Dill, 1983; Moraga and Anzaldua, 1981; Roberts, 1997; White, 1990). While intersectional analysis was developed not only by activists of color, they were the leading proponents of theory and organizational practices that recognized how racism, gender inequality, and class together shaped health outcomes, the salience of particular health issues, and the failure of the health care system to meet the particular health needs of women, communities of color, and the poor and the uninsured.

In the late 1970s and the 1980s, several critical issues underscored the value of emerging intersectional frameworks, including the campaign against sterilization abuse; congressional passage of the Hyde Amendment in 1976, effectively limiting poor women's access to abortion; and the AIDS crisis. I will discuss the first two of these briefly to suggest the critical role that activists played in developing the intersectionality framework. In the mid-1970s, the Committee to End Sterilization Abuse (CESA) was formed under the able leadership of Helen Rodriguez-Trias, a Puerto Rican physician in New York City. CESA sought to expose and curb hospital practices that led to disproportionately high rates of sterilization of women of color (Shapiro, 1985). CESA attributed these rates (as high as one-third of Puerto Rican and at least 25 percent of Native American women of childbearing age) to unjust and discriminatory health care practices that resulted in procedures being performed on women without their informed consent (Rodriguez-Trias, 1978).

After an intensive organizing campaign, CESA succeeded in forcing New York City to develop guidelines regulating sterilization in city hospitals. In 1979, it got the U.S. Department of Health, Education and Welfare to issue national guidelines requiring hospitals to secure informed consent in the language of the patient, with clear information about the operation's irreversibility and alternative birth control methods. This issue divided feminists: some predominantly white women's health organizations failed to support the campaign vigorously, and others opposed it, believing the guidelines would reduce access for white middle-class women, who often faced considerable difficulty getting physicians to sterilize them (Roberts, 1997).

Understanding sterilization abuse as a product of racist eugenic policies, disregard for women's right to control their reproductive lives, the reliance of poor women on public teaching hospitals or the Indian Health Service, and the exclusion of women, especially poor women, from health policy decision making did more than provide a strong foundation for the political campaign to reform sterilization policies. It also foreshadowed an analysis of women's health and reproductive rights that grew from the embodied experiences of poor women of color. Decentering the perspectives and needs of white middle-class women fostered a broader understanding of what reproductive freedom and health encompassed. In this way, the needs and perspectives of women who are marginalized because of racism and class inequality were foregrounded, creating the potential for a more inclusive social movement with a sharper, more comprehensive theoretical understanding of reproductive rights and health.

The Hyde Amendment, which Congress passed in 1976 to halt the use of federal Medicaid dollars to pay for abortion, was one of a series of restrictions on abortion that the antiabortion movement won in the courts and legislatures in the years following *Roe* v. *Wade* (1973). While some predominantly white feminist clinics and advocacy groups joined the unsuccessful campaign to overturn the Hyde Amendment, the response of the larger movement was "too little, too late," from the perspective of women of color within and outside the movement (Roberts, 1997). Women of color activists inside and outside the movement developed an analysis that went beyond the discourse of "rights" to show how capitalist social relations effectively prevent the poor from exercising fundamental rights (Davis, 1981; Roberts, 1997).

Given the emerging conflicts and divisions over race and class in the movement, a growing discourse on racism within the women's health movement, and a resulting effort to create more diverse organizations (by race, class, and sexuality), some local and national groups attempted to change the practices and political visions responsible for the hegemony of "white feminism" in women's health movement organizations (Morgen, 2002). And these political differences set the stage for a process that, beginning in the early 1980s, led to the formation of a number of independent women of color health organizations.[2] Some of the women who founded these new organizations had been involved in the predominantly white middle-class health movement organizations, but many had not. Their visions of a health agenda for poor women and women of color were nourished from multiple root stalks, including feminist health and reproductive rights, civil rights, community health, welfare rights and racial identity movements, and from their own experiences as health consumers and providers (Ross, 1998).

For example, Byllye Avery, an African American woman who founded the National Black Women's Health Project (NBWHP) in 1984, had been a cofounder of a feminist health clinic and a feminist birth center in Gainesville, Florida, in the 1970s. As a board member of the National Women's Health Network, Avery (1982) initiated a project on black women's health. She developed a network of African American women professionals, community women, and students to work for change in health care for black women; pursued research about African American women's health; organized self-help groups in communities across the country to provide a forum for discussion and mutual assistance for black women; and organized a national conference on black women's health that was held at Spelman College in 1983. The conference led to the founding of the NBWHP in 1984.

The NBWHP differed from many sister women's health movement organizations in important ways (Gary-Smith, 1989). Based on Avery's research suggesting an alarmingly high incidence of heart and cardiovascular disease and depression in African American women, the NBWHP moved beyond the reproductive health emphasis prevalent in the larger movement to include work on chronic disease, pioneering innovative health prevention programs, and other self-help and educational activities (Morgen, 2002). They located a health clinic in a housing project in Atlanta, opened a health policy office in Washington, D.C., and fostered the development of other women of color health groups in the United States and the African Diaspora. The organization developed an analysis of health rooted in understandings about racism, sexism, and economic inequality, and that analysis expanded to specify the particular needs of lesbians, older women, the disabled, and women living in public housing (Villarosa, 1994).

The NBWHP also helped nurture the development of other women of color health organizations over the next decade. Luz Alvarez Martinez, one of four cofounders of the National Latina Health Organization (NLHO), had attended the 1983 conference on black women's health in Atlanta and returned dedicated to founding a similar organization for Latinas. That dream became reality in 1986 in Oakland, California. In addition to health education and health services and participation in health advocacy, the NLHO offered bilingual and Spanish-language programs and services, identified and worked to serve the specific needs of immigrant, including undocumented, women, and mobilized their communities in support of a reproductive rights agenda inclusive of the needs and perspectives of Latinas.

Another women of color health organization, the Native American Women's Health Education Resource Center (NAWHERC), was founded by Charon Asetoyer (Comanche), who lived with her husband (Dakota Sioux) on his reservation. Their work began with informal conversations about the many health problems they and their families faced. Then a small group formed a nonprofit organization to develop education and health service programs to address the specific concerns of the women on the reservation. Their first project concerned fetal alcohol syndrome, a health issue that was not on the radar screen of most women's health organizations.

In 1988, NAWHERC opened its doors, the first women's health organization located on a reservation in the United States. Its activities have included community organizing and leadership development, a domestic violence project, AIDS prevention, child development, adult learning, assistance to groups working on toxic waste issues, cancer prevention, a food pantry and nutrition programs, scholarships for Native American women, and an information clearinghouse. NAWHERC helped to mobilize other Native American women around reproductive rights, with an agenda that drew on the particular histories, needs, and issues facing Native American women (Asetoyer, 1990, 1994). It also worked on research and advocacy projects reflecting their concern about the promotion of Norplant and Depo-Provera by the Indian Health Service, combining research and advocacy in an effort to influence federal health policy toward Native women.

In September 1993, the National Asian Women's Health Organization (NAWHO) was founded in Oakland, California. Acknowledging that the needs and concerns of Asian women are "at the same time specific and diverse, and that they must be addressed within community, cultural, and linguistic contexts," NAWHO conducts research, supports and provides health education and health services, and works to influence health policies that affect Asian women and families, including Asian Americans and Asian immigrants (National Asian Women's Health Organization, 1993–1994). They specifically related health to the "increasingly hostile developments in immigration, welfare and health policies [that] threaten to undermine the extent to which Asian American women and girls feel comfortable and safe in accessing and utilizing health education and services, particularly in the area of reproductive and sexual health" (National Asian Women's Health

Organization, 1995, p. 4). In addition to a number of high-profile policy-related conferences, NAWHO had worked closely with the Centers for Disease Control and Prevention to coordinate programs on diabetes, immunization, and tobacco control. In 1998, it organized a Women of Color Policy Briefing for media representatives, foundations, and advocates, taking its place among those groups sustaining linkages among women's health organizations and between these organizations, health professionals, and public policymakers.

By the early 1990s, the politics and landscape of the women's health movement had changed significantly, spurred largely by the work and analysis of these and other women of color health organizations. These groups provided the base from which women of color could offer services to women and families in their own racial and ethnic communities; challenge their marginalization in the U.S. women's health and reproductive rights movements; and represent the concerns of U.S. women of color nationally and at international conferences, such as the International Conference on Population and Development in 1994 and the United Nations conference in Beijing in 1995. Their work powerfully influenced the predominantly white women's health movement, which increasingly paid attention to organizational diversity and developing programs and services based on an intersectional understanding of women's health.

FOCUSING ON FEDERAL HEALTH POLICY AND HEALTH INEQUITIES

During the 1980s, women's health activism expanded beyond reproductive health, extending to breast cancer, AIDS, chronic disease, health financing, health insurance, and the politics and procedures of biomedical research (Batt, 1994; Norsigian, 1994; Ruzek, Olesen, and Clarke, 1997; Schneider and Stoller, 1995; Weisman, 1998). Many movement organizations, especially those representing women of color, became more inclusive and focused more on the unmet concerns of women of color and low-income women. These changes took place as the country was lurching politically to the right, resulting in a powerful backlash and decreased funding for the movement (Morgen, 2002).

Despite setbacks, the grassroots women's health movement, in coalition with "professionalized" women's health organizations (Ruzek and Becker, 1999), scored a series of victories that fostered changes in national health policy. These changes included the creation of offices for minority and women's health within some federal health agencies; changes in biomedical research protocols to require inclusion of women and minorities; some improvement in medical school admissions (especially for white women); increased funding for particular health problems affecting people of color and women; and growing attention by policymakers to what is now referred to as health "disparities" by gender and race.

In 1985, a major task force report criticized the U.S. Department of Health and Human Services (DHHS) for failing to respond adequately to women's health needs (U.S. Public Health Service, 1985). That year, the *Report of the Secretary's Task Force on Black and Minority Health,* published by DHHS, documented racial and ethnic "health disparities," measured by "disparate disease prevalence, progression and health outcomes, including excessively high mortality rates, for minorities from many conditions that affect all segments of the United States population" (Pinn, 1998, p. iii). In response to these reports and the political fallout that followed, the National Institutes of Health (NIH) developed a policy to foster the inclusion of women in clinic research and, some months later, in September 1987, a policy to foster the inclusion of racial minorities in clinical studies. But several years later the General Accounting Office (GAO) showed that there had been only limited changes in clinical trials. This led to more political pressure on Congress, ultimately resulting in passage of the Women's Health Equity Act establishing the NIH Office of Research on Women's Health in 1990. In 1991, Bernadine Healy, the first woman to head the NIH, announced the Women's Health Initiative, a major research initiative allocating hundreds of millions of dollars to research on breast cancer, cardiovascular disease, and osteoporosis.

While offices for minority and women's health were established in different federal health agencies, these were separate offices with distinct missions. Women of color were subsumed under the category of either "woman" or "minority," a move that intersectionality scholars argue produces invisibility and marginalization.

A rare exception was the *Women of Color Health Data Book: Adolescents to Seniors* (Leigh and Lindquist, 1998), published by the Office of Research on Women's Health in the Office of the Director of the NIH. In 1998, Surgeon General David Satcher announced the Initiative to Eliminate Racial and Ethnic Disparities in Health, and, in 1999, Congress commissioned a study on racial and ethnic disparities in health from the prestigious Institute of Medicine. These developments amplified attention to racial and ethnic disparities in health and health care both within the federal health bureaucracy and outside it, including research, symposia, conferences, and publications by public health and other researchers.

In the early 1990s, health care reform became a significant political issue, figuring prominently in Bill Clinton's 1992 presidential campaign. Feminist health organizations were among the more than one hundred organizations that formed the Campaign for Women's Health, with the goal of "redress[ing] many of the inequities women have faced securing health care for themselves and their families" as part of the larger effort at health care reform (Campaign for Women's Health, 1993, p. 7). Despite the failure of health reform during the Clinton administration, the now more audible discourse about inequities in health policy did not fade. Both professionalized and grassroots women's health organizations stepped up their advocacy activities concerning federal health policy. The NBWHP took their message, that vast inequities characterize the health of African Americans compared to white Americans, to highly visible and influential forums, including a March 1993 forum at the Harvard School of Public Health. Organizations such as the National Women's Health Network, the National Black Women's Health Project, and the National Asian Women's Health Organization kept up the pressure on federal agencies and Congress to redress the inequalities in health and health care that continued to plague white women and men and women of color.

I have argued that grassroots women's health movement organizations were among the earliest and most vocal advocates of analyzing how inequitable power relations translate to poorer health outcomes for women, communities of color, the poor, and immigrants. The definition of the health issues facing women of color as inextricably linked to the operation of systems of power—of racism, sexism, and class inequalities, as well as homophobia—was developed, reiterated, and echoed by women of color health movement organizations and activists across the country and, increasingly, by other women's health movement organizations. Scholars and activists affiliated with the movement promoted a discourse and research about health inequities that recognized the importance of specifying the particular health needs of different groups of women (for example, by race, ethnicity, class, age, sexuality, and citizenship status) and analyzing convergences and differences in health status, access to treatment, health outcomes, and quality of health care enjoyed by these groups as rooted in racism, sexism, and economic polarization. Individually and collectively, women's health movement organizations played a key role in getting the issue of racial, ethnic, and gender disparities in health on the public policy table nationally.

COMPARING INTERSECTIONAL AND POSITIVIST BIOMEDICAL APPROACHES

For scholars and activists concerned about the relation between health and inequality, and specifically the intersection of racism, sexism, and class relations in shaping differential health status and access to health care, the relatively recent attention of federal health policymakers to "health disparities" represents an important policy victory. Federal health policy currently at least nominally recognizes the existence of racial and ethnic disparities in health and health care (Cain and Kington, 2003). For example, the Department of Health and Human Services's "Initiative to Eliminate Racial and Ethnic Disparities in Health" and the "Healthy People 2010 Initiative" identify the reduction of racial and ethnic disparities in health as a major goal. However, there are significant differences between the discourse and agenda of the federal initiatives concerning racial and ethnic health disparities and the needs of women of color as these have been understood and articulated by researchers and activists associated with the women's health movement, especially those whose work derives from intersectional theory and analysis.

In this section, I examine two recent reports on racial and ethnic disparities in health. The first is *Unequal Treatment: Confronting*

Racial and Ethnic Disparities in Health Care (Smedley, Stith, and Nelson, 2003), released by the Institute of Medicine in 2002 and published by the National Academy of Sciences in 2003. The second publication was prepared for the National Colloquium on Black Women's Health, an event and publication (2003) cosponsored by the NBWHP, the Congressional Black Caucus Health Brain Trust, and the U.S. Senate Black Legislative Staff Caucus (National Black Women's Health Project, 2003). I use these two documents to examine some key differences between intersectional analysis and the positivist biomedical scholarship that informs the vast majority of health research. Given the breadth of and differences within the literatures informed by each of these paradigms, my goal is to underscore epistemological, theoretical, and methodological differences that need to be understood and discussed if scholars who work within these different paradigms are to have more fruitful exchanges and collaborations.

Unequal Treatment was commissioned by the U.S. Congress in 1999. The Institute of Medicine (IOM) prepared the report using its standard process: the selection of a committee of experts to prepare the report with the assistance of IOM staff, the commissioning of background research papers by renowned experts in the field, and extensive review of the committee report to ensure that it "meets institutional standards for objectivity, evidence and responsiveness to the study charge" (Smedley, Stith, and Nelson, 2003, p. vii). The report is the most comprehensive treatment of racial and ethnic disparities in health care yet published by such a prestigious body. It is important to point out that the congressional charge to the committee was to "assess the extent of racial and ethnic differences in health care that *are not otherwise due to known factors such as access to care, e.g., ability to pay or insurance coverage*" (2003, p. 3, emphasis added). In effect, Congress took off the table the issue of differential access to health care, which is itself one determinant of disparities in health and often serves as a proxy for (and coexists with) larger socioeconomic processes, such as inequitable access to jobs, income and food security, health insurance, and decent housing. To be fair, the committee acknowledged that this was problematic: "To a great extent, attempts to separate the relative contribution of these factors [access and non-access-related] risks presenting an incomplete picture of the complex relationships between racial and ethnic minority status, socioeconomic differences, and discrimination in the United States. . . . The committee therefore stresses that attempts to 'parcel out' access-related factors from the quality of health care for minorities remains an artificial exercise, and that policy solutions must consider the historic and contemporary forces that contribute to differences in access to and quality of health care" (2003, pp. 34–35).

The report concluded that racial and ethnic disparities in health care exist and have serious health outcomes for communities of color. However, the report also illustrates that the ways these disparities are defined, conceptualized, and studied by mainstream health policy experts and researchers wedded to the positivist biomedical model often result in research and a policy discourse that are comparatively impoverished in their ability to understand causes and experiences of or solutions to health disparities. There are at least three significant problems with the positivist biomedical paradigm in the IOM report, each of which distinguishes this approach from an intersectional one: (1) the extraction of race/ethnicity from the complex matrix of power relations that characterize and shape inequality in the United States; (2) the reduction of structural/systemic inequalities to individual-level problems of bias, stereotyping, and discriminatory behavior; and (3) framing issues in a putatively objective, scientific manner that also tends to mute the urgency and mask the human costs of social injustice.

First, rather than analyzing the intersectional relations among race, ethnicity, gender, and class as these shape and are reflected in racial and ethnic disparities in health, the IOM report focused exclusively on race and ethnicity, extracting race/ethnicity from its enmeshment in a complex system of power and inequality and sidelining questions about gender and class differences within and between racial and ethnic groups. Indeed, neither gender nor class is used as an analytical category in presenting or discussing research findings or policy recommendations. Given that the report focuses on racial disparities, why do I believe this is a problem? Because people of color are not simply racialized beings. They are men and women, they vary in their economic and other circumstances, and their lives as people of color diverge along gender and class lines. The background scholarly papers published along with the committee report were more likely than the committee report, and the committee report was more likely than the executive summary, to pay attention to either the gender specificities of health disparities or how gender and class pattern disparities in health care.[3] This became clear from the content analysis of the report I conducted.

Using a keyword search of the document available on the Web version of the report, I searched each reference to gender, race, racism, ethnicity, and class mentioned in the report.[4] I found very little discussion of women, gender, or class in the twenty-seven-page executive summary, the most widely read part of the report. The majority of the thirteen hits concerning women or gender in the executive summary were merely words in bibliographical references. The results for the term *class* (or surrogates for class) are similar. The word appears once in the executive summary and about twenty other times in the committee report. But *class* is used much more often and analytically in the scholarly background papers (for example, thirteen times by Geiger, 2003; seventy-three times by Byrd and Clayton, 2003; fifty-five times by Cooper and Roter, 2003). A search for *socioeconomic* turns up many more hits; it is used ten times in the summary and twenty-eight times in the introduction and literature review, and is scattered throughout other sections. Notably, however, as with gender, the analysis of socioeconomic status or class was not a major theme of the report. Indeed, the most common references to socioeconomic status occur when the term is used to explain that a study controlled for socioeconomic class in order to establish a causal relationship between race/ethnicity and health disparities.

The committee defined as the best evidence of racial and ethnic disparities those differences that were significant when studies controlled for gender and class. Because racial and ethnic disparities were determined to be scientifically valid only once they were separated from their enmeshment in other social relations of power that also affect health status and health care, the committee, by definition, could not develop an intersectional analysis. Because positivist biomedical research operationalizes gender, race, ethnicity, and class as discrete variables and controls one or more of these in order to determine correlational or causal relationships, the definitions and practices of what is perceived to be rigorous "science" work against intersectional analyses. Moreover, as I have already indicated, some of the most compelling evidence for the existence of class inequalities in health care and the ways these are related to racial and ethnic disparities concerns differential access to health care. Yet the committee was compelled to define access as outside its charge, resulting in what they themselves defined as an "artificial exercise" that hampers real understanding.

The second problem with the IOM report concerns the way racial and ethnic disparities are conceptualized, not only in relation to gender or class but in relation to the dynamics of discrimination and racism. Given that this report self-consciously focuses on racial and ethnic disparities, the paucity of analysis of racism is particularly problematic. Once again the keyword search showed that the background scholarly papers were far more likely than the report or the executive summary to name racism as a cause of racial and ethnic health disparities. Of the only four references to the term *racism* in the executive summary, three are buried in the references cited. The term *racism* is found fewer than twenty other times in the 243 pages of the report's main text. This compares to the use of the concept eighteen times in Geiger's background research article (2003), sixty-two times in the background paper by Byrd and Clayton (2003), thirty-one times in an article on the culture of medicine (DelVecchio Good, James, Good, and Becker, 2003), and a few times in the other research articles. Instead of the more systemic and dynamic analysis permitted by the concept "racism," the committee discusses discrimination, prejudice, and stereotypes, which appear fourteen, thirteen, and sixteen times, respectively, in the executive summary and hundreds of times after in the report.

It may not be surprising that the report avoids examining racial and ethnic disparities in the context of racism or the intersecting systems that position women of color at the bottom of the socioeconomic order given the nature of mainstream health policy discourse. Clearly the committee understood and even occasionally acknowledged racism: "Racial and ethnic disparities in health care emerge from an historic context in which health care has been differentially allocated on the basis of social class, race and ethnicity. Unfortunately, despite public laws and sentiment to the contrary, vestiges of this history remain and negatively affect the current context of health care delivery. And despite the considerable economic, social and political progress of racial and ethnic minorities, evidence of racism and discrimination remain in many sectors of American life" (Smedley, Stith, and Nelson, 2003, p. 123).

But notice how mention of racism disappears when this argument is presented in the executive summary: "Racial and ethnic disparities in health care occur in the context of broader historic and contemporary social and economic inequality, and evidence of persistent racial and ethnic discrimination in many sectors of American life" (Smedley, Stith, and Nelson, 2003, pp. 6–7).

There are analytical and theoretical differences between examining racism and examining bias, discrimination, prejudice, or stereotyping. The former locates the problem deep within the structures, institutions, and practices of social, political, and economic institutions; the latter locates the problem at the level of individual attitudes or in social interactions between providers and patients. Moreover, calling racism a "vestige" of the past that continues to inform the present differs from understanding racial oppression as a core aspect of our culture and economy.

Public health scholars Nancy Krieger (2003) and Sherman James (2003), among others, have recently argued that it is important to name racism as a health problem and as a cause of racial and ethnic disparities. James put it eloquently: "Because racism, operating through varied interpersonal and institutional pathways, is a fundamental cause of racial/ethnic health disparities, the elimination of these disparities—the magnificently democratic goal of Healthy People 2010—cannot be achieved without first undoing racism" (James, 2003, p. 198).

Clearly, if racism has to be undone before racial and ethnic disparities are eliminated, the report's recommendations should have been far more systemic and hard-hitting than they were.[5] Moreover, the failure to recognize that men and women of color experience the burdens of racism differently, and that poor women of color are among the most vulnerable and marginalized people in our society, means that the report not only fails to examine women of color as an analytical category but that the particular issues facing women of color are, for the most part, effaced.

The substitution of concepts such as discrimination, stereotyping, and bias for a structural analysis of racism has both epistemological and political sources. On the one hand, as Weber discusses eloquently (Chapter Two, this volume), the positivist biomedical model investigates race and ethnicity primarily as attributes of individuals and bias and discrimination as dimensions of behavior, focusing almost exclusively on empirical manifestations of these processes, something that is harder to do with a concept such as racism. Moreover, the validity of people's experiences or interpretations of racism, or even discrimination, is equivocated and, as below, defined merely as circumstantial evidence. In discussing focus groups filled with evidence of "health care inequity that participants attributed directly to racial or ethnic discrimination, their lack of English-language proficiency or both" (Grady and Edgar, 2003, p. 392), the authors concluded: "Overall participants felt that racial discrimination could not easily be separated from other forms of discrimination . . . the link between one's race or ethnicity and poor treatment can be very complex. While the underlying issues (e.g., economics, improper diagnosis) mentioned here parallel those discussed in an earlier section, the claims made in the following quotes only suggest that a lower quality of health care stems from racial or ethnic discrimination. The evidence for this causal relationship tends to be circumstantial" (p. 399).

Clearly it is important to understand the larger political and institutional contexts in which this report was prepared and disseminated. The IOM represents itself as committed to "objective, impartial evidence-based decision-making" (Berkowitz, 1998, p. iii). A recent history of the IOM argues that the past and current leadership of the institute endeavored to stay "independent of partisan politics" in order to promote their own legitimacy (Berkowitz, 1998, p. 258). But avoiding the appearance of partisanship is not the same as being uninfluenced by partisan politics, as Berkowitz shows in his history. In referring to the 1980s, he shows that after Reagan's election, the IOM reports shifted from an examination of "health care in the context of civil rights" to concern with "the growth of for-profit investment in health care" (p. 151).

While, for scholars who adopt a critical intersectional paradigm, racism is understood as a powerful analytical concept that recognizes systemic historical and contemporary power relations among racial groups, mainstream national politics often shuns attention to the language of racism. To introduce racism as a topic in policy circles in the current political climate is to evoke a series of tensions and meanings that those in power prefer to avoid. Getting issues of race on the table is facilitated by steering clear of a structural analysis of racism. However, there are high costs to this strategy, especially the reproduction of analyses of race and racism that remain mired in individual and behavioral rather than institutional and political-economic dynamics.

Finally, the tone of the IOM report is, like other IOM reports, objective, scientific, and dispassionate. This is consistent with the norms for positivist research, which valorize detachment and objectivity as signals of scientific rigor. The closest example of any sense of urgency was when committee chair Alan Nelson called racial/ethnic disparities "unacceptable" and eschewed further debate, calling instead for action at a public briefing held in March 2002. The norms of scientific discourse highly value language that sounds objective, that is, language that grants authority to the writer or speaker because of a presumption of professional distance and the absence of bias. While there is nothing wrong with this language, it does tend to sacrifice a sense of urgency to the requirements of dispassionate science.

In April 2003, one year after the IOM report was released, the NBWHP held the day-long National Colloquium on Black Women's Health in Washington, D.C., in collaboration with the Congressional Black Caucus Health Brain Trust and the U.S. Senate Black Legislative Staff Caucus. The background papers prepared for the conference were published as a report by the same name (National Black Women's Health Project, 2003). The program was organized "to explore issues impacting the unequal burdens in health, health care access and quality of care borne by African American women; to facilitate dialogues and public policy recommendations relative to those issues toward the elimination of racial and gender health disparities among African American women; and to generate a national sense of urgency to address the unequal burden of health issues borne by African American women" (p. 8). Conference speakers used the language of racial and ethnic disparities, but they articulated these issues quite differently from the IOM report, often drawing on and developing an intersectional analysis.

The examination of "unequal burdens in health, health care access and quality of care borne by African American women" (NBWHP, 2003, p. 22) refocuses the analysis to underscore the human effects of inequality, the experience of injustice. Both speakers and authors of the background research papers drew liberally on the embodied experiences of actual women, showing how the intersection of racism, sexism, and class inequalities shapes health outcomes. Unlike the scientific, bureaucratic discourse prevalent in the IOM report, the papers in the NBWHP publication move from the empirical evidence of health disparities to an analysis of how racial disparities are produced by the intertwined dynamics of racism, sexism, and the commodification and stratification of health in capitalist societies. This difference in discourse and analysis is not explained by the professional standing of the authors; they are all researchers with excellent academic credentials and expertise, including a medical writer–research fellow at Harvard Medical School, a professor at Northwestern School of Law, a senior research associate at the Joint Center for Political and Economic Studies, a board-certified internist who has also been a senior program officer at the Commonwealth Fund, a law professor at American University who has also worked at the National Women's Law Center, and a specialist in tobacco prevention and control and maternal and child health and youth services. Rather, intersectional scholarship does not eschew either structural analysis or political conclusions to empirical reality.

Like the IOM report, the colloquium provided strong evidence of ethnic and racial disparities in health status; the existence of discriminatory attitudes and practices by health care providers, including but not limited to physicians; the consequences of de facto segregated sources of health care; and barriers to communication and understanding across racial and ethnic borders. But these are all examined using an analytical framework that recognizes that black women's health experiences are shaped by the multiple realities of race, gender, and class as experienced in their lives as members of families and communities, as workers, health consumers, and the targets of multiple social policies. And, pointedly, black women are the focus of the analysis.

For example, Dr. Marsha Lillie-Blanton, vice president of the Kaiser Family Foundation, argued that health inequalities are part of the "larger and often longstanding inequities linked to race, to income, and in our case, to gender" (NBWHP, 2003, p. 34).[6] Dr. Maya Rockeymoore, a senior resident scholar for health and income security at the National Urban League Institute for Opportunity and Equality, defined health disparities as evidence that "there is a war being waged against African-American women and our families. It can also be interpreted as a war against poor, working class and middle class families" (p. 66). She argued that the unequal health burden borne by black women has its sources in a host of converging social policies that have effectively reduced the economic, health, and social safety net in this society, including changes in welfare, food stamps, and Supplemental Security Income, issues that are not (or rarely) addressed in the IOM report because access issues were disregarded. What distinguished these presentations from the IOM report was the way they used evidence from the scholarly literatures on health disparities—their own and other research from both the positivist biomedical and intersectionality literatures—to recognize the structural relationship between inequality and differential health and access to health care for African American women and their families. Their papers suggest that it is possible to work within the biomedical paradigm and analyze power, structural inequality, and racism.

Speaker after speaker presented evidence about the consequences of inequitable access to affordable, high-quality health care. For example, Dr. Wilhelmina Leigh showed how gender, race, and class intersect in shaping access to health care on a number of levels: differential rates of insurance coverage, how different types of health insurance shape quality of care, and how changes in public assistance have undermined both coverage and satisfaction with coverage in the era of Medicaid managed care. While Leigh argued that understanding racial and ethnic health disparities for women of color requires the examination of gender, race, ethnicity, and class together, she also recognized that it is difficult to do this precisely because much available data examines "differences separately by either race/ethnicity or by gender, but not by race/ethnicity and gender jointly" (NBWHP, 2003, p. 77). Her concern about how health data are collected and reported was echoed by Dora Hughes, M.D. and M.P.H., who argued that "the paucity of studies reporting data separately for African-American women makes it difficult to assess the true scope and magnitude of problems in health care quality" (p. 128).

Dr. Harriet Washington, author of the lead background paper, "Black Women and the Unequal Burden of Health Problems," concluded that the available empirical evidence leads not simply to a conclusion that there are racial and ethnic health disparities; she goes further, arguing that the evidence is of a "deep racial fissure" in American health care (NBWHP, 2003, p. 24). Washington went beyond the conventional discourse that labels inequities between whites and people of color as disparities, or a "health care gap"; she sees evidence of a "deep chasm separating African-Americans from the most advanced health care system in the world" (p. 24). Similarly, Dorothy Roberts examines black women's reproductive health in the context of a variety of social policies—eugenics, family planning, welfare "reform," and the differential opportunities dictated by types of (public versus private) or lack of access to health coverage—developing an analysis of gender, race, class, and religious tradition as converging determinants of black women's reproductive options and health care.

The final address was delivered by NBWHP founder Byllye Avery, who dispensed with the objective, technical language policymakers tend to use, urging the audience to be angry in the face of so much evidence that "we [black women] have been the ones at the bottom that capitalism feeds on" (2003, p. 117). She defines the health care system as laced with "institutionalized racism." At different points during the conference, Avery invoked the lived reality of inequitable access to and experiences of health care with narratives about actual women whose lived experiences personalize the profound policy issues at stake. For example, she talked about Ida, a fifty-three-year-old mother of four living with AIDS, and Ally, who until the year before worked full time and received health insurance but lost that insurance when her health failed and a disability prevented her from working full time. Ally, without health insurance, faced mounting bills and a myriad of health problems. Other speakers also incorporated the experiences of real individuals, not merely to personalize the problem of health disparities but because these women's lives demonstrated the inextricability of gender, race/ethnicity, and class. It is this kind of analysis that scholars and advocates articulate as they move from the realities and experiences of the lives of women to issues such as access to health care; relationships with health providers; the caretaking required when family members are sick; the health risks disproportionately borne by people who live in poor neighborhoods; the reasons for differential treatment for men and women and for whites and racial and ethnic minorities in physician offices, clinics, and hospitals; the impact of public health, immigration, welfare, and employment policies; and so much more.

My intent in comparing the intersectional and positivist biomedical paradigms as they shed light on health disparities is not to argue that one paradigm should supplant the other. Instead, by counterposing these analytical frameworks, I aim to encourage greater dialogue between scholars who work from these different perspectives and call into question the presumption that research in the positivist, biomedical tradition is, by definition, superior, more authoritative, or should be more influential for health policymakers. Given the institutional and political realities that shape the production of knowledge, it is almost certain that in the immediate future, the positivist biomedical framework will continue to be favored by policymakers, the primary funders of health research, and editors and reviewers of the journals in which much influential health research will be published. However, the intersectional framework is an exciting, viable alternative paradigm that calls into question the conventional positivist practice of extracting race and ethnicity from the complex social relations of power that shape the "unequal burden" of health and health care that disproportionately affects women of color.

The goal of eliminating or even significantly reducing racial, ethnic, gender, or class disparities in health will undoubtedly take a serious political commitment to changing a wide variety of medical practices, health care institutions, medical training, and public policies. Donna Christian-Christiansen, the chair of the Congressional Black Caucus Health Brain Trust, has argued that "the elimination of health disparities is the civil rights issue of the 21st century" (NBWHP, 2003, p. 23). Intersectional scholarship is a paradigm firmly rooted in principles of social justice, principles that are neither in conflict with good science nor central to the positivist biomedical model. It is the intent of this book to suggest that there is much to be gained from a robust dialogue among researchers whose work is rooted in positivist biomedical and intersectional paradigms. Such dialogue will not be productive unless scholars who work from these different paradigms understand the strengths and limitations of the epistemological, theoretical, and methodological premises of these different analytical frameworks.

It is also important to recognize the valuable role that political activists, in this case from the women's health and civil rights movements, have played in posing questions and articulating analyses about the complex relationship between social, economic, and political inequality and health, questions that need serious attention if our nation is to eliminate health disparities or even to make significant progress toward greater health equity. The women's health movement is an excellent example of the value of including women—whether as clients or consumers of health care or as health care providers or researchers or as constituents with a stake in health policy—in health care decision making and research. Efforts to change a health care system that for much of our nation's history has marginalized and subordinated women of all races, men of color, and the poor depend on forging alliances, collaborations, and partnerships based on mutual respect among those who see the system from their different vantage points and paradigms. My hope is that this chapter contributes to that worthy goal.

Notes

1. For a full discussion of both my methodology and a comprehensive treatment of the women's health movement, see Morgen (2002).
2. Silliman, Fried, Ross, and Gutierrez (2004), on the history of women of color health organizations, provides the best overview of these developments.
3. Interestingly, almost all the background papers produced by scholars for the IOM committee and published after the final committee report would fit squarely within the positivist, biomedical research tradition. Yet some of these papers draw conclusions or suggest concerns that overlap considerably with intersectional scholarship. Indeed, to my mind, the papers by Jack Geiger and Michael and Linda Byrd have much in common with some of the presentations at the National Black Women's Health Conference, perhaps more in common than they do with the committee report. In choosing the IOM report to represent the positivist, biomedical model, I do not mean to suggest that all research in this paradigm shares all the weaknesses (or strengths) of this report; rather, the IOM report is the epitome of the paradigm.
4. Using the search engine at http://www.nap.edu/books/030908265X/html, I read every hit for the keywords I used to examine the analysis

of gender, race, ethnicity, and class in the report. The keywords I used included *women, gender, class, race, ethnicity, racism, socioeconomic, prejudice, discrimination, stereotype, immigrant, Black women, African-American women, Latina, Native American, American Indian, Asian-American, Asian-Pacific Islander, lesbian, gay, minority women, gender inequality/inequity, differential treatment, gender bias,* and *class bias.*

5. The analysis of racism was even more muted in the report initially released by the Department of Health and Human Services on racial and ethnic disparities in health care, which was based on the IOM report. Clearly, the politics of the Bush administration are inconsistent with calling attention to systemic racism, let alone the convergence of racial, gender, and class oppression. When DHHS first released the report, it made significant changes in the executive summary, including removing the report's troubling conclusion: that differences in the health care treatment of various racial and ethnic groups were a "national problem" and were "pervasive" in the system (Beck, 2004). The definition of *health disparity* itself was removed, and the term was used only twice in the revised summary, a drastic change from the initial version, in which the term was used more than thirty times (Waxman, cited in Beck, 2004). Moreover, a new, upbeat introductory paragraph about dramatic improvements in our nation's health replaced the somber appraisal about the severity of racial and ethnic health disparities in the first lines of the DHHS executive summary (Beck, 2004). Following concerted negative publicity about these changes, DHHS director Tommy Thompson admitted that this editing was problematic and released a new summary without their deletions.

6. In this section, I use "Dr." to specify medical doctors. I have not indicated degrees in other cases.

References

Anzaldua, G. *Making Face, Making Soul: Haciendo Caras: Creative and Critical Perspectives by Women of Color.* San Francisco: Aunt Lute, 1990.

Asetoyer, C. "First There Was Smallpox." In M. Banzhaf and others (eds.), *Women, AIDS and Activism: Act Up New York Women and AIDS Group.* Boston: South End Press, 1990.

Asetoyer, C. "From the Ground Up." *Women's Review of Books,* 1994, *11,* 10–11, 22.

Avery, B. "Black Women's Health Project: Network Launches New Project." *Network News,* Feb. 1982, p. 1.

Bair, B., and Cayleff, S. E. (eds.). *Wings of Gauze: Women of Color and the Experience of Health and Illness.* Detroit: Wayne State University Press, 1993.

Batt, S. *Patient No More: The Politics of Breast Cancer.* London: Scarlet Press, 1994.

Beale, F. "Double Jeopardy: To Be Black and Female." In R. Morgan (ed.), *Sisterhood Is Powerful: An Anthology of Writings from the Women's Liberation Movement.* New York: Random House, 1970.

Beck, E. "Analysis: Disparities Report in Dispute." Jan. 15, 2004. http://www.upi.com/view.cfm?StoryID=20040114-025957-5999r.

Berkowitz, E. D. *To Improve Health: A History of the Institute of Medicine.* Washington D.C.: National Academy Press, 1998.

Boston Women's Health Book Collective. *Our Bodies, Ourselves: A Book by and for Women.* New York: Simon & Schuster, 1973.

Boston Women's Health Book Collective. *Our Bodies, Ourselves: A Book by and for Women.* (2nd ed.) New York: Simon & Schuster, 1984.

Byrd, M. W., and Clayton, L. "Racial and Ethnic Disparities in Health Care: A Background and History." In B. D. Smedley, A. Y. Stith, and A. R. Nelson (eds.), *Unequal Treatment: Confronting Racial and Ethnic Disparities in Health Care.* Washington, D.C.: National Academy Press, 2003.

Cade, T. *The Black Woman: An Anthology.* New York: New American Library, 1970.

Cain, V., and Kington, R. "Investigating the Role of Racial/Ethnic Bias in Health Outcomes." *American Journal of Public Health,* 2003, *93*(2), 191–192.

Campaign for Women's Health. *A Model Benefits Package for Women in Health Care Reform.* Washington, D.C.: Older Women's League, 1993.

Collins, P. Hill. *Black Feminist Thought: Knowledge, Consciousness, and the Politics of Empowerment.* New York: Routledge, 1990.

Combahee River Collective. "The Combahee River Collective Statement." In B. Smith (ed.), *Home Girls: A Black Feminist Anthology.* Latham, N.Y.: Kitchen Table Women of Color Press, 1983.

Cooper, L. A., and Roter, D. L. "Patient-Provider Communication: The Effect of Race and Ethnicity on Process and Outcomes of Health Care." In B. D. Smedley, A. Y. Stith, and A. R. Nelson (eds.), *Unequal Treatment: Confronting Racial and Ethnic Disparities in Health Care.* Washington, D.C.: National Academic Press, 2003.

Corea, G. *The Hidden Malpractice: How American Medicine Treats Women as Patients and Professionals.* New York: Morrow, 1977.

Davis, A. Y. *Women, Race, and Class.* New York: Vintage, 1981.

Davis, A. Y. "Sick and Tired of Being Sick and Tired: The Politics of Black Women's Health." In E. C. White (ed.), *The Black Women's Health Book.* Seattle, Wash.: Seal Press, 1990.

DelVecchio Good, M. J., James, C., Good, B., and Becker, A. "The Culture of Medicine and Racial, Ethnic, and Class Disparities in Health care." In B. D. Smedley, A. Y. Stith, and A. R. Nelson (eds.), *Unequal Treatment: Confronting Racial and Ethnic Disparities in Health Care.* Washington, D.C.: National Academic Press, 2003.

Dill, B. T. "Race, Class and Gender: Prospects for an All-Inclusive Sisterhood." *Feminist Studies,* 1983, *9,* 131–149.

Dreifus, C. *Seizing Our Bodies: The Politics of Women's Health.* New York: Vintage Books, 1977.

Fried, M. G. (ed.). *From Abortion to Reproductive Freedom: Transforming a Movement.* Boston: South End Press, 1990.

Gary-Smith, S. "Self-Help: Our Past, Present and Future." *Vital Signs,* 1989, *6*(1).

Geiger, J. "Racial and Ethnic Disparities in Diagnosis and Treatment: A Review of the Evidence and a Consideration of Causes." In B. D. Smedley, A. Y. Stith, and A. R. Nelson (eds.), *Unequal Treatment: Confronting Racial and Ethnic Disparities in Health Care.* Washington, D.C.: National Academy Press, 2003.

Grady, M., and Edgar, T. "Racial Disparities in Health care: Highlights from Focus Group Findings." In B. D. Smedley, A. Y. Stith, and A. R. Nelson (eds.), *Unequal Treatment: Confronting Racial and Ethnic Disparities in Health Care.* Washington, D.C.: National Academy Press, 2003.

Hughes, C. "Black Women and Quality of Care." In National Black Women's Health Project, Congressional Black Caucus Health Brain Trust, and U.S. Senate Black Legislative Staff Caucus. *National Colloquium on Black Women's Health.* Washington, D.C.: Congressional Black Caucus Health Brain Trust and U.S. Senate Black Legislative Staff Caucus, Apr. 2003.

James, S. "Confronting the Moral Economy of U.S. Racial/Ethnic Health Disparities." *American Journal of Public Health,* 2003, *93*(2), 189.

Krieger, N. "Does Racism Harm Health? Did Child Abuse Exist before 1962? On Explicit Questions, Critical Science, and Current Controversies: An Ecosocial Perspective." *American Journal of Public Health,* 2003, *93*(2), 194–199.

Leigh, W. A., and Lindquist, M. A. *Women of Color Health Data Book: Adolescents to Seniors.* Bethesda, Md.: Office of Research on Women's Health, Office of the Director, National Institutes of Health, 1998.

Leigh, W. A., and Lindquist, M. A. "Black Women and Access to Health Care." In National Black Women's Health Project, Congressional Black Caucus Health Brain Trust, and U.S. Senate Black Legislative Staff Caucus. *National Colloquium on Black Women's Health.* Washington, D.C.: Congressional Black Caucus Health Brain Trust and U.S. Senate Black Legislative Staff Caucus, Apr. 2003.

Moraga, C., and Anzaldua, G. (eds.). *This Bridge Called My Back: Writings by Radical Women of Color.* Watertown, Mass.: Persephone Press, 1981.

Morgen, S. *Into Our Own Hands: The Women's Health Movement in the U.S., 1969–1990.* New Brunswick, N.J: Rutgers University Press, 2002.

National Asian Women's Health Organization. *Report.* San Francisco: National Asian Women's Health Organization, 1993–1994.

National Asian Women's Health Organization. *Perceptions of Risk: An Assessment of the Factors Influencing Use of Reproductive and Sexual Health Services by Asian American Women.* San Francisco: National Asian Women's Health Organization, 1995.

National Black Women's Health Project. "Eliminating Racial and Ethnic Disparities in Health." 2001. http://www.nationalblackwomens healthproject.org.

National Black Women's Health Project, Congressional Black Caucus Health Brain Trust, and U.S. Senate Black Legislative Staff Caucus. *National Colloquium on Black Women's Health.* Washington, D.C.: Congressional Black Caucus Health Brain Trust and U.S. Senate Black Legislative Staff Caucus, Apr. 2003.

National Colloquium on Black Women's Health. "Opening and Welcome," "Unequal Burden," "Access to Care." 2003. http://www. kaisernetwork.org/health_cast/uploaded_files/041103_nbwhp_morning.pdf.

Nelson, J. "Abortions Under Community Control: Feminism, Nationalism, and the Politics of Reproduction Among New York City's Young Lords." *Journal of Women's History,* 2001, *13*(1), 157–180.

Norsigian, J. "Women and National Health Care Reform: A Progressive Feminist Agenda." In A. Dan (ed.), *Reframing Women's Health: Multidisciplinary Research and Practice.* Thousand Oaks, Calif.: Sage, 1994.

Pinn, V. W. "Foreword." In W. A. Leigh and M. A. Lindquist, *Women of Color Health Data Book: Adolescents to Seniors.* Bethesda, Md.: Office of Research on Women's Health, Office of the Director, National Institutes of Health, 1998.

Roberts, D. *Killing the Black Body: Race, Reproduction, and the Meaning of Liberty.* New York: Pantheon Books, 1997.

Roberts, D. "Black Women and Reproductive Health." In National Black Women's Health Project, Congressional Black Caucus Health Brain Trust, and U.S. Senate Black Legislative Staff Caucus. *National Colloquium on Black Women's Health.* Apr. 2003. Washington, D.C.: Congressional Black Caucus Health Brain Trust and U.S. Senate Black Legislative Staff Caucus, Apr. 2003.

Rodriguez-Trias, H. "Sterilization Abuse." *Women and Health,* 1978, *3,* 10–15.

Ross, L. "African American Women and Abortion." In R. Solinger (ed.), *Abortion Wars: A Half-Century of Struggle, 1950–2000.* Berkeley: University of California Press, 1998.

Ruzek, S. B. *The Women's Health Movement.* New York: Praeger, 1978.

Ruzek, S. B., and Becker, J. "The Women's Health Movement in the U.S.: From Grassroots Activism to Professional Agendas." *Journal of the American Medical Women's Association,* 1999, *54*(1), 4–8, 40.

Ruzek, S. B., Olesen, V. L., and Clarke, A. E. *Women's Health: Complexities and Differences.* Columbus: Ohio State University Press, 1997.

Schneider, B., and Stoller, N. (eds.). *Women Resisting AIDS: Feminist Strategies of Empowerment.* Philadelphia: Temple University Press, 1995.

Seaman, B. *The Doctor's Case Against the Pill.* New York: Wyden Books, 1969.

Shapiro, T. *Population Control Politics: Women, Sterilization and Reproductive Choice.* Philadelphia: Temple University Press, 1985.

Silliman, J., Fried, M. G., Ross, L., and Gutierrez, E. *Undivided Rights: Women of Color Organize for Reproductive Justice.* Cambridge, Mass.: South End Press, 2004.

Smedley, B. D., Stith, A. Y., and Nelson, A. R. (eds.). *Unequal Treatment: Confronting Racial and Ethnic Disparities in Health Care.* Washington, D.C.: National Academy Press, 2003.

Smith, S. L. *Sick and Tired of Being Sick and Tired: Black Women's Health Activism in America, 1890–1950.* Philadelphia: University of Pennsylvania Press, 1995.

U.S. Department of Health and Human Services. *Report of the Secretary's Task Force on Black and Minority Health.* Washington, D.C.: U.S. Government Printing Office, 1985.

U.S. Public Health Service. *Women's Health: Report of the Public Health Service Task Force on Women's Health Issues.* Washington, D.C.: U.S. Public Health Service, 1985.

Villarosa, L. (ed.). *Body and Soul: The Black Women's Guide to Physical Health and Emotional Well-Being.* New York: HarperCollins, 1994.

Washington, H. "Black Women and the Unequal Burden of Health Problems." In National Black Women's Health Project, Congressional Black Caucus Health Brain Trust, and U.S. Senate Black Legislative Staff Caucus. *National Colloquium on Black Women's Health.* Washington, D.C.: Congressional Black Caucus Health Brain Trust and U.S. Senate Black Legislative Staff Caucus, Apr. 2003.

Weisman, C. *Women's Health Care: Activist Traditions and Institutional Change.* Baltimore: Johns Hopkins University Press, 1998.

White, E. *The Black Women's Health Book: Speaking for Ourselves.* Seattle, Wash.: Seal Press, 1990.

Name Index

INDEX

CPSIA information can be obtained at www.ICGtesting.com
Printed in the USA
BVOW03s0043200813

328886BV00007B/93/P